THE PIH GUIDE TO

Chronic Care Integration for Endemic Non-Communicable Diseases

RWANDA EDITION
CARDIAC, RENAL, DIABETES, PULMONARY, AND PALLIATIVE CARE

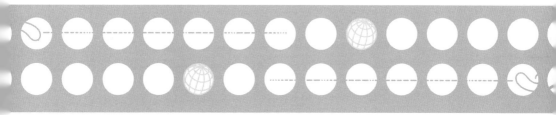

Partners In Health

Harvard Medical School
Department of Global Health and Social Medicine
Program in Global Non-Communicable Disease and Social Change

Brigham and Women's Hospital
Division of Global Health Equity

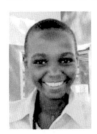

Jeanette Niyonsaba died from rheumatic heart disease at the age of fourteen. Jeanette fought her disease with bravery and determination. This guide is dedicated to her memory.

About the Cover

Butaro District Hospital is a 150-bed public facility that sits on a mountaintop in northern Rwanda's Burera District. In addition to serving the district's 350,000 people, the majority of whom still survive on about a dollar a day, Butaro will also serve as a national teaching hospital and clinical center of excellence. Led by Partners In Health, in collaboration with the Rwandan government, the hospital was built by 3500 men and women from the local community using local materials. This world-class facility was inaugurated on January 24th, 2011. At the inauguration ceremony, Rwandan President Paul Kagame said, "Butaro is more than a hospital. It is a unique story of exceptional people with the desire to see positive change in the world and in communities like the one hosting us today. ... It is also a story about strong and mutually benefiting partnerships and the fact that when we come together and join forces, commendable results can be achieved."

In the years to come, Rwandan clinical leaders based at this flagship teaching hospital will train the next generation of nurses and physicians tackling the long tail of endemic non-communicable disease throughout Rwanda, and the world.

PHOTO CREDIT: Matthew Craven and Peter Drobac

CONTRIBUTORS AND ACKNOWLEDGEMENTS

Editors-in-Chief

Gene Bukhman, MD, PhD
Alice Kidder, MD, MPH

Principal Authors

Alice Kidder, MD, MPH
Gene Kwan, MD
Corrado Cancedda, MD, PhD
Gene Bukhman, MD, PhD

Special Contributors

Eric Krakauer, MD, PhD (Chapter 2: Palliative Care)

Joseph Mucumbitsi, MD and Ralph Morton Bolman III, MD
(Chapter 5: Cardiac Surgery)

Andrea Braun, MD and Sharon Su, MD (Chapter 6: Renal Failure)

Charlotte Bavuma, MD and Anand Vaidya, MD (Chapter 7: Diabetes)

Nancy Lange, MD and Sanctus Musafiri, MD
(Chapter 10: Chronic Respiratory Disease)

Vanessa Wolfman, MD, MPH and Sara Stulac, MD (Pediatric Content)

Contributors

Patrick Almazor, Cheryl Amoroso, Ellen Ball, Amy Banham, Anne Beckett, Didi Bertrand Farmer, Agnes Binagwaho, Gilbert Biraro, Corrado Cancedda, Chadi Cortas, Jonathan Crocker, Maros Cunderlik, Felix Cyamatare, Peter Drobac, Symaque Dusabeyezu, Henry Epino, Paul Farmer, Ildephonse Fayida, Hamish Fraser, Bonnie Frawley, Amber Gaumnitz, Jill Hackett, Christiane Haeffele, Emily Hall, Michael Herce, Lisa Hirschhorn, Louise Ivers, Darius Jazayeri, Waking Jean-Baptiste, Joanel Joasil, Keith Joseph, Jules Kabahizi, Emmanuel Kamanzi, Shashi Kants, Vanessa Kerry, Salmaan Keshavjee, Tracy Kidder, Frances Kidder, Felicia Knaul, Meera Kotagal, Mike Landzberg, Patrick Lee, Jennifer Lewey, Natalie Lorent, Alishya Mayfield, Joia Mukherjee, Megan Murray, Emmanuel Musbeyezu, Francis Mutabazi, Cadet Mutumbira, Gedeon Ngoga, Jean Paul Ngiruwera, Victor Nkulikiyinka, Emilen Nkusi, Joseph Ntarindwa, Fabrice Usenga, Alice Nyirimana, Bonaventure Nzeyimana, Daniel Palazuelos, Lindsay Palazuelos, Manisha Patel, Ceeya Patton-Bolman, Giuseppe Raviola, James Rawn, Michael Rich, Robert Riviello, Elizabeth Riviello, Jean Louis Romain, Valens Rudakubana, Emmanuel Rusingiza Kamanzi, Jacklin Saint-Fleur, Sachita Shah, Aaron Shakow, Lawrence Shulman, Amy Sievers, Neo Tapela,

Kate Thorson, Mariam Uwase, Anand Vadivel, Ashwin Vasan, Loune Viaud, Alexandra Vinograd, David Walton, Charlotte Wu, Justin Zachariah.

Acknowledgements

We would like to thank the following reviewers for their comments on parts of this text at an earlier stage in its development: Ana Olga Mocumbi (Chapter 4: Heart Failure), Geoffrey Gill and John Yudkin (Chapter 7: Diabetes), Bongani Mayosi (Chapter 9: Rheumatic Heart Disease Prevention). We would like to thank Tracy Kidder for his editorial assistance. We thank the Doris Duke Charitable Foundation for implementation support for the handbook use.

We particularly wish to thank the Rwandan Ministry of Health for its exceptional leadership and support, as well as the people of Rwanda who continually inspire us.

This project was funded through a grant from the Medtronic Foundation to Partners In Health.

Design: Flanders + Associates

ISBN: 978-0-6154548-9-4

NOTICE
....

This guide was designed for use by advanced nurses, clinical officers, physicians, and policy makers dealing with endemic non-communicable diseases in rural Rwanda and similar settings. The chronic care integration guide has been prepared by Partners In Health with the assistance of various contributors and authors, including, without limitation, each of the following parties: the Department of Global Health and Social Medicine, Harvard Medical School; the Division of Global Health Equity, Brigham and Women's Hospital; and each of their affiliates, divisions, directors, officers, trustees, agents and employees (collectively, with Partners In Health, the "Contributors and Authors"), for general informational purposes only. It is not intended as and should not be regarded or relied upon as medical advice or opinion, or as a substitute for the advice of a medical practitioner. You should not rely on, take any action or fail to take any action based upon the chronic care integration guide.

Mention of specific drugs or products within the guide does not constitute endorsement by any of the above-named individuals or entities. With regard to specific drugs or products, medical practitioners are advised to consult their normal resources before prescribing to their patients.

Every possible effort has been made to ensure that the material presented herein is accurate, reliable, and in accord with current standards, but none of the contributors and authors represents or warrants that the information contained herein is complete or accurate or free from error. Wherever possible, the material has been harmonized with clinical algorithms currently employed by the national ministry of health. However, as new research and experience expand our knowledge and geographic reach, recommendations for care and treatment will change accordingly. As such, it is the responsibility of the individual clinician to use his/her best medical judgment in determining appropriate care and treatment based on individual patient needs, as well as relevant guidelines and constraints of the country and facility in which he/she works.

As between Partners In Health and you, Partners In Health or its licensors at all times owns and retains all right, title and interest in and to the chronic care integration guide, including all intellectual property rights therein and thereto. You may use and copy the chronic care integration guide, or portions of the guide, provided that you (i) promptly notify Partners In Health via email at **harvardncd@pih.org** of any such use; and (ii) reproduce all copyright notices, claims or reservation of rights appearing on the chronic care guide, as delivered to you, on all copies made pursuant to this sentence.

TABLE OF CONTENTS

CHAPTER 5
Cardiac Surgery Screening, Referral, Anticoagulation, and Postoperative Management   119

CHAPTER 9
Rheumatic Heart Disease Prevention

APPENDIX C
Indicators for Monitoring and Evaluation   297

APPENDIX D
Forms   307

Figures

CHAPTER 9

Tables

∙∙

CHAPTER 5

CHAPTER 6

Protocols

FOREWORD 1
Agnes Binagwaho

The Government of Rwanda views health care as a basic human right and, as such, our health care delivery model aims to serve all Rwandans, especially the most vulnerable. This rights-based approach is at the root of Rwanda's health strategy. It is articulated in Rwanda's Economic Development and Poverty Reduction Strategy, Rwanda's Vision 2020, and the United Nations' Millennium Development Goals. Our objective is to engage the nation in a participatory effort to eradicate poverty and the many ills it brings.

This guide has been developed in line with the overall health care strategy of the Ministry of Health of Rwanda in the regulation of development partner initiatives, and in the promulgation of policies and the execution of programs.

Over the past decade, Rwanda has seen child mortality under age 5 drop by half. We have achieved universal access to HIV therapy and now are able to address HIV/AIDS as a chronic disease. More women than ever are delivering their babies in health facilities, and more than 95% of Rwanda's 11 million people have health insurance. Rwanda's successes in preventing and treating the top killers—malaria, tuberculosis, HIV/AIDS, respiratory infections, and diarrheal diseases—have led to a dramatic increase in life expectancy. With over 400 health centers, 42 district hospitals, and 45,000 community health workers providing care at the village level, Rwanda has created a system to bring health care to both its urban and rural populations. This system has improved financial and geographic access to all Rwandans, even the poorest. And our accomplishments represent the strength of the Government's stance on health care and human rights and the support of its development partners.

Achievements such as these are pivotal. In another decade, Rwanda will undoubtedly continue to see its people living longer, healthier lives. The gross domestic product per capita will also likely increase, and Rwanda's population will be in better economic shape.

However, by fighting the current top killers we are only able to increase the life expectancy to approximately 54 years, since infectious diseases do not account for all of the country's disease burden. Regretfully, there remains a serious gap in Rwanda's current health care system. Non-communicable diseases (NCDs)—probably accounting for about 25% of the national burden of disease—have yet to be addressed in a strategic and systematic way.[1] These diseases include cardiovascular disease, cancer, epilepsy, pulmonary disease, and diabetes, among others. These are global diseases and yet, more often than not, NCDs are thought to be problems of middle- and high-income countries. In such countries, risk factors for NCDs include obesity, tobacco use, and other factors termed poor lifestyle choices. However, in Rwanda and other developing countries, this is not the case. NCDs are instead linked to malnutrition, infection, congenital abnormalities, and toxic environments. All of these factors are ultimately exacerbated by poverty. On top of that, HIV/AIDS, tuberculosis, malaria, and neglected tropical diseases further contribute to risk factors for NCDs, whether treated or untreated.

Rwanda is acutely aware of the need to both treat and protect its population from emerging risk factors that accompany urbanization. Over the next 5 years, the country anticipates expanding access to integrated chronic care by building on the existing health care platforms established by programs fighting infectious diseases. Expanded access and improved options for preventing and treating chronic illnesses and NCDs would have a tremendous impact on morbidity and mortality. Currently, there are many disease-specific advocacy groups in Rwanda fighting for advanced care for conditions such as cardiovascular illness, diabetes, epilepsy, and hemophilia. The challenge for Rwanda is to identify and execute the right set of integrated strategic plans for preventing and treating NCDs. Chronic care integration is one such plan.

Inshuti Mu Buzima (IMB)—the sister organization to the Harvard-affiliated nonprofit Partners In Health (PIH)—was invited to work in partnership with the Ministry of Health of Rwanda at the end of 2003. We appreciate that IMB-PIH is committed to supporting Rwanda's vision for health care and that it devotes itself to the needs of the entire populations of three districts. In particular, IMB-PIH has made a unique contribution in the area of chronic care and NCDs. This approach has led to joint undertakings between the Ministry of Health and IMB-PIH, including a conference in January 2010 focused on how to tackle non-communicable diseases in Rwanda. Through such discussions, chronic care integration has been identified as an indispensable part of strategic planning to improve the health of the Rwandan population. Other areas of planning for NCDs include gynecologic care at district hospitals; improving the quality of generalist physician care at district hospitals; histopathology; cancer care; cancer surgery; cardiac surgery, and neurosurgery. Now, in January 2011, Rwanda finds itself equipped with a health care system capable of launching chronic care integration; and IMB-PIH finds itself prepared to support the effort.

Many Rwandans are able to afford the prevention and treatment of uncomplicated cases of common diseases such as malaria or pneumonia,
but most cannot afford the costs of chronic care of HIV/AIDS, heart disease, diabetes, epilepsy, or cancer. Therefore, chronic lifelong treatment
and managed care for NCDs must be rooted in a publicly sponsored, tac-
tical, and efficient plan to achieve accessibility and affordability. Already
Rwanda has taken steps to tackle some of the prevention issues unique
to NCDs, including the improvement of household cooking stoves and
access to treatment for streptococcal pharyngitis, among myriad other
steps. But we have much work to do. We will never achieve our development goals if we don't take seriously the non-communicable ailments
of our patient populations—ailments which most of our citizens must
simply endure since they cannot pay for treatment. Without decreasing
the attention we currently have on combating communicable diseases,
the Ministry of Health affirms our unwavering dedication to preventing and treating non-communicable diseases, and making chronic care
available to all. It is in this context that I am proud to be collaborating on
this publication by Inshuti Mu Buzima–Partners In Health.

Thank you.

Agnes Binagwaho, M.D.
Minister of Health
Government of Rwanda

June 2011

References
· ·

1   Mathers C, Boerma T, Fat DM. The Global Burden of Disease: 2004 Update.
     Geneva: World Health Organization; 2008.

FOREWORD 2
Bongani Mayosi
....

2011 is the year of chronic non-communicable diseases (NCDs). The United Nations General Assembly will hold a Special Session on NCDs in September 2011 to galvanize the global community to address the scourge of NCDs, which is on the rise even in sub-Saharan Africa, the only region of the world where NCDs are not yet the leading cause of death. The countries and communities of sub-Saharan Africa are heterogeneous in terms of stage of economic development and their position in the epidemiologic transition from diseases of famine and pestilence (associated with poor socio-economic status) to diseases of affluence and plenty (associated with advanced economic development). Contrary to conventional wisdom, NCDs are as relevant to poor countries and communities as they are developed countries and wealthy communities.

This book by Dr. Gene Bukhman and his colleagues from Partners In Health at Harvard University in Boston is timely and represents a unique achievement in the manner in which it addresses politicians, health planners, policy makers, and clinicians with clear messages that are relevant and feasible in resource-poor settings. The first chapter on the integration of chronic care services in Rwanda deals with the central ingredient for success in developing services for NCDs—which is to build on existing services for communicable diseases and to extend them to achieve full coverage for all health conditions. It is followed by chapters on Palliative Care and Chronic Care (Chapter 2) and the Role of Community Health Workers, Family Planning, Mental Health, and Social Services (Chapter 3). These first three chapters are essential reading for senior officials in the Rwandan Ministry of Health and for all managers of health services and clinical leaders.

The last seven chapters of the handbook are aimed at the clinician who practices at all levels of care. The information contained in these sections highlights the unique epidemiology of NCDs among the "bottom billion" of the poorest people in the world. The information in these sections will be of great interest to all students and practitioners of the emerging field of global health.

This handbook is a model for the development of integrated services for NCDs in Rwanda. I look forward to the adaptation of this model to other countries, and to the assessment of its impact on quality of care and health outcomes where it is used.

Bongani M Mayosi, OMS, DPhil, FCP(SA)
Professor and Head, Department of Medicine
Groote Schuur Hospital and University of Cape Town
Cape Town, South Africa

May 2011

ABBREVIATIONS

ACE	Angiotensin-converting enzyme
ACE-I	Angiotensin-converting enzyme inhibitor
AFB	Acid-fast bacilli
AIDS	Acquired immune deficiency syndrome
ARV	Antiretroviral
ASD	Atrial septal defect
ASO	Anti-streptolysin O
BMI	Body mass index
BP	Blood pressure
CCC	Chronic care clinic
CHUB	University Teaching Hospital of Butare
CHUK	University Teaching Hospital of Kigali
CKD-EPI	Chronic Kidney Disease Epidemiology Collaboration
CKD	Chronic Kidney Disease
cm	Centimeter
CMP	Cardiomyopathy
COPD	Chronic obstructive pulmonary disease
Cr	Creatinine
CRD	Chronic respiratory disease
CRP	C-reactive protein
CXR	Chest x-ray
d4T	Stavudine
DBP	Diastolic blood pressure
DKA	Diabetic ketoacidosis
dL	Deciliter
EF	Ejection fraction
ESR	Erythrocyte sediment rate
GDP	Gross domestic product
GFR	Glomerular filtration rate
GINA	Global Initiative for Asthma
gm	Gram
GOLD	Global Initiative for Chronic Obstructive Lung Disease
HAART	Highly active antiretroviral therapy
HbA1c	Hemoglobin A1c
HCTZ	Hydrochlorothiazide
HHNW	Healing Hearts Northwest
HHV-8	Human herpesvirus 8
HIV	Human immunodeficiency virus
HIVAN	HIV-associated nephropathy
HONKC	Hyperosmolar non-ketotic coma

HTN	Hypertension
IM	Intramuscular
IMAI	Integrated Management of Adult Illnesses
IMB	Inshuti Mu Buzima
IMCI	Integrated Management of Childhood Illnesses
IMPAC	Integrated Management of Pregnancy and Childbirth
INR	International normalized ratio
IU	International units
IUATLD	International Union Against Tuberculosis and Lung Disease
IV	Intravenous
IVC	Inferior vena cava
JVP	Jugular venous pressure
K	Potassium
kg	kilogram
L	liter
μmol	micromole
mg	milligram
mL	milliliter
MOH	Ministry of Health
NCD	Non-communicable disease
NGO	Nongovernmental organization
NSAID	Nonsteroidal anti-inflammatory drug
OOH	Operation Open Heart
OPD	Outpatient department
PAL	Practical Approach to Lung Health
PDA	Patent ductus arteriosus
PEF	Peak expiratory flow
PIH	Partners In Health
PT	Prothrombin time
PTT	Partial thromboplastin time
RF	Rheumatic fever
RHD	Rheumatic heart disease
SACH	Save a Child's Heart
SBP	Systolic blood pressure
SC	Subcutaneous
TB	Tuberculosis
TMP-SMX	Trimethoprim-sulfamethoxazole
TOF	Tetrology of Fallot
VSD	Ventricular septal defect
WHO	World Health Organization

CHAPTER 1
Integration of Chronic Care Services in Rwanda
. . . .

1.1   The Long Tail of Endemic Non-Communicable Diseases in Rwanda

Non-communicable disease among the poor in Rwanda has a very different face than that seen in middle- or high-income populations. While Rwanda has enjoyed rapid economic growth and political stability in recent years, it remains one of the poorest countries in the world, with a per capita GDP of less than $1000. Only a quarter of its 10 million inhabitants are 30 or older, and more than 80% live in rural areas. According to the 2005 demographic and health survey (DHS), only 10% of adult women were overweight and more than 20% were severely underweight.[1,2] Most of the population survives on subsistence agriculture, and food insecurity is a perennial problem. Adjusted data from the 2005 DHS showed that 52% of children under age 5 were chronically malnourished (stunted).[3] Within this setting, chronic non-communicable diseases more often result from untreated infections and undernutrition than from the adoption of the unhealthy lifestyles available to poor people in rich countries (see **TABLE 1.1**).

The rural Rwandan health system includes village-based community health workers, nurse-staffed health centers, and district hospitals with generalist physicians. Most districts spend between $5 and $15 per capita for health services. On average, patients travel 2 hours to reach the nearest health center. Access to specialists (including internists and pediatricians) is largely limited to facilities in the capital, Kigali, and to the two university hospitals.

In 2005, the government of Rwanda invited Partners In Health (PIH), a Boston-based non-governmental organization, to support the country's initiative to strengthen rural health services. This effort, financed in part by the Clinton Foundation, included building and renovating health infrastructure, supplementing operational budgets, and providing training to local staff. By 2010, the project had reached three rural districts serving more than 750,000 people, and it had increased per capita health spending in those districts to around $27. During the same period, the government of Rwanda had achieved tremendous improvements in population health. These include extending health insurance to more than 90% of the population, reducing by half the mortality among young children, extending antiretroviral access to more than 80% of

HIV patients in need of treatment (universal access), and increasing the rates of facility-based deliveries.

At the time of PIH's engagement, chronic non-communicable diseases (NCDs) accounted for as much as 30% to 40% of adult hospitalization time in supported facilities. These diseases were over-represented because the patients tended to linger for weeks and months in hospitals—in part because of the lack of reliable outpatient follow-up. These conditions included cardiac, endocrine, renal, respiratory, and hematologic/oncologic disorders.

TABLE 1.1   Burden of Non-Communicable Diseases in Rwanda Linked to Conditions of Poverty

	Condition	Risk factors related to poverty
Hematology and oncology[4-7]	Cervical cancer, gastric cancer, lymphomas, Karposi's sarcoma, hepatocellular carcinoma	HPV, *H. Pylori*, EBV, HIV, Hepatitis B
	Breast cancer, CML	Idiopathic, treatment gap
	Hyperreactive malarial splenomegaly, hemoglobinopathies	Malaria
Psychiatric[8]	Depression, psychosis, somatoform disorders	War, untreated chronic diseases, undernutrition
	Schizophrenia, bipolar disorder	Idiopathic, treatment gap
Neurological[9-11]	Epilepsy	Meningitis, malaria
	Stroke	Rheumatic mitral stenosis, endocarditis, malaria, HIV
Cardiovascular[12-14]	Hypertension	Idiopathic, treatment gap
	Pericardial disease	Tuberculosis
	Rheumatic valvular disease	Streptococcal diseases
	Cardiomyopathies	HIV, other viruses, pregnancy
	Congenital heart disease	Maternal rubella, micronutrient deficiency, idiopathic, treatment gap
Respiratory[14,15]	Chronic pulmonary disease	Indoor air pollution, tuberculosis, schistosomiasis, treatment gap
Renal[16]	Chronic kidney disease	Streptococcal disease
Endocrine[17]	Diabetes	Undernutrition
	Hyperthyroidism and hypothyroidism	Iodine deficiency
Musculoskeletal[18,19]	Chronic osteomyelitis	Bacterial infection, tuberculosis
	Musculoskeletal injury	Trauma
Vision[20]	Cataracts	Idiopathic, treatment gap
	Refractory error	Idiopathic, treatment gap
Dental[21]	Caries	Hygiene, treatment gap

By non-communicable disease, we mean illnesses that may or may not have an infectious origin but persist despite eradication of the infection itself. NCDs pose a special challenge for governments in resource-poor settings. The data on disease burden for young adults and adolescents in sub-Saharan Africa is weak.[22,23] However, it is likely that conditions that probably account for three-quarters of the disease burden overall are largely infectious (see **TABLE 1.1** and **TABLE 1.2**).[24] The remaining quarter of disease burden is distributed in a kind of long tail of NCDs not dominated by any one condition (see **FIGURE 1.1**).

TABLE 1.2 Leading Causes of Death and Disability in Rwanda in Disability-Adjusted Life Years (DALYs)[24]

Disease	DALYs ('000)	Fraction of total DALYs	
Lower respiratory infections	843	15.6%	
Diarrheal diseases	633	11.7%	
HIV/AIDS	557	10.3%	
Maternal conditions	278	5.2%	
Malaria	277	5.1%	
Neonatal infections and other conditions	252	4.7%	
Birth asphyxia and birth trauma	237	4.4%	
Tuberculosis	187	3.5%	**74%**
Other infectious diseases (meningitis, STDs excluding HIV, childhood-cluster diseases, upper respiratory infections, Hepatitis B, Hepatitis C)	180	3.3%	
Tropical-cluster diseases	170	3.2%	
Prematurity and low birth weight	155	2.9%	
Protein-energy malnutrition	128	2.4%	
Nutritional deficiencies	102	1.9%	

FIGURE 1.1   The Long Tail of Endemic NCDs in Rwanda

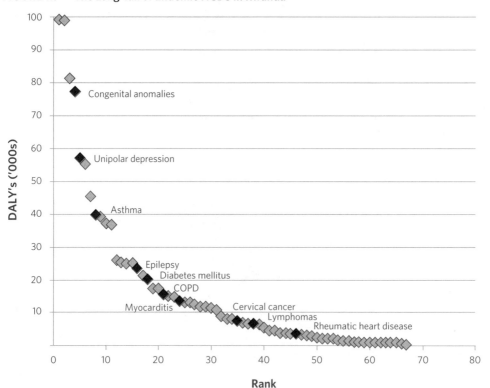

1.2   A Framework for Strategic Planning for Endemic Non-Communicable Disease

There is increasing evidence that vertical funding for major infectious diseases such as HIV has strengthened health systems around the world.[25] However, the problem with vertical planning for endemic NCDs in a country like Rwanda, is that, viewed individually, each non-communicable disease is relatively uncommon. In many ways, the advocacy dilemma associated with endemic NCDs is similar to that faced and addressed by the neglected tropical disease movement, which tackled a multitude of individually low-prevalence parasitic infections through a bundled approach.[26,27]

The planning issues for endemic NCDs are different from those faced by these infectious diseases, however, because of the heterogeneity of the interventions required to address NCDs. At the same time, entirely disease-specific approaches to individual NCDs threaten to cause more harm than good because they can divert precious manpower and funds from more prevalent health problems.

For this reason, it is crucial to link disease-specific advocacy for these conditions with a parsimonious strategic planning framework. From a policy and planning perspective, it is important to identify the right way to fill the treatment and prevention gaps.

Chronic care integration is one of the units for strategic planning that probably makes sense in some of the poorest health systems. There are many other units that are crucial to care and control of endemic NCDs (see **FIGURE 1.2**). These include referral-level functions such as histopathology and cardiac surgery, as well as district hospital–level service bundles such as integrated gynecologic services (including cervical and breast cancer screening). This handbook focuses on chronic care integration specifically.

FIGURE 1.2   Units of Planning for the Long-Tail Endemic NCDs

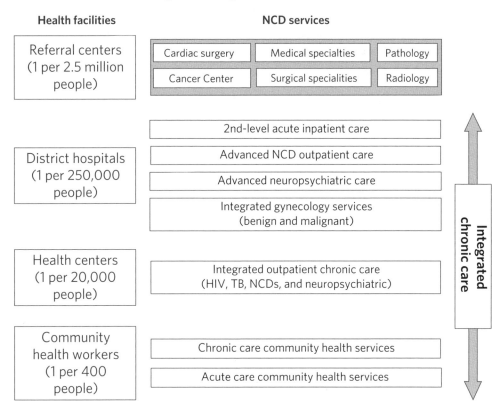

1.3 Decentralization and Integration of Chronic Care for Non-Communicable Disease in Rwanda

The process of building chronic care infrastructure has generally involved an incremental decentralization of services, first from the referral center to the district hospital, then from the district hospital to the health center, and finally from the health center to the community health worker. In general, as services are extended away from the referral center, they must become both more simplified and more integrated with other, similar services.

Rwanda began this process in the late 1990s with the decentralization of neuropsychiatric services to district hospitals. By 2005, chronic care for HIV, including antiretroviral therapy, was decentralized to the district level as well. By the end of the decade, chronic HIV care was available at most health centers in the country. Chronic care for NCDs, however, remained an obvious gap in the system. In 2006, the Rwandan Ministry of Health (MOH) began initial efforts to decentralize NCD services from the referral center to the district hospital. This handbook describes the strategy employed.

Other important pilot projects in low-income countries have tackled the problem of providing continuous care for patients with chronic diseases. These approaches have typically not addressed common advanced chronic conditions, such as heart failure, malignancies, and insulin-dependent diabetes.[28-30] However, scale-up of anti-retroviral therapy for HIV has generated strategies for decentralizing the delivery of complex health interventions for chronic conditions to large populations in resource-poor settings. Rwanda was among the countries that embraced these efforts early and now boasts a robust national HIV diagnosis, treatment, and prevention program.[31,32]

The Rwandan MOH has worked to adapt this effective model of decentralized HIV care to other complex chronic diseases. The MOH designed approaches to the diagnosis and treatment of endemic non-communicable diseases for use by advanced nurses, clinical officers, or generalist physicians. The protocols use simplified diagnostic techniques based on local epidemiology to place patients into broad categories of disease, corresponding with appropriate clinical pathways. These algorithms do not replace the need for certified specialist evaluation to confirm diagnoses, ensure quality control, and assess the need for surgery. However, the system does allow for more judicious use of scarce specialist time.

At the time of publication, Rwanda had three district level NCD clinics and four health center integrated chronic care clinics, located at PIH-supported sites. The clinics collectively followed about 2,300 patients with chronic diseases.

This handbook describes protocols for the diagnosis and treatment of chronic cardiovascular, endocrine, and respiratory diseases in the rural Rwandan setting. We hope that it will serve as a resource for both health system planners and clinicians engaged in the delivery of chronic care services. The topics covered mirror those in a forthcoming endemic NCD Training Manual, which addresses in greater detail the pathophysiology of these conditions, as well as pharmacology and examination techniques. Other chronic non-communicable diseases, such as hematologic/oncologic and neuropsychiatric illnesses, will be addressed in future volumes.

1.4   Which Chronic Diseases?

The types of chronic diseases treated and the desirable degree of integration across infectious, non-infectious, and neuropsychiatric conditions depend upon the epidemiology of the local setting as well as the number and prior training of existing health workers. In Rwanda, we have found that HIV, tuberculosis, hypertension, chronic respiratory diseases, diabetes, hyperreactive malarial splenomegaly, malignancies, chronic renal failure, epilepsy, mental health problems, rheumatic heart disease, and heart failure constitute the major chronic diseases presenting at the district-hospital and health-center level. By the late 1990s, Rwanda had already invested in a separate mental health and epilepsy nurse training program and had well-developed HIV and TB programs. In this context, continuity clinics for non-infectious conditions filled a recognized gap in existing chronic care infrastructure. In other settings, it may make sense to have a greater or lesser degree of integration across conditions.

1.5   The District Hospital as a Source of Clinical Leadership

In Rwanda, initial efforts around care of non-communicable diseases were focused at the district-hospital level. This approach provided a mechanism for dissemination. It also ensured that the needs of the sickest patients would be addressed first.[33]

In many countries, including Rwanda, the district hospital leaders work closely with the staff of health centers, providing in-service training, clinical mentorship, monitoring, and evaluation. Additionally, provision of high-quality services at district hospitals can help reduce transfers to referral centers. Investment in the development of clinical program leaders at the district level of the health system can move the management of more advanced conditions away from tertiary facilities, while at the same time creating a pathway for further decentralization of uncomplicated chronic care to sites located closer to the homes of patients. During this period of district strengthening, patients may well require direct subsidies to pay for transportation.

In some contexts, physicians might staff district-level continuity clinics entirely on their own. In Rwanda, nurses run the clinics because of a shortage of doctors. The scarce physician pool is, however, large enough to provide oversight. The physician role includes confirmation of new diagnoses and consultation on the management of complex cases. This approach mirrors Rwanda's chronic care infrastructure for HIV.[31]

Each PIH-supported district hospital in Rwanda has an advanced chronic care clinic for non-infectious diseases. These clinics see patients four to five days a week. They are staffed by two to three nurses who see 10 to 20 patients per day. Physicians supervise initial consultations, consult on complex cases, and meet regularly with the nurse program leader to discuss work plans, budgets, and program evaluation. Specialists from referral centers visit the clinic every one to two months to confirm diagnoses and provide ongoing training.

At first, when the number of patients was small, people with different conditions were seen on the same day. However, once patient volume increased, we found it useful to designate specific days of the week for particular diseases. This approach streamlined patient care and education and allowed for more focused interactions between nurses, district hospital physicians, and visiting specialists from referral centers. This approach also created a platform for more organized clinician training on specific diseases.

Initially, we trained advanced nurses at district clinics through daily, direct patient management with physicians. As the program grew, we formalized this process into a three-month-long training curriculum in advanced chronic disease management and basic echocardiography. The program includes both didactic and practical training by physicians and previously trained advanced nurses.

At the same time, an effort to develop a training strategy for health center–level clinicians required greater coordination of chronic care services. In this model, program leaders in NCDs, neuropsychiatry, and infectious diseases (HIV and TB) form a chronic care team that trains and mentors a group of health-center clinicians in the basic management of these conditions (see **FIGURE 1.3**). **TABLE 1.3** provides a sample schedule of the clinical and training duties of district-level clinicians.

FIGURE 1.3   Integration of Human Resources for Chronic Care

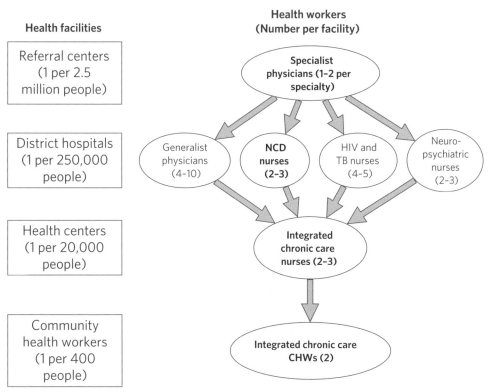

TABLE 1.3   Sample District Hospital-Based Clinician Schedule

	Monday	Tuesday	Wednesday	Thursday	Friday
Nurse 1	Preceptorship of health center nurses	Teaching (didactics)	District hospital heart failure clinic and preceptorship	Teaching (didactics)	Administration
Nurse 2	District hospital hematology/oncology and preceptorship	District hospital chronic respiratory disease and preceptorship	Teaching (didactics)	District hospital advanced diabetes and hypertension clinic and preceptorship	Teaching (didactics)

1.6   District Inpatient Care

A functional system of outpatient management of chronic disease relies in part on adequate inpatient services. District hospital physicians and nurses require education on inpatient management of non-communicable diseases, such as treatment of decompensated heart failure and diabetic ketoacidosis. For generalist physicians working at district level, this training can take place either in medical school or as a part of a post-graduate program. This guide does not address inpatient management specifically, but we have contributed to the World Health Organization's (WHO) forthcoming Integrated Management of Adult and Adolescent Illness District Clinician Manual for hospital care, and we refer interested readers to that guide.

High-quality inpatient care also requires good communication between outpatient and inpatient clinicians. At PIH-supported district hospitals in Rwanda, we have adopted several strategies to encourage this practice, particularly at the time of patient admission and discharge. When a patient is admitted to the district hospital, the outpatient clinician completes a transfer note and verbally discusses the case with the receiving physician. Depending on the complexity of the case, the inpatient physician is encouraged to discuss the case with other district and specialist physicians who have helped manage the patient in the ambulatory setting. At discharge, the inpatient physician completes a discharge form with pertinent information such as discharge medications and lab values, and the form is placed in the patient's chart and returned to the clinic. The patient receives education, assignment of a community health worker if indicated, and an outpatient clinic appointment prior to discharge.

1.7   Health Centers: Case Finding, Initial Management,
and Chronic Care

As the chronic NCD program develops, district-based clinical leaders should begin to train clinicians at the health-center level to provide basic services for common non-communicable diseases. Given the smaller number of clinicians working at health-center level and the smaller volume of patients, chronic care services may require a higher level of integration with other services, such as HIV treatment and neuropsychiatric care. Depending upon the number of staff available, health centers may want to train health care workers in basic management in broad clinical areas, such as chronic care, acute care, and women's health. This would constitute an in-country adaptation of WHO integrated management protocols such as Integrated Management of Childhood Illnesses, Integrated Management of Adult and Adolescent Illness, and Integrated

Management of Pregnancy and Childbirth. District-based clinical leaders are well poised to facilitate these trainings, which should include a mix of didactics and supervised clinical work with ongoing, on-site mentorship, monitoring, and evaluation. This process requires district-hospital staffing to include built-in time for clinician leader travel and training activities. Decentralization of clinical services also requires establishment of drug supply chains that include the health-center facilities. Because expansion of services to the health-center level has significant budgetary implications, decentralizing services may require strategies for additional financing developed by the MOH in partnership with other stakeholders.

1.8   Referral Centers

Historically, concerns about consumption of public health care budgets for services at the referral-center level have dominated much of the discourse around non-communicable disease prevention and treatment in resource-poor settings.[34] However, in the treatment of chronic conditions, only tertiary centers can provide certain diagnostic and therapeutic interventions efficiently and safely. As district hospitals improve delivery of acute and chronic care for patients with non-communicable diseases, referral centers can focus on those activities best provided at the tertiary level. These include specialty consultation for complex endocrine cases; echocardiography and cardiac surgery for rheumatic and congenital heart disease; pathologic diagnosis, surgery, chemotherapy, and radiation for malignancies; and computerized tomography and bronchoscopy for chronic respiratory disease. We have tried to finance outreach by specialists from referral centers to district hospitals in such a way as to promote public and governmental support for strengthening the national health system.

This guide does not cover the important and complex process of establishing essential specialty services such as cardiac surgery and oncologic care at referral centers. An individual country's human resources, health budgets, and epidemiology should guide decisions about how to prioritize investments in national referral services. We believe there is an ethical obligation to care for salvageable patients with advanced conditions, and we suspect that such services can often provide good value for money. At the same time, achieving good outcomes from advanced interventions often requires a system that provides decentralized follow-up and continuing care. This guide addresses these issues with regard to post–cardiac surgery follow-up in chronic care clinics.

1.9   Out-of-Country Referral

Among our chronic care patients, a subset require services not available nationally, such as cardiac surgery or radiation oncology. In Rwanda, the MOH has developed relationships with several regional cardiac surgery centers. PIH in Haiti has built similar relationships with a regional cardiac center. Increasingly, regional centers in low- and middle-income countries have begun to provide these services far more efficiently than facilities in the United States or Europe.

1.10   Screening

In some settings, community-based screening for common chronic diseases may be a reasonable approach to increase case finding. At the very least, community health workers engaged in acute care should be trained in recognizing the symptoms and signs of decompensated chronic diseases. Screening only makes sense, however, in a setting with established and effective chronic care services.

1.11   Principles of Patient Follow-Up and Retention: Community Health Workers and the Electronic Medical Record

Chronic care services in any setting struggle to achieve good patient follow-up and retention. While directly observed therapy for HIV treatment remains controversial, PIH-supported HIV programs have achieved exceptional patient retention and clinical outcomes.[35] In this system, community health workers, or *accompagnateurs*, visit patients on a daily basis to provide psychosocial support, administer medications, ensure adherence, and facilitate medication refills and clinic appointments. We have adopted a similar model for patients with other advanced chronic conditions, such as heart failure, insulin-dependent diabetes, and malignancies. The health workers also serve as a link between the health facility, finding patients who are lost to follow-up, and in some instances referring new or decompensated cases. Community health workers are becoming increasingly involved in wider case-finding activities, in patient education, and in the provision of acute, chronic, and palliative care for a range of conditions.

Good patient follow-up also relies on an organized system of record-keeping. Rwanda has adopted an electronic medical record system to store patient information, track visits, and monitor clinical progress. Clinicians record visits on standardized intake and follow-up forms that collect key patient demographic and clinical characteristics. Data officers in turn enter information into an electronic medical record that facilitates both patient follow-up and program evaluation and monitoring.

We have developed modules for the OpenMRS electronic medical record system, an open-source platform initiated collaboratively by PIH and the Regenstrief Institute. These modules are made publicly accessible at **http://modules.openmrs.org/modules**.

1.12   Equipment, Medication Procurement, and Costs

The WHO Essential Drug list includes most of the medications used in our programs. However, regional, district, and health center formularies may not include all of these drugs. Even when medications are on local formularies, the supply chain systems in place for antiretroviral (ARV) therapy or antituberculous medications have not yet extended to other chronically administered medications. Increasing access to these medications requires clinician training on their use as well as supplemental funding. Chronic disease already poses a large burden on patients in the form of lost income and the expense of clinic visits. In this context, patients cannot reasonably take on the full cost of medications that they must take over long periods of time. Chronic care programs should adopt the approach of ARV programs; they should provide chronically administered medications free or at minimal charge to patients at the point of care. **APPENDIX B** provides specific information on our modeled program costs for each condition.

Chapter 1 References

· ·

1   MEASURE DHS OM. Rwanda Demographic Health Survey III. 2005: Rwanda; 2005.

2   MEASURE DHS OM. Interim Rwanda Demographic Health Survey. 2007-08: Rwanda; 2009.

3   Ministry of Health. National Nutrition Summit Report. Investing in Nutrition as a Foundation for Sustainable Development in Rwanda. Kigali: Government of Rwanda; 2010 February.

4   Parkin DM, Sitas F, Chirenje M, Stein L, Abratt R, Wabinga H. Part I: Cancer in indigenous Africans—burden, distribution, and trends. Lancet Oncol 2008;9:683-92.

5   Newton R, Ngilimana PJ, Grulich A, et al. Cancer in Rwanda. Int J Cancer 1996;66:75-81.

6   Bedu-Addo G, Bates I. Causes of massive tropical splenomegaly in Ghana. Lancet 2002;360:449-54.

7   Weatherall DJ, Clegg JB. Inherited haemoglobin disorders: an increasing global health problem. Bull World Health Organ 2001;79:704-12.

8   Patel V, Prince M. Global mental health: a new global health field comes of age. JAMA 2010;303:1976-7.

9   Simms V, Atijosan O, Kuper H, Nuhu A, Rischewski D, Lavy C. Prevalence of epilepsy in Rwanda: a national cross-sectional survey. Trop Med Int Health 2008;13:1047-53.

10 Birbeck GL, Molyneux ME, Kaplan PW, et al. Blantyre Malaria Project Epilepsy Study (BMPES) of neurological outcomes in retinopathy-positive paediatric cerebral malaria survivors: a prospective cohort study. Lancet Neurol 2010;9:1173-81.

11 Edwards T, Scott AG, Munyoki G, et al. Active convulsive epilepsy in a rural district of Kenya: a study of prevalence and possible risk factors. Lancet Neurol 2008;7:50-6.

12 Commerford P, Mayosi B. An appropriate research agenda for heart disease in Africa. Lancet 2006;367:1884-6.

13 Mocumbi AO, Ferreira MB. Neglected cardiovascular diseases in Africa: challenges and opportunities. J Am Coll Cardiol 2010;55:680-7.

14 Bukhman G, Ziegler JL, Parry EH. Endomyocardial Fibrosis: still a mystery after 60 years. In: PLoS Neglected Trop Dis; 2008:e97.

15 Salvi SS, Barnes PJ. Chronic obstructive pulmonary disease in non-smokers. Lancet 2009;374:733-43.

16 White SL, Chadban SJ, Jan S, Chapman JR, Cass A. How can we achieve global equity in provision of renal replacement therapy? Bull World Health Organ 2008;86:229-37.

17 Mbanya JC, Motala AA, Sobngwi E, Assah FK, Enoru ST. Diabetes in sub-Saharan Africa. Lancet 2010;375:2254-66.

18 Atijosan O, Rischewski D, Simms V, et al. A national survey of musculoskeletal impairment in Rwanda: prevalence, causes and service implications. PLoS One 2008;3:e2851.

19 Stanley CM, Rutherford GW, Morshed S, Coughlin RR, Beyeza T. Estimating the healthcare burden of osteomyelitis in Uganda. Trans R Soc Trop Med Hyg 2010;104:139-42.

20   Mathenge W, Nkurikiye J, Limburg H, Kuper H. Rapid assessment of avoidable blindness in Western Rwanda: blindness in a postconflict setting. PLoS Med 2007;4:e217.

21   Petersen PE, Bourgeois D, Ogawa H, Estupinan-Day S, Ndiaye C. The global burden of oral diseases and risks to oral health. Bull World Health Organ 2005;83:661-9.

22   Obermeyer Z, Rajaratnam JK, Park CH, et al. Measuring adult mortality using sibling survival: a new analytical method and new results for 44 countries, 1974-2006. PLoS Med 2010;7:e1000260.

23   Jamison DT, World Bank. Disease and mortality in Sub-Saharan Africa. 2nd ed. Washington, D.C.: World Bank; 2006.

24   Mathers C, Boerma T, Fat DM. The Global Burden of Disease: 2004 Update. Geneva: World Health Organization; 2008.

25   Samb B, Evans T, Dybul M, et al. An assessment of interactions between global health initiatives and country health systems. Lancet 2009;373:2137-69.

26   Hotez PJ, Fenwick A, Savioli L, Molyneux DH. Rescuing the bottom billion through control of neglected tropical diseases. Lancet 2009;373:1570-5.

27   Hotez PJ, Daar AS. The CNCDs and the NTDs: blurring the lines dividing noncommunicable and communicable chronic diseases. PLoS Negl Trop Dis 2008;2:e312.

28   Kenge AP, Sobngwi E, Fezeu L, et al. Setting-up nurse-led pilot clinics for the management of non-communicable diseases at primary health care level in resource-limited settings of Africa. The Pan African Medical Journal 2009;3.

29   Janssens B, Van Damme W, Raleigh B, et al. Offering integrated care for HIV/AIDS, diabetes and hypertension within chronic disease clinics in Cambodia. Bull World Health Organ 2007;85:880-5.

30   Coleman R, Gill G, Wilkinson D. Noncommunicable disease management in resource-poor settings: a primary care model from rural South Africa. Bull World Health Organ 1998;76:633-40.

31   Shumbusho F, van Griensven J, Lowrance D, et al. Task shifting for scale-up of HIV care: evaluation of nurse-centered antiretroviral treatment at rural health centers in Rwanda. PLoS Med 2009;6:e1000163.

32   Lowrance DW, Ndamage F, Kayirangwa E, et al. Adult clinical and immuno-logic outcomes of the national antiretroviral treatment program in Rwanda during 2004–2005. J Acquir Immune Defic Syndr 2009;52:49-55.

33   Daniels N. Just health: meeting health needs fairly. New York: Cambridge University Press; 2008.

34   Feachem RG, World Bank. The health of adults in the developing world: a summary. Washington, D.C.: World Bank; 1993.

35   Farmer P, Leandre F, Mukherjee JS, et al. Community-based approaches to HIV treatment in resource-poor settings. The Lancet 2001;358:404-9.

CHAPTER 2
Palliative Care and Chronic Care
. . . .

Palliation is the aspect of healthcare concerned with the prevention and relief of suffering rather than treatment of specific diseases. Palliative treatments aim primarily to improve the quality of life, but may also include life-extending therapies. Chronic diseases fall along a spectrum of symptom burden and risk of death. Palliative care is an integral component of treating patients with many chronic diseases, particularly in their more severe manifestations. These diseases and their treatments can cause distressing symptoms, such as pain, dyspnea, and nausea. The suffering due to these symptoms usually remains unrelieved under conditions of extreme poverty and is exacerbated by the terrible financial and psychosocial burden of illness in rural sub-Saharan African villages. In this setting, palliation becomes an essential task for the family and the health care provider, one that tests the limits of our commitment to another person's well-being. Palliative care should be provided throughout the course of a disease and not just at the end of a patient's life (see **FIGURE 2.1**). The balance of disease-specific and palliative therapies depends on the nature of the underlying pathology.

FIGURE 2.1   Diagram of Palliative Care throughout the Course of Illness and Bereavement (Adapted from WHO)[1]

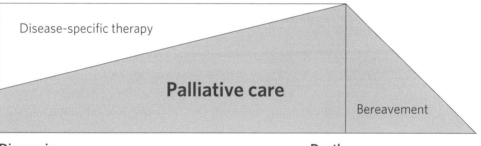

Disease-specific therapy

Palliative care

Bereavement

Diagnosis   Death

In this chapter, we describe the essential role palliative care plays in delivering effective chronic care for non-communicable diseases in resource-poor settings. In other sections of the handbook, we have attempted to incorporate palliative treatments into each disease-specific approach. Rwanda has recently approved palliative care policies designed to make pain control widely available. However, this effort is still in a nascent stage. We have based our material on our team's palliative care experiences in Vietnam and Uganda, which have well-developed programs.[2-5] Rwanda aims to make palliative care a fully integrated part of chronic care services.

2.1 History and Philosophy of Palliative Care Efforts in Resource-Poor Settings

To many, palliation has become synonymous with end-of-life care. This is because, in wealthy nations, palliative care has developed as an alternative to disease-modifying treatments of unlikely benefit for patients with advanced disease. It is often the path chosen at the end of a long battle with an illness at a time when aggressive measures to extend life clearly seem inappropriate.

However, in any setting, attention to symptom relief throughout the disease course should complement efforts to modify the disease and extend life. In fact, recent data suggests that early palliative care can improve both the longevity and the quality of life of some cancer patients.[6] A narrow conception of palliation is even less relevant in places where patients have had access to neither life-prolonging treatment nor palliation.[7]

Palliative care should never be considered an alternative to disease-modifying treatments for patients reasonably likely to benefit from them. Efforts to provide palliative care to AIDS patients, for example, without simultaneous efforts to provide HIV prevention, diagnosis, and antiretroviral (ARV) treatment, are never justified. The reverse is true as well. Programs that offer only one or the other do not provide optimum care and create an unjustifiable dichotomy between palliative and disease-modifying or curative treatments. In fact, the two approaches are interdependent—ARVs are often the most effective means of relieving the symptoms of HIV-related disease, and at the same time palliation of HIV-related symptoms and ARV side effects can increase ARV adherence and extend life. Moreover, HIV remains a chronic disease with significant morbidity and mortality even with therapy, and ARV therapy itself is associated with serious health problems over time. Policies to ensure comfortable and dignified deaths are widely viewed as a human right.[7-9]

Although there is no longer debate about the need for universal access to ARVs, there are still many treatments for non-communicable diseases that are not readily available in resource-poor settings. Of course, there are limits. All medical interventions fall within a spectrum both in terms of cost and efficacy. When do we say a therapy is too expensive in light of the expected benefit? Even in high-resource settings, there are debates about the cost and benefits of specific interventions and whether there is a societal obligation to provide them. Countries like the United Kingdom have attempted to answer this question through formal cost-effectiveness analyses and have developed national guidelines.[10] Similar efforts have been undertaken for resource-poor settings.[11]

As we have learned from the global experience with ARVs, it is often possible to decrease the price of effective therapies through advocacy and collective bargaining. This observation has made effectiveness a more important criterion than cost in determining the appropriate scope of services for a population. Furthermore, the total cost of high-impact, high-cost interventions may not be very significant at country level, if the prevalence of the disease is low. At the same time, the total price of low-cost, low-impact therapies may be very high if the condition is very prevalent (see **TABLE 2.1**). In Rwanda, the Ministry of Health has worked to increase access to high-impact therapies. In some instances, such as renal transplant and dialysis, this has been particularly challenging. Low-impact, high-cost treatments, on the other hand, are controversial even in very wealthy countries. We have not worked to make such treatments available in the Rwandan setting.

TABLE 2.1   Cost/Impact Matrix of Medical Interventions, with Examples

	High impact of therapy	Low, marginal impact of therapy
High cost	• Anti-tuberculosis drugs for multidrug-resistant TB • ARVs for HIV • Cardiac surgery • Renal transplant • Dialysis	• Erlotinib for metastatic pancreatic cancer • Implantable cardioverter defibrillators for cardiomyopathy • Tiotroprium bromide for COPD • Long-acting, patented preparations of shorter-acting medications
Low cost	• Morphine for pain • Bed nets for malaria prevention • Oral rehydration therapy for diarrhea	• Hydrochlorothiazide for Stage 1 or 2 hypertension without high-risk features

Organizations such as the WHO recognize palliative care as an essential component of the treatment of chronic diseases such as cancer and HIV/AIDS. A recent WHO study in five sub-Saharan African countries found that roughly 1% of their populations were in need of end-of-life palliative care each year.[1] They also concluded that because of patient preference and cost considerations, home-based palliative care was the most appropriate model for most patients. The WHO has developed a Palliative Care Guideline Module as part of its package of Interim Guidelines for First-Level Facility Health Workers in Low-Resource Settings.[12] It covers in detail how to treat various common symptoms.

2.2   Community Health Workers and Common Palliative Care Interventions in the Treatment of Chronic Disease

Vertical palliative care programs have attempted to fill an unmet need for palliative services in some African countries. These programs often acknowledge the benefits of integration into existing health systems, but frequently find that this is difficult to achieve. Rwanda has sought to break this pattern by integrating palliative care into chronic care services at the district-hospital, health-center, and community level.

In this model, a central palliative care unit will provide oversight, including training, monitoring, and supervision. It also will ensure both that opioid pain medication is accessible by anyone in need and that the risk of opioid diversion for illicit purposes is minimized. This unit may be located within university teaching hospitals. At district level, palliative care will be integrated into existing functions of physicians and advanced NCD nurses. Physicians will perform initial evaluations of patients in need of home-based palliative care and prescribe medications, including oral morphine. NCD nurses will then be charged with monitoring these patients and with providing oversight of health center–based nurses. At the health-center level, nurses will adjust prescriptions and provide oversight and training to the community health workers. All essential palliative care medications should be available at the health-center level in order to maximize patient access. At the community level, each village in the country will be staffed by community health workers devoted to treating patients with chronic disease. These community health workers will provide adherence support as well as palliative care for patients with chronic disease. Palliative interventions will include providing clinical care and emotional support to patients throughout the course of their chronic illnesses, as well as helping to provide home-based end-of-life care for patients and their families. This community-based work complements efforts to address palliative needs in the clinic and hospital setting and will make possible a continuum of palliative care from the hospital to the home that is essential but rarely available in the developing world.

2.2.1 Assessment of Symptoms

True integration of palliation within a model of chronic disease care includes a thorough assessment of physical and psychosocial distress at the time of disease diagnosis. These elements should be reviewed on each return visit as part of the assessment of disease control. The needs of the family members helping to care for the patient also should be assessed intermittently. Often, palliative efforts will include delivering material support to families impoverished by the patient's illness, including help with housing, food, and school fees. Addressing the social needs of these patients and their families requires coordination with government ministries engaged in agriculture, education, and social welfare.

Palliative care researchers have developed a validated questionnaire, which has been tested in rural sub-Saharan African settings (see **TABLE 2.2**).[13] These questions will not be applicable for all patients with chronic illness, such as those with mild asthma or hypertension. We have incorporated these questions into our clinical forms where appropriate in the Rwandan NCD clinics. We are in the process of developing more simplified tools for assessment of home-based symptom management by community health workers.

TABLE 2.2 Symptom Assessment Scale (Adapted from the African Palliative Outcomes Scale)[13]

Questions for patient:	
Q1. Please rate your pain during the last 3 days	0 (no pain) – 5 (worst/overwhelming pain)
Q2a. Have any other symptoms (e.g., nausea, coughing, or constipation) been affecting how you feel in the last 3 days? **Q2b.** If so, please rate each symptom during the last 3 days: Dyspnea? Nausea or vomiting? Constipation? Diarrhea? Others? (specify)	0 (no, not at all) – 5 (overwhelmingly) 0 (no, not at all) – 5 (overwhelmingly) 0 (no, not at all) – 5 (overwhelmingly) 0 (no, not at all) – 5 (overwhelmingly) 0 (no, not at all) – 5 (overwhelmingly) 0 (no, not at all) – 5 (overwhelmingly)
Q3. Have you been feeling worried about your illness in the past 3 days?	0 (no, not at all) – 5 (overwhelming worry)
Q4. Over the past 3 days, have you been able to share how you are feeling with your family or friends?	0 (no, not at all) – 5 (yes, I've talked freely)
Q5. Over the past 3 days, have you felt that life was worthwhile?	0 (no, not at all) – 5 (yes, all the time)
Q6. Over the past 3 days, have you felt at peace?	0 (no, not at all) – 5 (yes, all the time)
Q7. Over the past 3 days, have you had enough help and advice for your family to plan for the future?	0 (no, not at all) – 5 (as much as wanted)
Questions for family caregiver:	
Q8. Over the past 3 days, how much information have you and your family been given?	0 (none) – 5 (as much as wanted) N/A
Q9. Over the past 3 days, how confident has the family felt caring for the patient?	0 (not at all) – 5 (very confident) N/A
Q10. Has the family been feeling worried about the patient over the last 3 days?	0 (not at all) – 5 (severe worry) N/A

2.2.2 Symptom Management

A wide array of chronic diseases afflicts our patients. Many cause one or more common, distressing symptoms. Therapies aimed at these nonspecific symptoms are an important component of chronic disease treatment algorithms. Here we touch on some of the principles outlined in the Integrated Management of Adult and Adolescent Illness Palliative Care Guideline Module, the Vietnam Ministry of Health Guidelines on Palliative Care for Cancer and AIDS Patients, and the Hospice Africa Uganda Palliative Medicine Guide.[2,5,12] Chemotherapy and radiation therapy, both of which have important roles in relieving pain and other symptoms due to cancer, will be addressed in a forthcoming manual on cancer care and control.

2.2.3 Pain

Pain accompanies many chronic diseases and is a major cause of disability and suffering. However, access to pain relief typically is limited or nonexistent in resource-poor settings. Many countries severely restrict the use of morphine out of fear of opioid diversion or the creation of addiction among patients. A 2004 study by the International Narcotics Control Board revealed that countries with 80% of the world's population comprised only 6% of the world's total opioid consumption.[14] However several countries in sub-Saharan Africa, including Uganda, South Africa, and Rwanda have adopted policies to increase access to opiates.[15,16]

There are two major categories of chronic pain, which often require different therapies.

2.2.3.1 Nociceptive Pain

Nociceptive pain is caused by the stimulation of pain receptors at the end of normal sensory nerves that mediate pain. Nociceptive pain is further subdivided into somatic and visceral pain. Somatic receptors in the skin, soft tissues, muscle, or bone are stimulated, and the resulting pain usually is easy for the patient to localize and describe. Pain in the skin is often sharp, burning, or throbbing. Pain in the muscle is often gnawing or dull. Pain in the bone is also gnawing and dull, but can become sharp with movement. Visceral pain typically is not localized, but more diffuse, and may be referred to a site distant from the lesion. It may be dull or sharp and may produce a feeling of pressure. It is caused by stimulation of pain receptors in internal organs, including hollow viscera. It may be due to blockage, swelling, or stretching of the organs due to metastases, inflammation, or other causes.

2.2.3.2 Neuropathic Pain

Neuropathic pain is caused by damage to nerves or brain. Neuropathic pain is often described as burning or like an electric shock. There also can be numbness, tingling, or allodynia (pain resulting from a stimulus that normally is not painful, such as light touch) in the area innervated by the injured nerves. This type of pain is very common among our diabetic, cancer, and HIV/AIDS patients. Any kind of injury to nerve tissue can result in neuropathic pain, including compression or infiltration by tumor, ischemia from poor circulation (in diabetes mellitus), infection by varicella zoster or HIV virus, or neurotoxic medications, such as some cancer chemotherapy drugs and some ARVs, especially d4T (stavudine).

2.2.3.3 Principles of Pain Management

The following principles are important to successful treatment of pain:[1]

1. **WHO three-step pain-relief ladder.** Escalating therapy from a non-opioid (acetaminophen/paracetamol, ibuprofen, or aspirin) to a weak opioid (codeine or low-dose morphine), and finally to a strong opioid (standard-dose morphine). In Rwanda, a weak opioid such as codeine is not widely available, and we therefore substitute low-dose morphine. The WHO recommends a three-step approach to relief of pain.[1] According to the WHO, this simple method can relieve 80%–90% of cancer pain (see **FIGURE 2.2**). While designed for treatment of cancer pain, this approach is effective for pain of most causes. Patients with moderate or severe pain, or pain that is not relieved by non-opioids, can be given the standard 5-mg starting dose of oral morphine. If the pain is partially but still not adequately relieved after 60 minutes, the same dose can be repeated. If the patient has no relief after 60 minutes, a double dose should be given. This process can be repeated until adequate pain relief is achieved or until unacceptable side effects occur. In settings such as rural Rwanda, palliative care will take place primarily in the home. For this reason, we emphasize the use of oral over injectable morphine.

    A strong opioid such as morphine is first-line treatment for moderate or severe pain of any kind, including neuropathic pain. However, neuropathic pain sometimes is not relieved by opioid or non-opioid treatment. In this situation, adjuvant medications, such as amitriptyline or phenytoin, can be useful. In other situations, adjuvant medications can be used to reduce or eliminate the need for opioid therapy. For example, even severe pain caused by liver metastases sometimes can be relieved with a steroid, such as prednisolone or dexamethasone.

FIGURE 2.2   The WHO Three-Step Pain Ladder[1]

		Severe pain or pain persisting/increasing Strong opioid +/- non-opioid +/- adjuvant
	Moderate pain or pain persisting/increasing Weak opioid (or low-dose strong opioid) +/- non-opioid +/- adjuvant	
Mild pain Non-opioid (paracetamol or NSAID) +/- adjuvant		

2. **Dosing intervals.** For constant or chronic pain or pain that recurs frequently, pain medications should be given around the clock at appropriate intervals, rather than as needed, to help keep pain in check. Allowing pain to rebound between doses causes unneeded suffering and can also make the pain harder to control. The analgesic effect of immediate-release oral morphine lasts 4 hours. Therefore, the drug should be given at least this frequently to control chronic pain. A double dose can be given at bedtime to help eliminate the need for a dose in the middle of the night.

3. **Opioid tolerance.** Opioid tolerance is a normal phenomenon that occurs in many patients who take an opioid for chronic pain for at least a few months or more. It means that an increase in the dose may be required over time to achieve the same analgesic effect, even when the disease remains stable. This is something that should be anticipated as a normal part of treating pain and not as a sign of psychological dependence (addiction). All patients taking pain medication should be re-evaluated regularly and their medication regimen and doses adjusted according to their needs. Patients whose disease is worsening or who develop tolerance may need progressively higher doses, while others whose disease is responding to treatment may need lower doses. However, opioid therapy should not be stopped abruptly to avoid opioid withdrawal syndrome. Rather, when opioid therapy is no longer needed, the dose should be reduced gradually by no more than 50% every 2–3 days.

4. **Route of administration.** In most cases, oral rather than intravenous or subcutaneous medications should be used, given the limited inpatient capacity and relative difficulty of providing parenteral medications in the home. In Rwanda, liquid morphine preparations will be distributed by community health workers following initial prescription by a physician. Liquid morphine is made from powder in various concentrations depending on the patient's needs. (See **APPENDIX A** for oral morphine recipes.) When patients can no longer tolerate oral medications, buccal or rectal routes may be used. Because the absorption of morphine by these routes is unpredictable, higher doses may be required.

5. **Rescue doses.** Patients taking an opioid around-the-clock for pain may have occasional breakthrough pain: a flare-up of pain despite otherwise adequate pain relief. When breakthrough pain occurs, it should be treated with an extra dose of opioid. The rescue dose should be 10% of the total 24-hour dose of opioid. For example, if a patient taking morphine 10 mg orally every 4 hours has breakthrough pain, she should be given a 6 mg rescue dose.

6. **Opioid side effects.** Most patients taking an opioid develop constipation. Therefore, a low dose of a laxative should be prescribed for most patients when opioid therapy is initiated, and the dose should be adjusted at subsequent visits based on the patient's pattern of bowel movements. Opioid-induced constipation does not diminish with time, so laxative therapy is always important for patients taking opioids. Some patients develop nausea from opioid therapy. In most cases, the nausea is mild and resolves in a few days. When it is more severe or constant, it can be treated with a low dose of haloperidol (0.5 mg orally, intravenously, or subcutaneously). Sedation is a common side effect of opioids. This, too, is usually mild and usually diminishes with time. Patients who have been in pain for some time may fall asleep when opioid therapy is started not because the drug sedates them but because they are exhausted and finally able to sleep. Respiratory depression is a rare side effect of opioid therapy when guidelines are followed, and it never occurs before sedation.

TABLE 2.3 lists the essential pain medications (based on the Rwandan formulary) that should be available at the health-center level.

TABLE 2.3   Essential Medications for Pain Relief

Symptom	Medication	Dose	Notes
Mild pain/ fever reducers (non-opiates)	Acetaminophen/ paracetamol	**Adult:** 0.5–1 gram every 4 to 6 hours. Not to exceed 4 grams in 1 day **Child:** 10-15 mg/ kg (maximum 90 mg/kg/day divided every 4-6 hours)	Use maximum 2 grams per day in patients with enlarged livers or known liver disease. Very toxic to liver in overdose.
	Ibuprofen	**Adult:** 400–800 mg every 6-8 hours (maximum dose 2.4 gm/day) **Child:** 10 mg/kg every 6-8 hours	Particularly effective in bone pain. Anti-inflammatory at higher doses. Can cause digestive upset and gastrointestinal bleeding. Do not use in renal failure. Decrease doses in patients with severe liver failure. Prolonged prescription requires cimetidine or omeprazole for gastrointestinal prophylaxis.
	Diclofenac	**Adult:** 25–75 mg every 12 hours	Same as ibuprofen, but less expensive for long-term use, with simpler dosing.
Moderate to severe pain	Morphine, liquid preparation	**Adult:** 2.5–10 mg every 4 hours. May give double dose at bedtime. No maximum dose. Titrate to patient comfort. **Child:** 0.15 mg/ kg–0.3 mg/kg every 4 hours. Titrate as with adults.	Dose increases may be limited by oversedation. Should decrease the dose or increase the dosing interval in case of any renal failure. Constipation is a common problem and all patients should be placed on a bowel regimen prophylactically (see **TABLE 2.5**).
Neuropathic pain (burning pains or shooting)	Amitriptyline	**Adult:** 10–25 mg by mouth daily. **Child:** 0.1 mg/kg once a day at bedtime. Increase as needed by 0.2-0.4 mg/kg every 2-3 days to a maximum of 2mg/kg/day	Dose should be titrated upward every week to effect. May take weeks to work. Maximum dose in adults is 100 mg per day. Side effects include initial drowsiness, postural hypotension, dry mouth, mild tachycardia, constipation. Life-threatening cardiac toxicity with overdose.
	Phenytoin	**Adult:** 100 mg twice per day initially, increase up to 400 mg twice per day if needed **Child:** 2.5-5 mg/ kg twice per day (maximum 200 mg twice per day)	Can use instead of, or in addition to, amitriptyline if neuropathic pain persists. Avoid if on anti-retrovirals due to drug interactions.

Symptom	Medication	Dose	Notes
Muscle spasms	Diazepam	**Adult:** 2.5–10 mg by mouth 2 to 3 times per day **Child:** 0.05 mg/kg–0.1 mg/kg 3 to 4 times per day (maximum 0.8 mg/kg/day)	Drowsiness, ataxia.
Pain from swelling, inflammation, or neuropathy	Prednisolone	**Adult:** 20–80 mg by mouth daily **Child:** 1 mg/kg x 1–2x/day by mouth	May also improve nausea, fatigue, and appetite. Particularly helpful in the case of malignant lesions causing localized swelling in the muscle or bone. The dose should be decreased gradually over a period of 2–3 weeks and then stopped to avoid side effects.

2.2.4 Dyspnea

Many types of chronic disease can result in severe dyspnea. Heart failure and chronic respiratory disease can cause dyspnea even in early stages. Treatment protocols outlined in the following chapters will help to relieve this symptom. Patients with dyspnea due to advanced, untreatable cancers and those dying of respiratory compromise from any cause should be treated with an opioid such as morphine if other treatments are not effective. Morphine is very effective at relieving dyspnea. Dosage is the same as for pain (see **SECTION 2.2.3**). At the end of life, some patients develop secretions in the upper airway and throat. The sound that these secretions make when air passes through them can be disturbing for family members even when the patient is not short of breath. Counseling by a community health worker in this situation can be helpful. Hyoscine butylbromide, an anti-cholinergic medication, can also help dry secretions if needed. The typical dose for adults is 20 mg every 2–4 hours around the clock, or as needed. The medicine can be given either orally or rectally, as described below for anti-nausea medications.

2.2.5 Nausea/Vomiting

Nausea and vomiting occur with many chronic diseases, either as a result of the disease process itself or as a side effect of medications. Nausea may have many causes. For instance, in heart, liver and renal failure, the gut walls may become edematous and function poorly, a condition that leads to nausea and vomiting. Nausea-producing substances that are either taken into the body (such as medications or food toxins) or produced by the body (in liver or renal failure, for example) stimulate certain areas of the brain that control nausea and vomiting. **TABLE 2.4** indicates the appropriate therapy for nausea depending on the cause. When patients cannot tolerate oral medication, tablets may be ground up and mixed with water for rectal insertion via a syringe without a needle.

Haloperidol and promethazine occasionally may cause a dystonic reaction, characterized by muscle spasms. This is uncomfortable, but not dangerous, and should be treated with diphenhydramine.

TABLE 2.4   Essential Medications for Control of Nausea/Vomiting

Cause of nausea	Therapy
Liver failure, renal failure, metabolic derangement, drug side effect, or bacterial infection (nausea due to a toxin or inflammatory mediator)	**Haloperidol** **Adult:** 0.5-1 mg 2-4 times per day given orally, IV, or SC, around the clock or as needed **Child (≤ 40 kg):** 0.025-0.05 mg/kg/day in 2-3 divided doses. Increase by 0.25-0.5 mg/day every 5-7 days as needed to maximum dose 0.15 mg/kg/day
	Promethazine **Adult:** 12.5-25 mg every 4 hours orally, IV, IM, or by rectum **Child (≤ 40 kg):** 0.25-1 mg/kg 4 times a day orally, IV, IM, or by rectum. Maximum dose: 25 mg per dose
	Dexamethasone **Adult:** 8-20 mg once a day in the morning or 4-10 mg 2 times per day IV or IM, around the clock or as needed **Child (≤ 40 kg):** 0.5-1 mg/kg 2 times per day IV or SC around the clock or as needed. Maximum dose: 10 mg 2 times per day
Increased intracranial pressure, bowel obstruction, or distension of liver or of hollow viscus due to neoplasm	**Dexamethasone** **Adult:** 4-10 mg 2 times per day IV or IM, around the clock or as needed **Child (≤ 40 kg):** 0.5-1 mg/kg 2 times per day IV or SC around the clock or as needed. Maximum dose: 10 mg 2 times per day
Anxiety	**Diazepam** **Adult:** 2.5-10 mg 3 times per day, orally, IV, or SC, around the clock or as needed **Child (≤ 40 kg):** 0.05-0.1 mg/kg/day divided 3-4 times per day (maximum 0.8 mg/kg/day)
Gastroparesis	**Metoclopramide** **Adult:** 10 mg, 4 times per day, orally, IV, or SC, around the clock or as needed. **Child:** 0.1-0.2 mg/kg/dose 4 times per day, orally, IV or SC, around the clock or as needed
Stimulation of vestibular apparatus	**Chlorpheniramine** **Adult:** 4 mg orally every 4 hours, around the clock or as needed **Child (≤ 40 kg):** 1-2 mg by mouth every 4-6 hours. Maximum dose: 6 mg/day for 2-5 yo, 12 mg/day for 6-11 yo, around the clock or as needed
	Promethazine **Adult:** 12.5-25 mg every 4 hours orally, IV, IM, or by rectum **Child:** 0.25-1 mg/kg 4 times a day orally, IV, IM, or by rectum. Maximum dose: 25 mg
Adjuvants for nausea/ vomiting of any cause	**Chlorpheniramine** **Adult:** 4 mg orally every 4 hours, around the clock or as needed **Child (≤ 40 kg):** 1-2 mg by mouth every 4-6 hours. Maximum dose: 6 mg/day for 2-5 yo, 12 mg/day for 6-11 yo, around the clock or as needed

2.2.6 Constipation

Constipation frequently afflicts patients with chronic illness, either as a side effect of medications or due to the disease itself. In addition, chronically ill patients may not be very mobile or may be unable to tolerate fibrous diets, further slowing intestinal motility.

All patients with constipation should be assessed for fecal impaction with a digital rectal exam and disimpacted manually as needed. All patients should be encouraged to take fibrous foods and fluids, as tolerated. Laxatives and enemas may also be used to ease constipation (see **TABLE 2.5**). The most common types of laxatives are stimulants (bisacodyl), osmotic agents (lactulose), and lubricants (glycerine). In patients with constipation due primarily to opioid therapy, a stimulant laxative is first-line therapy. Osmotic laxatives should be used only in patients who are well hydrated. In severe cases of opioid-induced constipation, oral naloxone can be used to reverse the opioid effect on the gut.

TABLE 2.5   Essential Therapies for Treating Constipation

Treatment	Dose
Glycerin suppository	**Adult:** 4 gm suppository per rectum daily
	Child (≤ 40 kg): 2 gm suppository per rectum daily
Lactulose syrup	**Adult:** 15–45 ml 2–3 times per day orally, maintain 30–90 ml/day
	Child (≤ 40 kg): 7.5 ml 1 time per day orally
Bisacodyl	**Adult:** 10 mg once or twice daily, orally or per rectum
	Child (≤ 40 kg): 0.3 mg/kg once daily by mouth. Maximum dose: 10 mg. Can also be given per rectum
Naloxone	**Adult:** 1–2 mg every 8 hours. Should only be given orally for this indication

Patients with intermittent bowel obstruction due to a malignancy may benefit from steroid therapy (see prednisolone dosing in **TABLE 2.3**).

2.2.7 Diarrhea

Many chronic illnesses can lead to diarrhea. For instance, cancer treatments that can cause diarrhea include some chemotherapeutic drugs, or radiation. Patients with diarrhea who take a diuretic medication should be seen by a clinician for adjustment of therapy to avoid dangerous volume depletion. Patients with chronic illness are also more susceptible to infectious causes of diarrhea. In the case of accompanying fever or bloody stool, infectious causes should be considered as a possibility and treated appropriately. Conversely, antibiotics also can cause diarrhea by killing normal bowel flora.

All patients with severe diarrhea should have oral replacement of fluids and electrolytes, if possible and appropriate. When a patient taking a laxative develops diarrhea, the laxative should be discontinued until the diarrhea stops.

TABLE 2.6 outlines the evaluation and treatment of diarrhea not obviously due to infection. Narcotics and anticholinergic medications such as hyoscine butylbromide can help reduce diarrhea if loperamide is not available.

TABLE 2.6   Symptomatic Management of Diarrhea

Treatment	Dose
Loperamide	**Adult:** 4 mg orally initially, then 2 mg orally after every loose stool, up to a maximum of 16 mg per day **Child (weight 13–20 kg):** 1 mg orally 3 times per day **Child (weight 21–30 kg):** 2 mg orally up to 3 times per day
Morphine, liquid preparation (low dose)	**Adult:** 2.5 mg every 8 hours. May give orally, buccally, or rectally **Child (≤ 40kg):** 0.15 mg/kg, up to 2.5 mg every 4 hours. Administer as with adults
Hyoscine butylbromide	**Adults:** 10-20 mg every 6 hours orally or rectally

2.2.8   Delirium/Agitation

Patients with terminal illness may become delirious with or without agitation. Delirium and agitation are associated with significant morbidity and mortality and are distressing to both the patient and the family. Common causes of delirium include psychoactive medications (especially benzodiazepines), renal or liver failure, hypoxia or hypercapnia, metabolic derangements such as hypercalcemia, or central nervous system disorders such as infection, bleeding, or tumor. Sometimes there is an underlying permanent dementia that must be distinguished from reversible delirium, and often delirium has multiple causes.

Treatment of delirium includes trying to orient the patient, attempting to maintain normal sleep-wake schedules, and avoiding benzodiazepines. Patients may also be treated with haloperidol at a dose of 0.5–5 mg 2 to 4 times per day orally. It may be given more frequently for severe symptoms. Chlorpromazine, a more sedating medication, also can be used at 10–50 mg 2 or 3 times per day orally. Heavily sedating the patient is not recommended, except in extreme circumstances when the patient's safety is at risk.

2.2.9   Pruritus and Pressure Ulcers

Pruritus or itching is a common but often overlooked side effect of chronic illness that can cause severe distress. Renal failure often causes pruritus. Any patient with chronic illness is at risk for cholestasis, which also can cause itching. Opiates can also cause pruritus.

Treatment depends on the cause. Any allergenic medication or substance should be identified and removed. If morphine that is needed to treat pain or dyspnea appears to be the cause of pruritus and no other strong opioid is available, an antihistamine such as chlorpheniramine may provide relief. The lowest effective dose should be used due to this medication's sedating effect. Pruritus in the setting of renal failure is often due to dry skin and can be relieved by emollient lotions. See **TABLE 2.7** for treatment details.

Skin care of chronically ill, bedridden, malnourished, or incontinent patients is essential. Patients can quickly develop pressure ulcers, skin tears, and superficial fungal infections. The patient should be kept as clean and dry as possible. Intact skin can be cleansed with an antibacterial agent such as povidine-iodine. Open wounds should be cleansed gently with saline. A wet or bleeding wound can be packed with povidine-iodine gauze. Dry wounds should be packed and dressed with gauze or cotton coated with petroleum jelly. If the wound is malodorous, metronidazole powder should be sprinkled on the wound prior to applying the dressing. Metronidazole powder may be obtained either by opening metronidazole capsules, or by crushing the tablets.

TABLE 2.7 Management of Chronic Pruritus and Skin Care

Condition	Treatment
Pruritus due to dry skin, renal failure	Emollient lotion such as calamine
	Chlorpheniramine **Adult:** 4 mg orally every 4 hours, around the clock or as needed **Child (≤ 40 kg):** 1–2 mg orally every 4 hours, around the clock or as needed
Contact dermatitis (e.g., from tape used in hospitals)	Remove allergenic substance High-potency topical steroid such as 0.05% betamethasone valerate
Scabies	Permethrin lotion applied from head (avoid face) to toes. Leave lotion on for 8–14 hours, then wash off. The usual adult dose is 20–30 grams. Repeat in 1 week. Wash all clothes and bedding and dry in the sun. Do not use for babies less than 2 months old
Cholestasis	**Adult:** Prednisolone 10 mg per day. Cimetidine 400 mg twice per day.
Pruritus due to opioids	**Chlorpheniramine** **Adult:** 4 mg orally every 4 hours, around the clock or as needed **Child (≤ 40 kg):** 1–2 mg orally every 4 hours, around the clock or as needed
Foul odor from wounds	Keep wound clean. Crush metronidazole tables and sprinkle onto wound daily

2.2.10 Giving Bad News

Care should be taken whenever giving bad news to minimize emotional distress for the patient and family. The following is a list of general guidelines for giving bad news, however each cultural setting may require different techniques.

1. Determine in advance whom the patient would like to receive medical information and the most culturally appropriate way to give bad news.

2. Suggest that support persons such as family members or friends be present when bad news will be discussed.

3. Take the time to sit down.

4. First explore the patient's or family's understanding of the disease and gently correct misconceptions.

5. Pause frequently to give the patient or family a chance to absorb the news and ask questions.

6. Be prepared for strong reactions such as anger or grief.

7. Offer to see the patient or family soon again to answer questions and provide emotional support.

2.2.11 Psychosocial and Spiritual Issues

Patients with chronic diseases often experience significant social, financial, and spiritual distress. Often, this is the most difficult aspect of their disease. Community health workers can help provide support to these patients. They can also identify those in need of more intensive psychological, social work, or spiritual support. In Rwanda, almost all district hospitals have a neuropsychiatric health nurse who can see patients with symptoms of depression or anxiety. There is also a social work team that can make home visits and assess needs for housing, food, and educational support. In some cases, patient associations may serve as a source of support to patients. In Rwanda, patient associations have served as a platform for income-generating activities and have also provided a community for patients living with HIV.

Chapter 2 References

1   World Health Organization. A community health approach to palliative care for HIV/AIDS and cancer patients in sub-Saharan Africa: World Health Organization; 2003.

2   Palliative Medicine. Pain and symptom control in the cancer and/or AIDS patient in Uganda and other African countries. 4th edition. Entebbe, Uganda: Hospice Africa Uganda; 2006.

3   Palliative care for HIV/AIDS and cancer patients in Vietnam. Advanced training curriculum: Massachusetts General Hospital; 2008.

4   Palliative care for HIV/ AIDS and cancer patients in Vietnam. Basic training curriculum: Massachusetts General Hospital; 2007.

5   Guidelines on palliative care for cancer and AIDS patients. Hanoi, Vietnam: Ministry of Health; 2006.

6   Temel JS, Greer JA, Muzikansky A, et al. Early palliative care for patients with metastatic non-small-cell lung cancer. N Engl J Med;363:733-42.

7   Krakauer EL. Just palliative care: responding responsibly to the suffering of the poor. J Pain Symptom Manage 2008;36:505-12.

8   Gwyther L, Brennan F, Harding R. Advancing palliative care as a human right. J Pain Symptom Manage 2009;38:767-74.

9   Spence D, Merriman A, Binagwaho A. Palliative care in Africa and the Caribbean. PLoS Med 2004;1:e5.

10 Hawkes N. Health technology assessment. NICE goes global. BMJ 2009;338:b103.

11 Laxminarayan R, Mills AJ, Breman JG, et al. Advancement of global health: key messages from the Disease Control Priorities Project. Lancet 2006;367:1193-208.

12 World Health Organization. Integrated Management of Adolescent and Adult Illness. Guidelines for first-level facility health workers at health centre and district outpatient clinics. 2004.

13 Harding R, Selman L, Agupio G, et al. Validation of a core outcome measure for palliative care in Africa: the APCA African palliative outcome scale. Health Qual Life Outcomes;8:10.

14 Report of the international narcotics control board for 2004. Vienna, Austria: International Narcotics Control Board; 2004.

15 Harding R, Higginson IJ. Palliative care in sub-Saharan Africa. Lancet 2005;365:1971-7.

16 Anne Merriman RH. Pain control in the African context: the Ugandan introduction of affordable morphine to relieve suffering at the end of life. Philosophy, Ethics, and Humanities in Medicine 2010;5.

CHAPTER 3

Role of Community Health Workers, Family Planning, Mental Health, Pharmacy, Laboratory, and Social Services in the Treatment of Chronic Disease

· ·

An effective program for managing chronic disease cannot simply focus on physical ailments and disease states. An effective clinical intervention requires understanding the social background of patients along with their home, family, and financial situations. Disease has rendered many of our patients destitute and unable to pay for health care. Chronic disease has also led to depression in many of our patients, reducing their capacity to seek care. The chronic disease programs implemented through a collaboration between PIH and the Rwanda Ministry of Health work with a range of service providers to give patients the best chance at regaining health and quality of life.

3.1   Community Health Workers

Since 2007, Rwanda has implemented a national community health worker (CHW) program. Every village (around 100–250 households) has four CHWs. Two of these, a man and a woman, are called *binômes*, and they focus primarily on case identification and referral for a variety of diseases, as well as the treatment of childhood diseases like pneumonia, diarrhea, and malaria, and community support for malnutrition. Each village has a maternal health worker responsible for identification of pregnant women, antenatal care visits, and ensuring delivery at health facilities. The final health worker is in charge of social affairs in the community and is responsible for the compilation of performance-based financing reports. CHWs receive performance-based financing through cooperatives.

Districts supported by PIH have also introduced a cadre of community health workers focused on treatment and support for patients with chronic communicable and non-communicable diseases. The government of Rwanda has moved to introduce two of these chronic care CHWs, who work alongside the four mentioned above, in each village.

One key function of chronic care CHWs is to visit patients on a regular (usually daily) basis to provide adherence support. All patients on antiretroviral therapy for HIV or anti-tuberculosis treatment for TB are assigned a chronic care CHW. In the case of NCDs, there is a much greater range of severity within the chronic conditions. Most patients do not require such intensive support. NCD clinicians currently assign chronic care CHWs only to those patients with advanced conditions such as cancer, heart failure, rheumatic heart disease, or insulin-dependent diabetes. Occasionally patients with hypertension, chronic respiratory disease, or epilepsy may be assigned a CHW during a period when their disease is poorly controlled. CHWs are also used to help identify patients with less severe disease who have been lost to follow-up or who require refills of medications between visits. Among the roughly 2000 patients enrolled in the NCD program, only 500 have a chronic care CHW assigned. Patients with less severe conditions may ultimately need CHWs assigned to give less intensive adherence support.

In comparison with HIV and TB treatment, NCD management often requires more complex medication regimens along with more frequent clinic visits and changes in dosing. As part of comprehensive chronic care training, CHWs must learn about palliative care, proper inhaler technique, subcutaneous insulin administration and monitoring, diuretics, and signs of decompensation, among other topics. Some specific aspects of training for chronic care CHWs are mentioned in disease-specific chapters in this manual. Comprehensive training for chronic care CHWs will be discussed in a forthcoming revision of the *Partners In Health Accompagnateur Training Guide.*[1]

3.2 Housing Assistance

Many of the sickest patients live in marginal housing with dirt floors, inadequate roofing, and poor access to clean water. Post-cardiac surgery patients and patients receiving chemotherapy for cancer are at particular risk of developing life-threatening infections in these conditions. For this group of NCD patients, a social worker evaluates the patient's living situation and refers patients with inadequate housing to the POSER (Program on Social and Economic Rights) program to have their house repaired or rebuilt.

This program is currently available only in districts where there is a partnership between PIH and the Ministry of Health. It is an innovation that will require adaptation in order to be integrated into the national system.

Housing standards have been established at the district level throughout Rwanda, with short- and long-term goals already in place to help reach them. Allocations of housing aid should prioritize residents with chronic diseases as a particularly vulnerable group in need of additional support in order to adhere to new standards.

3.3   Nutritional Support

Malnutrition worsens most disease states. This risk is higher for certain groups of patients. Patients with diabetes who are on insulin may develop life-threatening hypoglycemia if their food supply is irregular. Malnutrition can also worsen severe heart failure and render many medical therapies ineffective. For these reasons, patients with severe heart failure or insulin-dependent diabetes at PIH-supported sites are evaluated by a social worker and, if necessary, are referred to the nutrition department for a therapeutic food supplementation.

This strategy presents several challenges. Direct provision of food is expensive and is likely beyond the budgets of most low-income countries. Furthermore, it does not address the root causes of food insecurity. PIH has adopted this strategy as an emergency stopgap measure, and considers it an essential part of medical therapy for certain chronic diseases. However, longer-term strategies such as promotion of household agricultural practices and income-generating activities are likely to be more helpful and more lasting over the long term.

3.4   Mental Health

This guide does not deal specifically with therapeutic approaches to mental illness. These issues will be addressed in a forthcoming volume on neuropsychiatric illness. Chronic physical illness, however, can be accompanied by chronic mental illness. Loss of functional ability can lead to an inability to work, to provide for a family, and to perform basic functions. Thus illness can result in deepening poverty. Depression and hopelessness can ensue. Stigmatization because of physical ailments and functional disabilities can also result in social isolation. Screening tools have been developed to evaluate for depression among the chronically ill. Patients who are found to have depression will be referred to the mental health clinic for counseling and treatment. Even when they do not meet clinical criteria for a diagnosis of depression, many patients suffering from chronic diseases can benefit from the assistance of a social worker or counselor.

3.5   Family Planning in Chronic Disease

By working to increase health facility–based deliveries and access to prenatal care, Rwanda has decreased its maternal mortality rate from 1400 maternal deaths per 100,000 live births in 2000 to 750 maternal deaths per 100,000 live births in 2005.[2] In spite of these improvements, pregnancy and childbirth still pose a high risk of maternal morbidity and mortality to the women of Rwanda and other poor countries.

Women with chronic diseases face an even greater risk of harm from childbearing. Almost any chronic disease increases the risk of maternal or fetal complications in pregnancy and childbirth. Some conditions, such as heart failure, make pregnancy potentially deadly. Other conditions require medications, such as warfarin and ACE inhibitors, that can lead to serious birth defects.

Every female patient of childbearing age (15–45 years) who presents to the NCD clinic for care is tested for pregnancy and asked about use of birth control. All patients are educated about the availability of family planning services at the health center nearest to where they live. Women at high risk of morbidity or mortality from pregnancy are strongly counseled to avoid pregnancy and are referred to the family planning clinic that day for advice on birth control. At each follow-up visit, clinicians ask patients about their use of birth control. Clinicians also keep track of when patients on long-acting family planning methods such as medroxyprogesterone injections require re-dosing.

All pregnant women are referred to their health center's prenatal clinic for pregnancy-related care. The NCD clinic continues to manage chronic conditions during pregnancy. In some cases, prenatal and NCD clinicians must closely work with each other to manage patients with a chronic illness and a pregnancy complication, such as preeclampsia.

3.6   Pharmacy Services

The pharmacy is an essential component of any health facility. In many resource-poor settings, stock-outs of essential medications leave health care workers helpless to provide appropriate therapies to their patients. Even available medications may be too expensive for impoverished patients to afford if co-payments are high. These problems are magnified when dealing with chronic diseases, which require a steady, uninterrupted supply of medication.

Rwanda has worked to mitigate these problems by improving supply chain organization, and by making medications more affordable through subsidized universal health insurance. Pharmacies have already developed strategies to avoid problems in procurement of ARVs. Treatment of chronic NCDs requires the same level of vigilance in procurement practices. As in the case of ARVs, co-payments for other chronic disease medications may need to be eliminated or minimized in order to reduce barriers to care.

Mistakes at the pharmacy level can be deadly. It is essential that pharmacists receive adequate training on the dangers and appropriate dosing of the medications they dispense. This becomes even more difficult in dosing medications for children. Many of the medications in this book will need to be crushed and diluted, or cut into halves or quarters to achieve appropriate dosing for children or small adults. Moreover, many of the medications used to treat chronic diseases can be deadly even in small doses. Pharmacists should take an active role in educating patients about these risks and ensuring that adults know to store all medications out of reach of children.

In the early days of new NCD programs, clinicians should double-check all medications dispensed from the pharmacy. NCD programs introduce new medications, often with multiple dosage preparations, that can be easily confused, with deadly consequences.

Pillboxes can be helpful for medication storage. However, they have the disadvantages of being time consuming to fill and leaving drugs unlabeled. Their use requires additional pharmacy staffing and training.

3.7   Laboratory

Many of the protocols in this handbook rely on laboratory testing to make diagnoses or guide treatment. Electrolytes can be particularly difficult to measure accurately. At PIH-supported facilities, we have found point-of-care testing for assessment of metabolic function to be useful at the district level. These machines are portable, can be used in the clinic (saving the patient from having to wait in line at the lab) and provide reliable results at a relatively low cost. The same machines can also be used to check INR in patients who are anticoagulated. Additional point-of-care technologies used at the district level include small, dedicated PT/INR, glucose, and HbA1c machines. In some cases, patients who live or travel far from a health facility may be given their own PT/INR machines to monitor anticoagulation.

3.8   Other Diagnostic Equipment

Ultrasound is becoming increasingly miniaturized and inexpensive. Many of our protocols rely on ultrasound to help guide diagnosis and therapy. Ultrasound is often available at the district level, but is used primarily for obstetric indications. We have found it useful to have a dedicated machine for use in the NCD clinic. This machine should be compatible with both cardiac and abdominal probes and be capable of color Doppler, but not necessarily spectral Doppler. Ideally, images should be archived. This allows an external reviewer to monitor the quality of image acquisition and interpretation, and serves as a teaching tool for clinicians.

Commonly available electrocardiographic (ECG) equipment is often cumbersome to use. Additionally, these machines frequently use consumables that are vulnerable to stock-outs. Portable, single-lead ECG machines may be useful in settings where the primary diagnoses of interest are arrhythmias. These machines typically also allow easy transmission of images to a cardiologist for confirmation of the diagnosis.

Automated blood pressure measurement machines are generally preferred to manual devices. These automated machines have been validated, and are more reliable in practice than manual measurement. They should be equipped with normal and small adult-size cuffs. They should also be able to use electrical power both from an outlet and from batteries. In our experience, semi-automated machines are unreliable and tend to slow down a busy clinic due to frequent inability to generate a reading. Manual machines should be available as a back-up and for small children.

Chapter 3 References

1   Mukherjee J, ed. Partners In Health Accompagnateur Training Guide. First Edition. Boston: Partners In Health; 2008.

2   MEASURE DHS OM. Rwanda Demographic Health Survey III. 2005: Rwanda NISR; 2005.

CHAPTER 4

Heart Failure

. . . .

Heart failure accounts for 5% to 10% of hospitalizations among adults throughout sub-Saharan Africa.[1-8] Surveys dating back to the 1950s show that these numbers have not changed substantially for at least the past half-century. In the 1980s and 1990s, the introduction of two-dimensional echocardiography helped clarify the causes of heart failure in this setting.[9] Reports from referral centers on the continent showed that most cases of heart failure were due to non-ischemic cardiomyopathies, congenital heart disease, rheumatic heart disease, or hypertensive heart disease rather than coronary artery disease (see **TABLE 4.1**). Even in urban centers with an increasing prevalence of vascular risk factors, non-ischemic etiologies of heart failure still dominated.[10-18]

TABLE 4.1   **Causes of Heart Failure Reported by Selected Echocardiographic Referral Centers in Sub-Saharan Africa**

Authors	Country	n	Age[†]	RHD* (%)	DCM[‡] (%)	EMF[§] (%)	HTN HD[††] (%)	ICM[‡‡] (%)	CHD[€] (%)
Amoah et al. 2000[19]	Ghana	572	42	115 (20)	65 (11)	22 (4)	122 (21)	56 (10)	57 (10)
Freers et al. 1996[9]	Uganda	406	N/A	58 (12)	40 (8)	99 (22)	38 (8)	4 (1)	75 (15)
Kingue et al. 2005[20]	Cameroon	167	57	41 (25)**	46 (27)	5 (12)	91 (55)	4 (3)	N/A
Thiam et al. 2002[21]	Senegal	170[§§]	50	76 (45)**	12 (7)	0 (0)	58 (34)	30 (18)	N/A

† Age = Mean Age; * RHD = Rheumatic heart disease; ‡ DCM = Dilated cardiomyopathies; § EMF = Endomyocardial fibrosis;
†† HTN HD = Hypertensive heart disease; ‡‡ ICM = Ischemic cardiomyopathy ; € CHD = Congenital heart disease
** These series reported total valvulopathies. §§ Patients were double counted if they had two etiologic processes.

In Rwanda, we have found a similar distribution of causes of heart failure at rural district hospitals (see **FIGURE 4.1**). Roughly half the cases are potential surgical candidates.

FIGURE 4.1   Distribution of Causes of Heart Failure in a
Rwandan NCD clinic (n = 134)

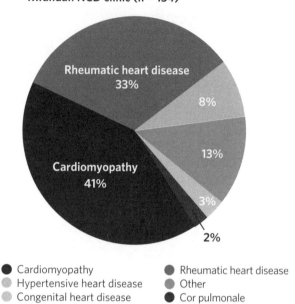

● Cardiomyopathy   ● Rheumatic heart disease
● Hypertensive heart disease   ● Other
● Congenital heart disease   ● Cor pulmonale

In the past decade, ultrasound has become increasingly available in sub-Saharan Africa. This has opened up the possibility of decentralizing heart failure diagnosis and treatment from the referral centers to district-level facilities. However, even where the technology is available, few district hospitals have personnel trained in echocardiography. One reason for this is the complexity of traditional cardiology training models.[22]

This chapter offers a simplified approach to heart failure diagnosis and medical management at the district-hospital and health-center levels. The approach is based on four years of experience with more than 300 patients in this setting. It relies on the fact that heart failure in this population is due to a limited number of causes that result in dramatic findings on physical examination or on echocardiography. The approach is designed for rapid training of advanced nurses, clinical officers, and generalist physicians. We have been using this model and teaching it to district-level clinicians in Rwanda since 2007. We have found that with some mentorship and training, Rwandan NCD nurses and district doctors have mastered the required skills quickly. District-level nurses acquire these skills through a three-month integrated training on diagnosis and management of NCDs. Our internal monitoring and evaluation has shown that in almost all cases, clinicians have been able to follow the algorithms, and with them, have been able to independently manage heart failure patients effectively.[23-25]

4.1   Defining Categories of Heart Failure

In resource-poor settings, it is often difficult to confirm a diagnosis of heart failure, let alone differentiate between the many different types of heart failure. This can lead to both over- and underdiagnosis of heart failure as well as initiation of inappropriate treatments.

Our approach teaches district-level clinicians to categorize heart failure into one of five different groups (see **TABLE 4.2**). We have designed these categories to be narrow enough to guide appropriate treatment, yet broad enough to require only minimal echocardiographic and diagnostic skills for classification. Groupings are based on the following findings: evidence of cardiomyopathy, mitral stenosis, a large right ventricle or dilated inferior vena cava (IVC) on echocardiography, or presence of a murmur, cyanosis (in a child or young adult), or severe hypertension on physical exam (see **TABLE 4.4** and **TABLE 4.5**). Each of the groupings created by this approach contain a variety of types of heart failure. However, within each group, the appropriate short-term medical management of the conditions is the same. This approach also identifies patients who may be surgical candidates and therefore prioritizes them for evaluation by a cardiologist.

In this model, heart failure treatment initially takes place at the district-level NCD clinic and not at health centers. One reason for this is that echocardiography should be available at district but not health center–level facilities. Furthermore, heart failure cases are often more complex than patients with other NCDs, requiring a greater level of clinician training for appropriate classification. In some cases, patients who are on stable therapy for many months may be referred back to the health center–level integrated chronic care clinic for routine follow-up.

The role of the cardiologist in this model is restricted to supervising and mentoring the district-level clinicians, and evaluating patients who are potential surgical candidates. Ideally, this secondary evaluation by a fully trained echocardiographer will happen within six months of initial diagnosis.

TABLE 4.2 lists the categories of heart failure important for medical management at the district hospital level. In the following sections, we explain in detail, first, how to recognize each diagnostic finding and, second, how to manage each category of heart failure.

Age is an important consideration in making a diagnosis of heart failure. Some types of heart failure, such as congenital or rheumatic heart disease (excluding mitral stenosis), are more common in children. Mitral stenosis often affects young or middle–aged adults. Hypertensive heart disease occurs more frequently in older adults and is virtually nonexistent in children. Cardiomyopathies and isolated right–sided heart failure can occur at any age, but are more common in the adult population. **TABLE 4.3** lists the most common cause of heart failure by age.

TABLE 4.2   Important Diagnostic Categories in Heart Failure

1. Cardiomyopathy	
Diagnostic criteria	1. Moderately to severely depressed left ventricular function (ejection fraction < 40%)
2. Hypertensive heart disease (not applicable to children)	
Diagnostic criteria	1. Severe hypertension
	2. Shortness of breath
	3. Normal to mildly depressed left ventricular function (ejection fraction ≥ 40%)
3. Mitral stenosis (rare before age 25)	
Diagnostic criteria	1. Mitral valve that doesn't open well with typical hockey-stick or elbow deformity
	2. Normal to mildly depressed left ventricular function (ejection fraction ≥ 40%)
4. Other valvular heart disease (including rheumatic and congenital)	
Diagnostic criteria	1. Normal to mildly depressed left ventricular function (ejection fraction ≥ 40%)
	2. No mitral stenosis
	3. Blood pressure ≤ 180/110 mmHg (in an adult)
	4. Dramatic heart murmur or cyanosis (in a child or young adult)
5. Isolated right heart failure	
Diagnostic criteria	1. Ejection fraction ≥ 40%
	2. No mitral stenosis
	3. Blood pressure ≤ 180/110 mmHg (in an adult)
	4. No heart murmur
	5. Large right ventricle or dilated inferior vena cava on echocardiography

TABLE 4.3 Common Causes of Heart Failure by Age

0–5 years	1. Congenital heart disease (most common)
	2. Cardiomyopathy (rare)
6–15 years	1. Congenital heart disease (most common)
	2. Acute rheumatic fever (peak age)
	3. Rheumatic heart disease (mostly regurgitant lesions, mitral stenosis very rare)
	4. Cardiomyopathy (rare)
16–30 years	1. Rheumatic heart disease (most common; regurgitant lesions more frequent than mitral stenosis)
	2. Cardiomyopathy (less common, mostly viral, HIV or peripartum)
	3. Congenital (less common)
31–40 years	1. Rheumatic heart disease (both mitral stenosis and regurgitant lesions)
	2. Cardiomyopathy (as common as rheumatic heart disease, multiple etiologies)
	3. Congenital (rare)
> 40 years	1. Cardiomyopathy
	2. Rheumatic heart disease (both mitral stenosis and regurgitant lesions)
	3. Hypertensive heart disease
	All etiologies roughly equal in prevalence
Isolated right–sided heart failure can occur at any age because of its many etiologies, but is more common in older patients.	

4.2 Physical Exam Findings for Classification of Heart Failure

Heart failure patients can have a wide variety of physical exam findings. Our diagnostic algorithms use only blood pressure (in adults) and the presence of dramatic murmurs or cyanosis (in a child) to classify patients. Other findings, such as signs of fluid overload, tachycardia, and increased respiratory rate, are important in determining medication adjustments and disposition within each diagnostic algorithm.

Blood pressure in our clinics is obtained with automatic machines. Providers are taught the importance of proper cuff size, and often small adult-sized cuffs are necessary for this low-BMI population. We define severe hypertension in adults as blood pressures greater than 180 mmHg systolic or 110 mmHg diastolic.

Murmurs can be difficult to detect, even with expensive stethoscopes and highly trained ears. However, we ask our clinicians to be able to recognize only the very obvious, loud murmurs, since these are the ones most likely to reflect serious valvular pathology aside from mitral stenosis. We also do not dwell on the characterization of the type or location of the murmurs.

Persistent or intermittent cyanosis in a child outside of acute respiratory illness is often a presenting sign of congenital heart disease. Some of these children will have lesions that do not cause murmurs.

TABLE 4.4 Physical Exam Findings in Classification of Heart Failure

1. Dramatic murmurs
2. Blood pressure ≥ 180 mmHg systolic or 110 mmHg diastolic (in adults)
3. Cyanosis (in a child or young adult)

4.3 Echocardiography for Classification of Heart Failure

Echocardiography is essential to confirm and characterize the diagnosis of heart failure. Our diagnostic and treatment algorithms rely on the clinician's ability to master two echocardiographic views of the heart: the parasternal long axis view and the subcostal view (see below). In those views, clinicians are asked to be able to recognize only four different abnormalities: (1) moderately to severely decreased ejection fraction (EF); (2) mitral stenosis; (3) a very large right ventricle; and (4) an enlarged inferior vena cava. The technical approach to obtaining ultrasound images is described in more detail in the *PIH Manual of Ultrasound for Resource-Limited Settings.*[24]

TABLE 4.5 Echocardiographic Findings in Classification of Heart Failure

1. Moderately to severely decreased EF (< 40%)
2. Mitral stenosis
3. Very large right ventricle (much larger than the aortic root or left atrium)
4. Clearly enlarged and non-collapsing vena cava (≥ 2.5 cm) in an adult

4.3.1 The Parasternal Long Axis View

The parasternal long axis view is obtained in the following manner: with the patient lying on the left side, the probe is placed to the left of the sternum, in the 4th or 5th intercostal space, with the probe marker pointed toward the right shoulder. The mitral valve and aortic valve should be clearly seen (see **FIGURE 4.2** and **FIGURE 4.3**).

FIGURE 4.2 Parasternal Long Axis View

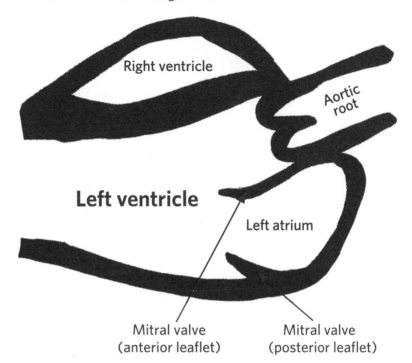

FIGURE 4.3   Normal Parasternal Long Axis View on Echocardiography
(Diastole, top; Systole, bottom)

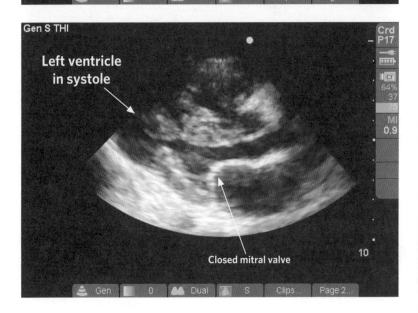

4.3.2   The Subcostal View

The subcostal view is obtained with the probe placed under the xiphoid process. The image generated is of the heart flipped upside down, with the liver seen at the top of the screen (see **FIGURE 4.4**). The IVC is seen as a black tube entering the right ventricle (see **FIGURE 4.5**). It should be measured 2 cm from its entrance into the right ventricle.

FIGURE 4.4 Subcostal View

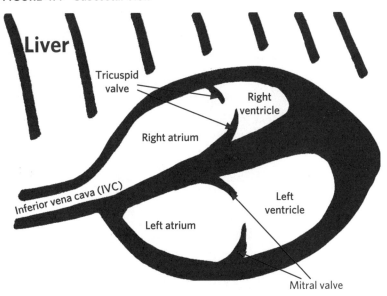

FIGURE 4.5 Subcostal View with Normal IVC (top) and Dilated IVC (bottom)

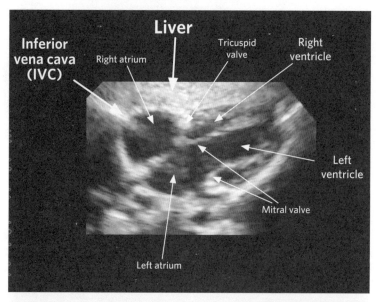

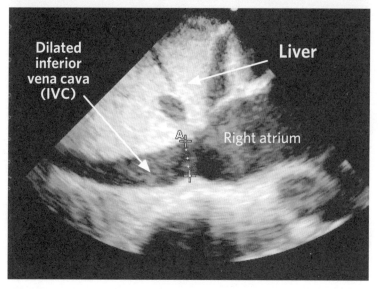

We have found that as clinicians become more adept at these views, many take it upon themselves to learn the other basic echocardiographic views and findings. This level of echocardiography may be helpful but is not essential in determining appropriate medical management of heart failure. For more in-depth instruction on echocardiography techniques, please refer to the *PIH Manual of Ultrasound for Resource-Limited Settings.*[24]

4.3.3   Ejection Fraction and Fractional Shortening

Evaluation of ejection fraction (EF) is the first and perhaps most important diagnostic skill in categorizing heart failure. EF refers to the amount of blood that the heart pumps out with each beat. Ejection fraction is a measure of the heart's systolic function: how well the heart works during the squeezing phase of the cardiac cycle. A normal EF is between 55% and 65%, meaning that the normal heart pumps about half of the blood in the left ventricle out into the aorta with each beat.

EF is generally classified as normal (≥ 55%), mildly reduced (40%–55%), and moderately to severely reduced (< 40%). A moderately to severely reduced EF means a patient has a cardiomyopathy, a failure of the heart muscle. While echocardiography machines can generate measurements of EF, qualitative visual assessment is more reliable. In a cross-sectional view, this translates into how much the walls of the ventricle are seen to move toward each other with each heartbeat. This distance is called the fractional shortening. A normal ejection fraction of 55% corresponds to a fractional shortening of about 25%. This means that when the normal heart squeezes in systole, the distance between the walls narrows by only 25%.

We teach our clinicians to evaluate EF in the parasternal long view. It can also be assessed in the parasternal short axis, and apical 4-chamber views.

FIGURE 4.3 shows the normal relationship between the heart in diastole (relaxation) and systole (contraction). Notice that the volume of the left ventricle decreases in systole, and the left ventricular walls become thicker as the ventricle contracts and squeezes the blood out into the aorta.

FIGURE 4.6 shows how the left ventricular walls do not move together very much in a heart with a cardiomyopathy—the left ventricle remains about the same size contracted as relaxed, and the walls do not thicken much. Compare this to the normal heart in **FIGURE 4.3**.

**FIGURE 4.6   Cardiomyopathy in Parasternal Long Axis View
(Diastole, top; Systole, bottom)**

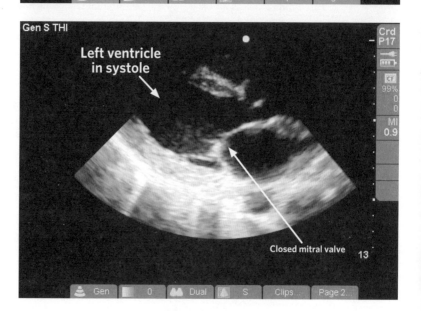

4.3.4   Assessment for Mitral Stenosis

In patients with rheumatic mitral stenosis, the mitral valve has a strikingly characteristic appearance in the parasternal long axis view (see **FIGURE 4.7**). The features of typical rheumatic mitral stenosis include: (1) a small opening of the mitral valve in diastole (see **FIGURE 4.3** and **FIGURE 4.6** for comparison); (2) the anterior leaflet of the mitral valve has a hockey stick or elbow deformity; (3) left ventricular function is typically normal.

FIGURE 4.7   Mitral Stenosis in Diastole

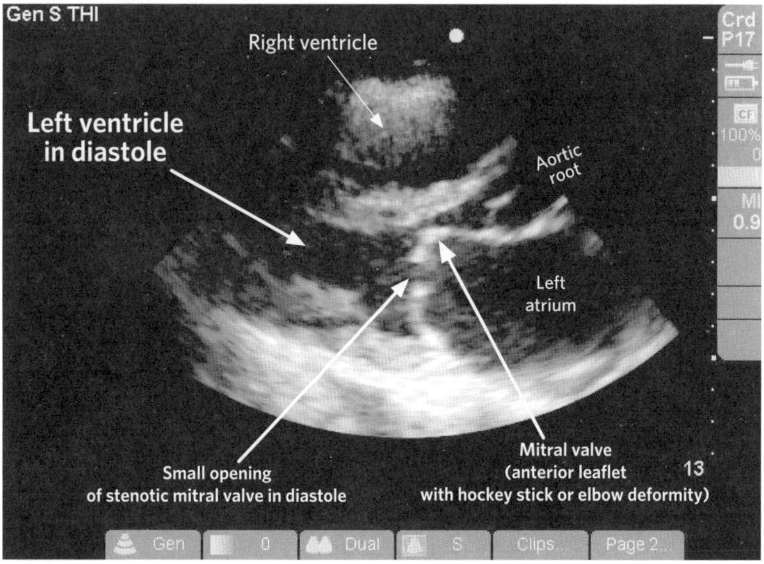

4.3.5   Assessment of Right Heart Size

In cases of right heart failure, the right ventricle may appear enlarged on the parasternal long axis view (see **FIGURE 4.8**). Normally, the right ventricle is roughly the same size as the aortic root and the left atrium.

FIGURE 4.8   Right Ventricular Enlargement (Parasternal Long View)

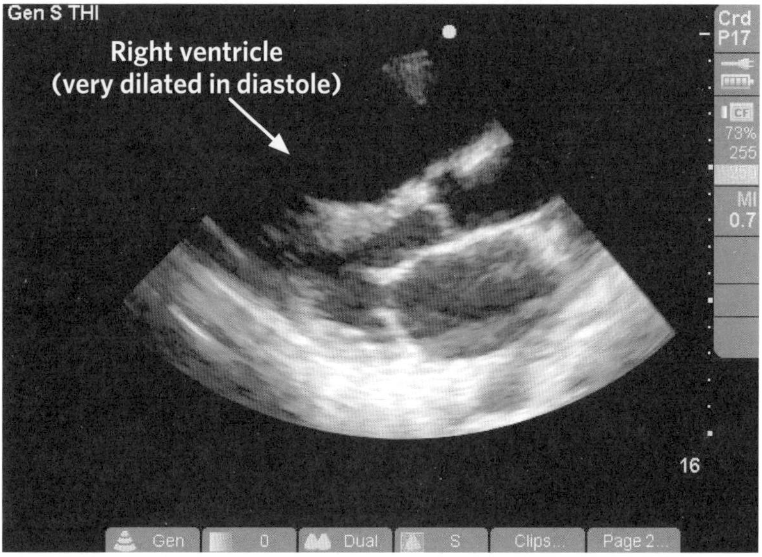

4.3.6   Assessment of the Inferior Vena Cava

The inferior vena cava in the subcostal view should be small and collapse by 50% with each inspiration. An IVC greater than 2 cm in adults that doesn't collapse is strongly suggestive of some element of right-sided heart failure (see **FIGURE 4.5**).

4.3.7   Assessment of Pericardial Effusion

Pericardial effusions can occur in many different types of heart failure. They can also occur in patients with no history of heart failure, such as those with cancer or renal failure. They are listed here as a key echocardiographic finding because recognition of a very large pericardial effusion (≥ 3 cm in diastole in an adult) in a patient with decompensated heart failure should prompt immediate admission to the district hospital for possible pericardiocentesis. It is not, however, one of the findings we use as a diagnostic criteria for heart failure categorization.

Since fluid appears black on ultrasound, pericardial effusions appear as an extra stripe of black around the heart. This can be seen best in the subcostal view, but can also be seen in the parasternal long axis view (see **FIGURE 4.9**). Many patients may have small pericardial effusions.

FIGURE 4.9   Pericardial Effusion (Parasternal View, top;
Subcostal View, bottom)

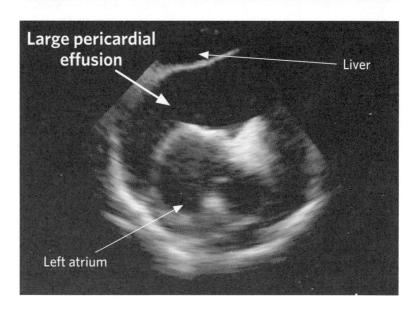

4.4   Initial Recognition and Referral of the Heart Failure Patient

Heart failure patients may present to any level of the health care system. All patients with suspected or confirmed heart failure should eventually be referred to the district NCD clinic.

At health-center level, heart failure patients often present with non-specific symptoms. In our anecdotal experience, most patients with clinically important heart failure in Rwanda will have shortness of breath at a decreased level of activity. Clinicians should refer patients to the NCD clinic who do not have an infectious process to explain their shortness of breath or who have any of the findings in **TABLE 4.6** (see below) that suggest an underlying cardiac etiology. **CHAPTER 10** outlines the acute care health center approach to shortness of breath.

TABLE 4.6   Common Signs and Symptoms of Heart Failure
(Usually Present in Addition to Shortness of Breath)

1. Lower-extremity edema
2. Loud murmurs
3. Orthopnea (shortness of breath when lying prone)
4. In children: otherwise unexplained cyanosis, lethargy, poor feeding, or poor weight gain

Another subset of patients will have dramatic edema or ascites without shortness of breath. These patients may have isolated right-sided heart failure. They may alternatively have renal or liver failure. All such patients should be referred to the district NCD clinic for echocardiography and lab testing to determine the cause of the edema.

Integrated chronic care providers at health centers may also see patients with symptoms that should prompt referral to the district NCD clinic, such as those with severe hypertension who develop shortness of breath or edema, or patients with wheezing who are not improving with asthma therapy. Triggers to refer to the district-level clinic are addressed in chapters covering these topics.

Very young children with heart failure will present with non-specific symptoms, such as poor feeding, cyanosis, irritability, hypotonia or poor growth. Most children with heart failure will have a valvular or congenital lesion accompanied by a loud murmur. A smaller subset will present with cyanosis without a murmur. Heart failure should be considered in any child with these signs or symptoms.

Another group of heart failure patients will be referred to the outpatient district NCD clinic from the district hospital inpatient units. Many patients with heart failure only seek medical care once they have become very ill and require hospitalization. Algorithms for recognition and management of heart failure patients in the inpatient district hospital are included in the WHO's forthcoming district clinician manual for adult and adolescent care. The WHO algorithms are similar to those presented here for use in the outpatient setting, with an added emphasis on stabilization of the severely decompensated patient. Patients are started on appropriate outpatient therapy prior to discharge and given a follow-up appointment in the district-level NCD clinic. In some cases, the NCD clinic nurses may see hospitalized heart failure patients together with their physicians to help ensure good continuity of care.

Suspected heart failure patients referred to the district NCD clinic should receive a complete history, physical exam, creatinine testing, and echocardiography. Patients will be classified into one of five heart failure diagnostic categories or receive an alternate, non-cardiac diagnosis.

Clinicians will then determine the initial treatment based on the treatment algorithm for that diagnostic category (see **PROTOCOL 4.1**).

Patients with unstable vital signs, severe symptoms, or dramatic fluid overload are classified as having decompensated heart failure and will be referred for admission to the district hospital for stabilization and diuresis (see **PROTOCOL 4.2**).

Patients are then assessed for the presence or absence of a cardiomyopathy. All patients with an estimated EF of less than 40% are defined as having a cardiomyopathy. Regardless of other abnormalities, these patients will be treated according to the cardiomyopathy treatment guidelines (see **SECTION 4.8**).

Once cardiomyopathy has been ruled out, patients are assessed for the presence of mitral stenosis on echocardiography. These patients are treated as having mitral stenosis, regardless of the presence of other valvular lesions (see **SECTION 4.10**).

Adult patients without cardiomyopathy or mitral stenosis are then assessed for presence of severe hypertension. If present, they are categorized as having hypertensive heart disease (see **SECTION 4.9**). Hypertensive heart disease is extremely rare in children.

Remaining patients are then assessed for presence of a heart murmur or cyanosis. Those with loud, obvious murmurs without cardiomyopathy, mitral stenosis, or hypertensive heart disease are categorized as having some variety of congenital or rheumatic valvular disease apart from mitral stenosis (see **SECTION 4.11**). Cyanosis with or without a murmur is a common presenting sign of congenital heart disease in children and young adults. Patients with cyanosis without another explanation (e.g., severe respiratory illness) are also placed in this heart failure category. In infants and toddlers, almost all heart failure will be due to congenital lesions. Rheumatic heart disease rarely affects children less than 5 years old.

The remaining patients are evaluated for signs of isolated right heart failure, such as a very large right ventricle or a dilated IVC on echocardiography. These patients are classified as having isolated right heart failure (see **SECTION 4.12**).

Patients with none of the preceding findings are evaluated for other non-cardiac causes of their symptoms, such as renal or liver failure.

PROTOCOL 4.1   Initial Diagnosis and Management of Heart Failure

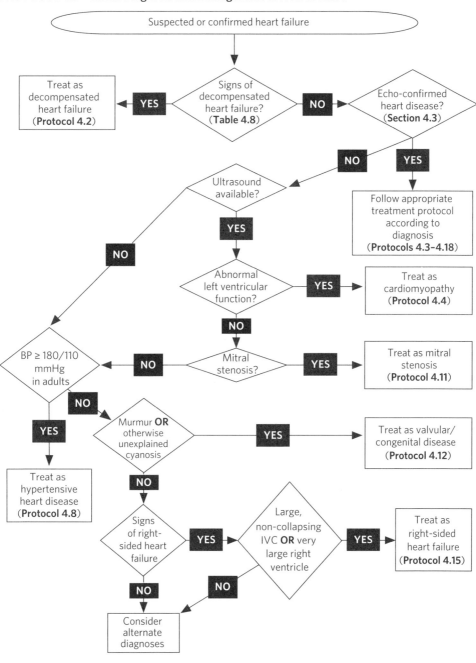

Next, all treatment algorithms begin with an assessment of the patient's symptom severity and volume status. This assessment will be discussed in the following sections.

4.5   Heart Failure Severity Classification

Patients with heart failure of any etiology fall along a common continuum of symptom severity. These are categorized into four groups, based on the New York Heart Association classification system (see **TABLE 4.7**). Understanding this classification system allows the NCD clinician to clearly document a heart failure patient's clinical course. Sometimes patients may fall between two classes. This classification system is not as useful for very young children.

Mild abnormalities of heart structures in many cases never lead to symptoms of heart failure. Patients with moderate to severe abnormalities may also be asymptomatic or mildly symptomatic (class I or II) for months to years, thanks to the body's compensatory mechanisms. However, as heart failure progresses, these compensatory mechanisms generally fail and patients develop more symptoms, placing them in a higher heart failure class. Heart failure treatment can slow and sometimes even reverse this progression, allowing some patients to move to a lower heart failure class.

TABLE 4.7   New York Heart Association Heart Failure Classification

Class I	Patients with cardiac disease but no resulting limitation of physical activity. Ordinary physical activity does not cause symptoms.
Class II	Patients with cardiac disease resulting in mild limitation of physical activity. Patients are comfortable at rest. Ordinary physical activity (farming, running, carrying water, climbing a hill) causes symptoms.
Class III	Patients with cardiac disease resulting in moderate limitation of physical activity. Patients are comfortable at rest. Less than ordinary physical activity (light housework, walking on flat ground) causes symptoms.
Class IV	Patients with cardiac disease resulting in severe limitation of physical activity. Patients have symptoms at rest. Any physical activity causes symptoms.

4.6   Decompensated Heart Failure

When a patient's body is no longer compensating well for the degree of heart dysfunction, volume status and functional ability will worsen. This is termed decompensated heart failure. Clues that a patient has entered this state are abnormal vital signs (such as low blood pressure and fast heart rate) and severe symptoms of dyspnea and orthopnea (see **TABLE 4.8**). Again, children may present with different signs and symptoms, such as lethargy, cyanosis, or hypotonia. Vital sign parameters are also different in children (see **APPENDIX E**). These patients are too sick to be treated in the community and require inpatient management of their fluid status and other symptoms. **PROTOCOL 4.2** provides guidance on how to evaluate and initiate treatment for patients with decompensated heart failure prior to transfer to the inpatient unit.

TABLE 4.8   Signs and Symptoms of Decompensated Heart Failure

Vital signs (if child, see **APPENDIX E** for normal vital sign ranges by age)	Blood pressure	Very low (SBP ≤ 80 mmHg in adults) Very high (SBP ≥ 180 mmHg in adults)
	Pulse	Very low (≤ 40 bpm in adults) Very high (≥ 120 bpm in adults)
	High respiratory rate	≥ 24 breaths/minute in adults
	Low oxygen saturation	Saturation ≤ 90% (note patients with a cyanotic congenital lesion may be stable at a low oxygen saturation)
Symptoms	Inability to lie down flat Severe dyspnea at rest **In children ≤ 5 years:** hypotonia, new or worsened cyanosis, lethargy, poor feeding	

Assessment of vital signs and the patient's overall condition is the first step in evaluating any heart failure patient. This initial assessment should determine whether or not the patient is decompensated and in need of hospitalization for treatment. Refer to **APPENDIX E** for a guide to normal vital signs by age in children.

The following vital signs should be collected on every visit: heart rate, blood pressure, and weight. Oxygen saturation, respiratory rate, and temperature should be checked if a patient seems ill or in distress.

Patients with heart failure can often be in a stable condition with low blood pressures (as low as systolic blood pressure of 80 mmHg in adults). If a patient feels well and is not tachycardic, a low blood pressure can be tolerated. However, these patients are more fragile than others and medication adjustments should thus be made even more carefully.

TABLE 4.9 lists some of the common reasons for acute worsening of a heart failure patient. A very high blood pressure (≥ 180/110 mmHg in an adult) can result in severe decompensation of the heart failure patient. Acute increases in blood pressure may cause the heart to stiffen and a subsequent backup of fluid into the lungs, resulting in acute pulmonary edema. Heart failure patients with signs of decompensation and very high blood pressures should receive immediate interventions to lower blood pressure (see **SECTION 8.4** and **TABLE 8.4**).

Large changes in vital signs or very abnormal values should trigger (1) investigation of the cause; (2) initial attempts to stabilize the patient; and (3) preparations for transfer to a higher level of care. See **PROTOCOL 4.2** for the algorithm for initial management of decompensated heart failure.

TABLE 4.9   Reasons for Acute Decompensation in Patients with Heart Failure

1. Medication nonadherence or recent changes in medications
2. Change in diet (e.g., increase in salt intake)
3. Acute illness (e.g., pneumonia, rheumatic fever, endocarditis)
4. Worsening valvular disease
5. Pregnancy Exacerbates all types of heart failure, but especially mitral stenosis (2nd and 3rd trimester) and peripartum cardiomyopathy.
6. Arrhythmia Especially common in patients with cardiomyopathies and valvular disease, particularly mitral stenosis.
7. Worsened hypertension Very high blood pressure can cause acute stiffening of the heart muscle and back up of fluid into the lungs (pulmonary edema).

PROTOCOL 4.2 Management of Decompensated Heart Failure

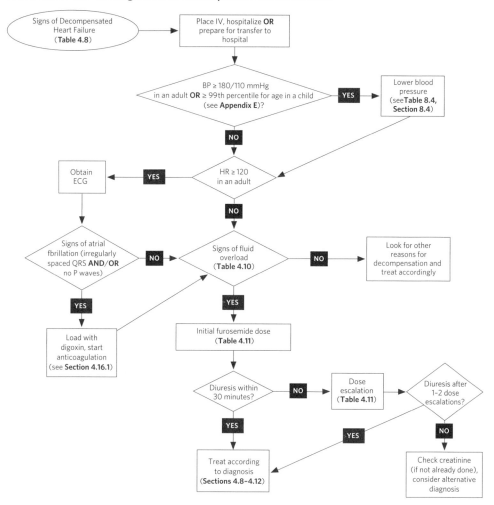

4.7 Fluid Status Assessment

After assessment of vital signs, assessment of fluid status is the next step in management of any patient with known or suspected heart failure.

Fluid retention occurs because the kidneys, to compensate for poor cardiac function, hold on to extra fluid to try to maintain adequate tissue blood flow. At a certain point, this compensatory mechanism fails, as the extra fluid leaves the blood and goes into tissue, leading to congestion of the lungs and/or the extremities and abdomen. This extra fluid results in many of the symptoms of heart failure. Moving this fluid out of the tissues and out of the body through the urine is called diuresis, and medications that promote this process are called diuretics. Furosemide (trade name Lasix) is the most commonly used diuretic in heart failure.

Assessing volume status accurately can be difficult. There is no one test or finding that accurately diagnoses volume imbalances, but rather a collection of physical findings and symptoms that need to be taken into consideration in determining the nature and degree of fluid imbalance. With practice, clinicians should be able to make a reasonable assessment of fluid status, with the warning that even experts sometimes get this assessment wrong. Here as in most of medicine, if a therapy does not produce the expected result, the diagnosis should be reconsidered.

Heart failure patients will fall into three broad volume status categories: (1) hypovolemic, meaning the patient has too little fluid in the body; (2) euvolemic, meaning the patient is in good fluid balance (neither too much nor too little) and is at a dry weight; or (3) hypervolemic, meaning the patient has an excess of fluid in the body.

Within the hypervolemic category, there are three subcategories based on severity of fluid overload: mild, moderate, and severe. Categorization is based on assessment of symptoms, physical findings, and comparison of current weight to the patient's dry weight, if known.

Assessing fluid status involves (1) asking the patient about symptoms of fluid overload (i.e., orthopnea, dyspnea); (2) examining the patient, making special note of whether the neck veins are distended, whether there are crackles on lung exam, and whether there is any lower-extremity edema or ascites; and (3) measuring creatinine if the patient is new to the clinic and on a regular basis thereafter.

TABLE 4.10 Volume Status Categories and Diuretic Adjustment

Category	Hypovolemic	Euvolemic	Hypervolemic		
			Mild	*Moderate*	*Severe (decompensated)*
Weight	Less than dry weight	At dry weight	≤ 5 kg above dry weight (in an adult)	≥ 5 kg above dry weight (in an adult)	≥ 5 kg above dry weight (in an adult)
Symptoms	Variable	Class I–II	Class I–II	Class II–III	Class III–IV
Vital signs	Tachycardia Hypotension	Normal	Normal	Mild tachycardia	Tachycardia, tachypnea, hypoxia, hypotension, or hypertension
Physical exam	Does not always correlate with severity. Signs of fluid overload include distended neck veins, lung crackles, louder murmurs, hepatomegaly, ascites, and lower-extremity edema. However, can be intravascularly hypovolemic and still have signs of hypervolemia in lungs, extremities, and abdomen.				
Creatinine	Increased	Stable or decreased	Stable or decreased	Can be increased (due to hypoperfusion of the kidneys), stable or decreased.	
Diuretic adjustment	Stop all diuretics	Reduce or maintain dose (if starting beta-blocker, do not reduce diuretic)	Maintain or increase dose	Increase dose	Start IV furosemide and prepare for transfer to hospital if possible

With diuresis, these symptoms and physical findings should improve (see **TABLE 4.10**). However, patients with low serum protein, significant right-sided failure, or renal failure may continue to have residual edema despite intravascular euvolemia. As a patient gets close to his dry weight, the creatinine may start to rise. This is one sign that it may be time to decrease a patient's diuretic dose. All patients with suspected heart failure should have a creatinine checked on the initial visit and then at least every three months if they are on diuretics. A creatinine should also be measured if there is a change in the patient's clinical status.

When a patient is deemed to be fluid-overloaded, the key clinical decision is whether the patient requires hospitalization for fast, intravenous diuresis, or whether the fluid can be taken off more slowly with oral diuresis as an outpatient. A patient who appears decompensated due to fluid overload should be hospitalized for intravenous diuresis. **PROTOCOL 4.3** presents an algorithm for appropriate management of diuretics according to fluid status assessment.

PROTOCOL 4.3   Volume Status Assessment and Diuretic Adjustment

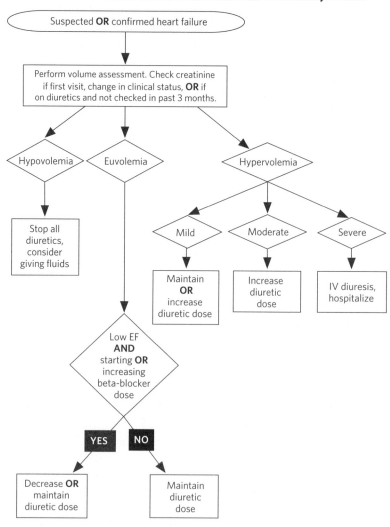

Patients with renal failure pose a special challenge for diuretic management. If a patient is very fluid-overloaded, removal of fluid can improve the heart's ability to pump and increase the amount of blood delivered to the kidneys. Renal function will improve, with a resulting drop in creatinine levels. However, if the patient is not fluid-overloaded or if too much fluid is removed, blood flow to the kidneys will decrease and renal function will decline, with a resulting rise in creatinine levels. Therefore, it is important to pay attention to the trend in creatinine as a clue to the patient's current volume status.

In fact, because the kidneys do not benefit from any of the fluid stored outside of the blood vessels and in the tissues, a patient can have too much fluid stored in the feet, abdomen, and lungs, yet not enough fluid in the blood. This situation will also lead to increased creatinine. For this reason, we generally recommend that clinicians err on the side of keeping patients slightly fluid-overloaded.

In this chapter, we use a creatinine cutoff of 200 µmol/L in adults or 2x normal creatinine for age in children as a definition of renal failure. These values should fall within class 3 kidney disease (CKD 3) and correspond with a glomerular filtration rate (GFR) between 30 and 60 mL/min. **CHAPTER 6** discusses the diagnosis and management of renal failure in more detail.

4.7.1   Guidelines for Initiating Intravenous Diuresis

All patients who are decompensated with any signs of hypervolemia will require intravenous diuresis. As the body becomes increasingly fluid-overloaded, the tissues become edematous. This includes the gut, which can lead to poor absorption of oral medications. For this reason, intravenous furosemide is the preferred medication for patients with severe fluid overload.

Intravenous diuresis should be initiated immediately upon diagnosis of severe fluid overload while preparing for transfer to the hospital. Furosemide should work quickly, with an average onset of 15 minutes from administration. If the patient does not respond, it may be that the threshold for diuresis has not been reached and a higher dose is needed. If the patient does not urinate within 30 minutes of the first dose, the dose can be doubled. **TABLE 4.11** provides suggested starting, escalation, and maximum doses of intravenous furosemide. Intravenous furosemide lasts about 2 hours and should be dosed 2–4 times per day.

TABLE 4.11   Intravenous Furosemide Dosing

Initial dosing		Escalation	Maximum dose
Patient does not already take furosemide	**Adult:** 40 mg IV 2x–3x/day	Double every 30 minutes until response or maximum dose achieved	**Adult:** 100 mg IV 2–4x/day
	Pediatric (≤ 40 kg): 0.5 mg/kg IV 2x/day		**Pediatric:** 4 mg/kg IV 2–4x/day
Patient already takes furosemide	Double effective outpatient dose and give as IV		

Furosemide is twice as effective when given intravenously as when given orally. It also acts faster and wears off more quickly. It is important to keep this in mind when transitioning patients from one form of the drug to another (see **TABLE 4.12**).

TABLE 4.12 Equivalent Oral and IV Furosemide Doses

Oral	IV
80 mg PO	40 mg IV

Once a patient has been diuresed effectively, it is very important to make note of the dry weight—the weight at which the patient is euvolemic. Any weight gain over that can be considered fluid gain, unless there is reason to believe that the patient has other reasons to gain weight (i.e., a growing child). When a patient is discharged from the hospital, this value should be communicated to the outpatient provider.

4.7.2 Guidelines for Initiating and Titrating Oral Furosemide at Health-Center Level

Most patients with heart failure will have a tendency to store too much extra fluid. It may be possible to wean some patients off all diuretics with proper therapy, but most will require a low long-term maintenance dose. This means that patients who were previously hypervolemic but become euvolemic after diuresis will still often require diuretics to prevent reaccumulation of fluid. In these patients and in those who are mildly hypervolemic, oral diuretics can be used to maintain good fluid balance and to control symptoms. **TABLE 4.13** outlines the recommended dosing of oral furosemide.

TABLE 4.13 Oral Furosemide Dosing

Dose adjustment				
Hypovolemia	Euvolemia	Mild hypervolemia	Moderate hypervolemia	Severe hypervolemia
Stop all diuretics, consider giving fluid	May attempt to decrease dose unless starting or increasing beta-blocker	Keep dose the same	Increase current dose (by no more than double)	Admission and intra-venous diuresis (see **TABLE 4.11**)

Adult dosing
Initial dose: 40 mg 1x/day.
Maximum dose: 80 mg 2x/day.

Pediatric dosing		Starting doses			
	< 10 kg	10 kg	15 kg	20 kg	30 kg
40 mg tablet	See mg/kg dosing*	10 mg ¼ tab 1x/day	10-20 mg ¼-½ tab 1x/day	20 mg ½ tab 1x/day	20-40 mg ½-1 tab 1x/day
Initial dose: 1 mg/kg 1x/day.					
Increase by: 0.5-1 mg/kg per dose or increase frequency of dosing.					
Maximum dose: 4 mg/kg 2-4x/day.					

* May require crushing pills and diluting to achieve appropriate dose. This should only be done under the supervision of an experienced clinician.

4.7.3   Guidelines for Use of Other Diuretics

Other oral diuretics besides furosemide may be used to help achieve and maintain euvolemia (see **TABLE 4.14**). These medications are generally added to furosemide to increase the strength of diuresis. While they may be very effective, these medications can also increase the chances of electrolyte abnormalities and other side effects of furosemide, and should be used with caution.

4.7.3.1   Spironolactone

Spironolactone (trade name Aldactone), like furosemide, acts on the kidneys to increase urination. While furosemide tends to cause hypokalemia, spironolactone will maintain or increase blood potassium levels. Spironolactone can be particularly effective in patients with ascites. Because spironolactone can increase blood potassium levels, it should only be used in the setting of normal renal function (defined here as a creatinine ≤ 100 µmol/L in adults or within the normal range for age in children (see **APPENDIX E** for pediatric ranges)).

4.7.3.2   Hydrochlorothiazide

Hydrochlorothiazide is a weaker diuretic than furosemide, but acts in much the same way. When taken 30 minutes prior to furosemide, hydrochlorothiazide can make furosemide work better, causing a larger diuresis. A very small number of patients should require this. This combination can cause massive diuresis and loss of vital electrolytes, and therefore should only be considered in consultation with a physician and with very close monitoring of electrolytes.

TABLE 4.14 Other Oral Diuretic Dosing

Drug	Initial dosing	Notes	Maximum dose
Spironolactone	**Adult:** 25 mg 1x/day	Add if patient has significant ascites and normal renal function	50 mg/day
	Pediatric (≤ 40 kg): 2.5 mg/kg 1x/day		3 mg/kg/day
Hydrochlorothiazide	**Adult:** 12.5 mg 1x/day	Can be used if furosemide is not available or added to furosemide if greater diuresis is desired.	25 mg/day
	Pediatric (≤ 40 kg): 1 mg/kg/day		12 mg/day

4.7.4   Dangers of Diuresis

Diuretics are powerful medications. If used in excess, they can cause excessive water loss and resulting damage to the kidneys. This in turn can cause dangerous electrolyte imbalances and even death.

For this reason, it is important to err on the side of using smaller doses and keeping patients slightly hypervolemic. Patients must be educated on the dangers of overdiuresis and instructed to stop their diuretic medications if they develop fever or diarrhea, which in combination with medications can lead to serious dehydration.

When adding two diuretics together, the effect on electrolytes is increased. Combinations should be used only in the setting of normal creatinine. If possible, sodium, potassium, and creatinine should be monitored at regular intervals in these situations.

4.8   Cardiomyopathy

The term cardiomyopathy encompasses several types of heart disease, all of which lead to a similar outcome of heart muscle dysfunction. The common feature of all these diseases is a low ejection fraction, usually less than 40% (fractional shortening less than 20%).

There are many different causes of cardiomyopathy (see **TABLE 4.15**). As stated above, some types of heart failure begin as a cardiomyopathy. Others, however, such as valvular or hypertensive heart disease, can progress to a cardiomyopathy over time. Any patient with an ejection fraction less than 40%, regardless of the cause, should be treated primarily as a cardiomyopathy. Cardiomyopathies affect patients of every age group but are rare in children.

TABLE 4.15   Etiology of Cardiomyopathy in Rwanda

Idiopathic	Most of the cases of cardiomyopathy are caused by an unknown process. Many may be due to a previous viral infection.
HIV cardiomyopathy	HIV can cause direct cellular damage to heart muscle. ARVs can delay or reverse this process.
Alcohol-related cardiomyopathy	Chronic alcohol use can be toxic to the heart muscle. If the patient stops drinking alcohol, the function may improve with time.
Peripartum	Women can develop a cardiomyopathy in the last month of pregnancy and up to six months postpartum. This often improves with appropriate management and avoidance of subsequent pregnancies.
Viral myocarditis	Many different viruses can infect the heart muscle and cause dysfunction. This often improves with time, but may be permanent.
Anemia	Severe anemia (sometimes due to cancer or poor nutrition) can lead to cardiomyopathy. This can improve when the anemia is treated.
Advanced valvular disease	Most valvular conditions causing abnormal flow of blood within the heart can lead to a cardiomyopathy. This is particularly true with regurgitant lesions. This is not the case for pure mitral stenosis, in which the left ventricle is protected, while the right ventricle ultimately suffers.

In many cases, identifying the cause of the cardiomyopathy is not important, because the clinical management will be the same. However, several causes can be corrected with proper additional therapy. Patients with anemia-induced cardiomyopathy may improve as their anemia is corrected. Likewise, ARV therapy may reverse some of the systolic dysfunction in patients with HIV-induced cardiomyopathy as well as prevent non-cardiac HIV-related complications. For these reasons, all patients with a newly diagnosed cardiomyopathy should have their hemoglobin and HIV serotest checked. In addition, all patients with a newly diagnosed cardiomyopathy should be asked about their alcohol intake. Cardiomyopathy is a rare cause of heart failure in children, but may occur as a result of a viral infection or from congenital or rheumatic valvular lesions.

All cardiomyopathies, regardless of etiology, are managed with diuretics and with medications, such as beta-blockers and ACE inhibitors, which have been proven in clinical trials to decrease risk of death in adults and improve symptoms over the long term. **PROTOCOL 4.4** provides an outline for cardiomyopathy management.

PROTOCOL 4.4   Cardiomyopathy Management

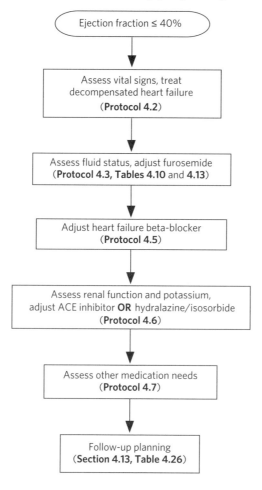

4.8.1   Vital Sign Assessment

As in all types of heart failure, cardiomyopathy management begins with an assessment of the patient's vital signs, weight, and overall condition. Patients with cardiomyopathies will often have low blood pressures. However, heart failure patients with systolic low blood pressures (below 80 mmHg in an adult or below normal range for age in a child), along with other signs of decompensation (tachycardia, respiratory distress, altered mental status), should be hospitalized.

4.8.2   Fluid Status Assessment

The next step in the management of cardiomyopathy is evaluation of fluid status and titration of diuretics. In the case of a cardiomyopathy, diuretic doses should not be reduced if beta-blockers are going to be added or increased at the same visit. This is because, in the short-term, beta-blockers can exacerbate fluid retention.

4.8.3   Titration of Mortality-Reducing Medications

Beta-blockers, ACE inhibitors, spironolactone, and the combination of hydralazine and isosorbide dinitrate have all been shown to decrease morbidity and mortality among adult cardiomyopathy patients when used at doses proven effective in large trials.[26] The provider's goal is to increase the doses of these drugs until reaching a target dose. However, this increase must be achieved gradually, and there are certain factors that make even small increases of these drugs dangerous. If side effects develop, the provider must be able to identify what drug is the culprit. Therefore, only one drug should be increased at each visit. In general, if the patient is euvolemic and stable, it is best to increase only the patient's beta-blocker at the first visit. If there are contraindications to increasing the beta-blocker, the ACE inhibitor can be increased first. At the second visit, the ACE inhibitor may be increased. In this manner, medications are increased one at a time until goal doses are achieved or dose-limiting side effects occur.

These medications are not as well–studied in children. It is difficult to conduct randomized trials for patients with a rare disease. However, there is reason to think that these medications may confer similar benefits in children as in adults. Additionally these medications have been found to be safe for use in childhood cardiomyopathy if appropriately low doses are administered.

There is no good data on the use of isosorbide and hydralazine in children. However, the clinician might consider its use in a child with cardiomyopathy who also has renal failure precluding the use of an ACE inhibitor. This should be done in close consultation with a pediatrician or cardiologist as the hemodynamic effects of these medications in children can be unpredictable.

TABLE 4.16   Mortality-Reducing Medications for Cardiomyopathy
                in Adults

Beta-blocker			
	Starting dose	Dose change	Target dose
Carvedilol	3.125–6.25 mg 2x/day	3.125–6.25 mg 2x/day	25 mg 2x/day
Atenolol*	12.5 mg 1x/day	12.5 mg 1x/day	50 mg 1x/day
ACE inhibitor			
	Starting dose	Dose change	Target dose
Lisinopril	5 mg 1x/day	5 mg 1x/day	20 mg 1x/day
Captopril	12.5 mg 3x/day	12.5 mg 3x/day	50 mg 3x/day
Enalapril	2.5 mg 2x/day	2.5 mg 2x/day	10-20 mg 2x/day
Hydralazine/isosorbide dinitrate **(Contraindications to beta-blocker and/or ACE inhibitor)**			
	Starting dose	Dose change	Target dose
Hydralazine	25 mg 3x/day	25 mg 3x/day	50 mg 3x/day
Isosorbide	10 mg 3x/day	10 mg 3x/day	30 mg 3x/day
Potassium-sparing diuretic			
	Starting dose	Dose change	Target dose
Spironolactone	12.5–25 mg 1x/day	12.5 mg 1x/day	25 mg 1x/day

* Only if no carvedilol or other heart failure beta-blocker available.

TABLE 4.17 Medications for Cardiomyopathy in Children (≤ 40 kg)

Beta Blockers					
Starting doses	**< 10 kg**	**10 kg**	**15 kg**	**20 kg**	**30 kg**
Carvedilol 6.25 mg tablet	See mg/kg dosing*	See mg/kg dosing*	See mg/kg dosing*	1.5 mg ¼ tab 2x/day	1.5 mg ¼ tab 2x/day
Initial dose: 0.05 mg/kg/dose 2x/day. **Maximum dose:** 0.4 mg/kg/dose 2x/day **OR** 25 mg 2x/day.					
Atenolol 50 mg tablet	See mg/kg dosing*	See mg/kg dosing*	12.5 mg ¼ tab 1x/day	12.5-25 mg ¼-½ tab 1x/day	25 mg ½ tab 1x/day
Initial dose: 0.5-1 mg/kg as one daily dose. **Maximum dose:** 2 mg/kg as one daily dose.					
ACE Inhibitors					
Starting doses	**< 10 kg**	**10 kg**	**15 kg**	**20 kg**	**30 kg**
Lisinopril 10 mg tablet	See mg/kg dosing*	See mg/kg dosing*	See mg/kg dosing*	2.5 mg ¼ tab 1x/day	2.5 mg ¼ tab 1x/day
Initial dose: 0.07 mg/kg/day as one daily dose. **Maximum dose:** 0.6 mg/kg/day or 20 mg as one daily dose. **Notes:** Do not use in children with a creatinine ≥ 2x the normal value for age (see **APPENDIX E** for normal ranges). Not safe for use in pregnancy.					
Captopril 25 mg tablet	See mg/kg dosing*	6.25 mg ¼ tab 2x/day	6.25 mg ¼ tab 3x/day	6.25-12.5 mg ¼-½ tab 2x/day	12.5 mg ½ tab 3x/day
Initial dose: 0.3-0.5 mg/kg/dose 2-3x/day. **Maximum dose:** 2 mg/kg/dose 2-3x/day. **Notes:** Do not use in children with a creatinine ≥ 2x the normal value for age (see **APPENDIX E** for normal ranges). Not safe for use in pregnancy.					
Hydralazine/Isosorbide Dinitrate** (Contraindications to B-blocker and/or ACE inhibitor)					
Starting doses	**< 10 kg**	**10 kg**	**15 kg**	**20 kg**	**30 kg**
Hydralazine 50 mg tablet	See mg/kg dosing*	See mg/kg dosing*	See mg/kg dosing*	See mg/kg dosing*	12.5 mg ½ tab 3x/day
Initial dose: 0.25-0.3 mg/kg/dose 3x/day. **Maximum dose:** 1.7 mg/kg/dose 3x/day or 25 mg 3x/day.					
Isosorbide dinitrate 10 mg tablet	See mg/kg dosing*	See mg/kg dosing*	2.25 mg ¼ tab 3x/day	2.25 mg ¼ tab 3x/day	5 mg ½ tab 3x/day
Initial dose: 0.15 mg/kg/dose 3x/day. **Maximum dose:** 0.5 mg/kg/dose 3x/day or 10 mg 3x/day.					

Potassium-Sparing Diuretic					
Starting doses	< 10 kg	10 kg	15 kg	20 kg	30 kg
Spironolactone 25 mg tablet	See mg/kg dosing*	12.5 mg ½ tab 1x/day	12.5–25 mg ½–1 tab 1x/day	25 mg 1 tab 1x/day	25–50 mg 1–2 tabs 1x/day

Initial dose: 1 mg/kg as one daily dose.

Maximum dose: 3 mg/kg/dose given once a day or 50 mg as one daily dose.

Notes: Do not use in children with a creatinine > the normal value for age (see **APPENDIX E** for normal ranges). Consider cutting the dose by half if patient is also on furosemide.

* Note that dosing medications for small children may require crushing pills and diluting. This should only be done under the supervision of an experienced clinician.

** There is no good evidence of the efficacy of this medication combination for the treatment of heart failure in children. We recommend initiating these medications only in consultation with a pediatrician or cardiologist.

4.8.3.1   Beta-Blockers in Heart Failure

Beta-blockers are a class of drugs that work on receptors in the heart to slow heart rate and reduce the work the heart muscle must do with each squeeze. In large randomized trials, certain types of beta-blockers have been shown to reduce the risk of death in adult patients with cardiomyopathies by around 30%.[27-31] Beta-blockers shown to prolong life in these heart failure patients include carvedilol, metoprolol succinate, and bisoprolol.

Atenolol is the beta-blocker most often available in low-resource settings. This drug is very inexpensive and is mentioned specifically in the 2008 WHO model drug formulary (though as a treatment for angina, not for heart failure).[32] Unfortunately, there is no prospective, randomized data to support its use in patients with cardiomyopathies.[33]

In comparing the price of heart failure beta-blockers (all generic at this point), we have found the price of carvedilol to be the lowest through our usual distributors (see **APPENDIX B**). We have judged that the benefits of carvedilol (or another heart failure beta-blocker) are probably significant enough to justify its addition to the national formulary. Atenolol can be used if no heart failure beta-blocker is available.

Beta-blockers should be used with caution in patients with cardiomyopathies. In the short-term, beta-blockers can actually cause fluid overload even though they stabilize volume status over the long term. Beta-blockers should be started only when a patient is euvolemic and should not be started or increased at the same time that diuretics are reduced. Likewise, they should not be started or increased in the setting of low heart rate (≤ 55 beats per minute or lower than normal range for age in a child (see **APPENDIX E**), or very low systolic blood pressure (≤ 80 mmHg or lower than normal range for age in a child (see **APPENDIX E**), or in the case of a patient with severe asthma. Side effects of beta-blockers include aggravation of asthma symptoms, bradycardia, and hypotension.

PROTOCOL 4.5 provides guidance on beta-blocker titration in cardiomyopathy.

PROTOCOL 4.5 Beta-Blocker Titration in Cardiomyopathy

4.8.3.2 ACE Inhibitors

ACE inhibitors are a class of medication that work on the kidneys, blood vessels, and heart muscle to decrease blood pressure, decrease fluid retention and prevent harmful remodeling of heart muscle. They have been shown to reduce mortality by around 30% in adult patients with cardiomyopathies.[34-37] Although all ACE inhibitors are acceptable for use, lisinopril has the lowest cost and requires only once per day dosing (see **TABLE 4.16** for adults and **TABLE 4.17** for children and **APPENDIX B**).

In the presence of renal failure, ACE inhibitors can cause a dangerous rise in potassium. Patients with an elevated creatinine (≥ 200 μmol/L (≥ 2.3 mg/dL) in adults) or ≥ twice the normal value for age in children (see **APPENDIX E**) should not be placed on an ACE inhibitor unless potassium levels can be easily monitored at regular intervals. ACE inhibitors also cause birth defects and should never be used in women who are pregnant. Like beta-blockers, ACE inhibitors can cause low blood pressure and should be avoided in patients with a low systolic blood pressure (less than 90 mmHg in adults or outside of the normal range for age in children).

PROTOCOL 4.6 provides guidance on titration of ACE inhibitors in cardiomyopathy.

4.8.3.3 Hydralazine and Isosorbide Dinitrate

Hydralazine is an arteriolar dilator, and isosorbide dinitrate is a venodilator. When used in combination, they have been shown in large clinical trials to decrease the risk of death in adult patients by about 30% and improve heart failure symptoms, although they are not as effective as ACE inhibitors.[38-40] Hydralazine and isosorbide have the advantage of affecting heart rate and renal function less than beta-blockers and ACE inhibitors. They are safe to use when bradycardia limits beta-blocker use and/or when renal function prohibits ACE inhibitor use. However, this drug combination is expensive, it requires inconvenient three-times-a-day dosing, and it can result in significant side effects such as headaches, which may limit patient adherence. For these reasons, we generally reserve the use of hydralazine/isosorbide dinitrate for patients with contraindications to beta-blockers and/or ACE inhibitors. Caution should be exercised when starting or increasing these medications in patients with low systolic blood pressure (less than 90 mmHg in adults or lower than normal range for age in children). As mentioned above, this drug combination is not well studied in the pediatric population and for this reason should be used with caution in children with cardiomyopathies.

PROTOCOL 4.6 also provides guidance on titration of hydralazine/isosorbide in cardiomyopathy.

PROTOCOL 4.6   ACE-Inhibitor Titration and Use of Hydralazine/Isosorbide in Cardiomyopathy

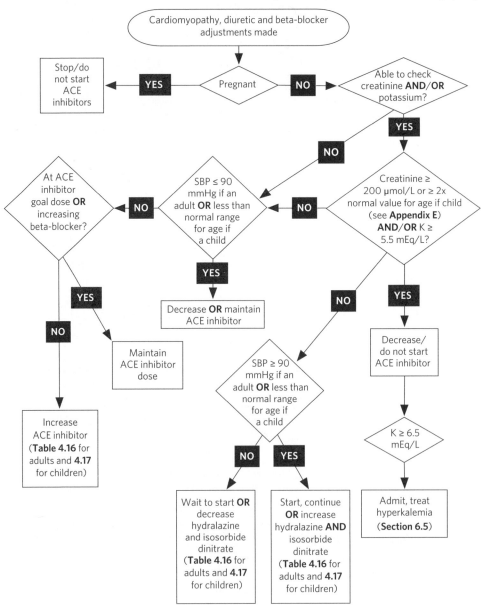

4.8.3.4   Spironolactone

As described in **SECTION 4.7.3**, spironolactone can be a useful adjunctive diuretic in cases of ascites. Like ACE inhibitors, spironolactone can cause a rise in serum potassium, especially in the presence of renal failure. It should only be used if the creatinine is normal (< 100 μmol/L or < 1.1 mg/dL in an adult or normal range for age in a child). On the other hand, it may be a useful adjunct in patients with chronically low potassium secondary to the use of furosemide or hydrochlorothiazide. Spironolac-tone has also been shown to reduce mortality by 30% in adult patients with left ventricular dysfunction who are already taking ACE inhibi-tors.[41,42] **TABLE 4.16** and **TABLE 4.17** show recommended dosing.

4.8.4 Other Medications in Cardiomyopathy Management

Depending on the suspected etiology of cardiomyopathy and/or disease cofactors, certain adjunctive medications may be indicated. **PROTOCOL 4.7** provides guidance on using these other medications.

PROTOCOL 4.7   Other Medication Needs for Cardiomyopathy Patients

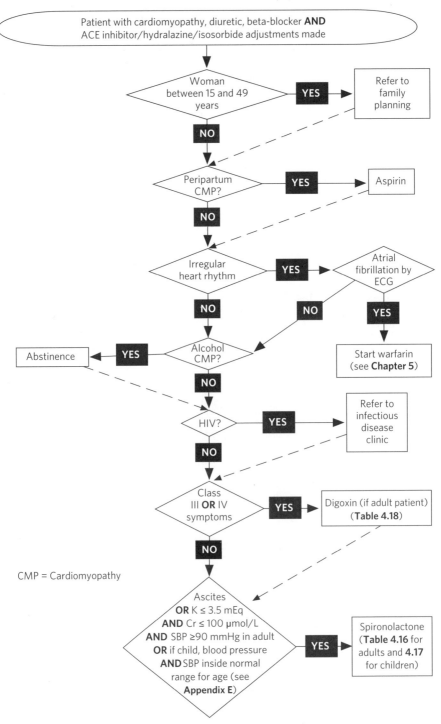

CMP = Cardiomyopathy

4.8.4.1 Digoxin (Digitalis)

Digoxin is one of the oldest and most widely available medications for the treatment of heart failure. It acts to increase the pumping function of the heart and can also slow down the heart rate if atrial fibrillation is present. Using digoxin can improve symptoms in patients with heart failure. However, in a large clinical trial, it did not decrease mortality.[43] Also, at high doses, toxicity can develop, which will result in visual changes, dizziness, or nausea, and can lead to dangerous arrhythmias. Toxicity will occur if digoxin is used in patients with renal failure, so this drug should be used only if the creatinine level is ≤ 100 μmol/L.[44] We reserve digoxin for patients with class III or IV heart failure symptoms. For patients with known atrial fibrillation, digoxin may be started to help with rate control. We do not discuss digoxin use in children. In Rwanda, we currently do not have dose formulations small enough for children available at district level and pills cannot be crushed.

TABLE 4.18 lists recommended digoxin dosing.

TABLE 4.18 Adult Digoxin Dosing

Starting dose	Maximum dose
0.125 mg/day	0.25 mg/day

4.8.4.2 Aspirin

When the heart does not pump well, blood tends to sit still inside the heart and may form clots, which can then embolize (travel to other parts of the body), causing stroke or other catastrophic events. Peripartum cardiomyopathy patients are at particularly high risk for this, as well as for venous clots. They should be started on 100 mg of aspirin daily to help thin the blood. Patients with evidence of an active clot will need stronger anticoagulation (see **CHAPTER 5**).

4.8.4.3 Birth Control

All female patients of childbearing age should be counseled on the dangers of pregnancy in the setting of a cardiomyopathy. The physiologic changes during pregnancy, including increased fluid retention and smaller lung volumes, mean that heart failure symptoms almost always worsen. In the case of peripartum cardiomyopathy, subsequent pregnancies can be lethal. All women should be advised to use birth control. Clinicians should work with family-planning staff to coordinate efforts and ensure that women at risk receive timely and appropriate birth control. See **CHAPTER 3** for further discussion of birth control for women with heart failure.

4.8.4.4   Antiretrovirals (ARVs)

Untreated HIV infection frequently leads to cardiomyopathy.[45,46] Predictors of HIV cardiomyopathy are opportunistic infection and length of time since HIV diagnosis. All patients with a newly diagnosed cardiomyopathy should be tested for HIV. If a patient is HIV positive, regardless of the CD4 count, the patient should be treated with ARVs according to local protocols.

4.9   Hypertensive Heart Disease Etiology and Diagnosis

Hypertension creates stress on the heart, which has to work harder to push blood into a high-pressure system. In response to this workload, the heart muscle gets thicker (hypertrophy) and stiffer. This change defines hypertensive heart disease. The thick, stiffened walls are not able to relax as normal heart walls do, making it difficult for the heart to fill with blood. The common echocardiographic finding is a thickened heart wall. Usually, patients with hypertensive heart disease will have normal or only mildly depressed systolic function (ejection fraction between 40% and 50%) with left ventricular hypertrophy, but some can progress to very low ejection fractions.

Hypertensive heart disease results from long-standing, severe hypertension. The hypertension itself may be idiopathic (which is most common) or secondary to another problem (such as a kidney or endocrine disorder). In young patients (≤ 40 years old) a secondary cause should be suspected—severe renal failure in particular—although hypertension itself can cause renal failure. As with all types of heart failure, new patients should be screened for renal failure with a creatinine.

Hypertensive heart disease is an extremely rare cause of heart failure in children. This chapter refers only to adult diagnostic criteria and medication dosing.

Treatment of hypertensive heart disease includes control of volume status and blood pressure. **PROTOCOL 4.8** provides an outline for hypertensive heart disease management.

PROTOCOL 4.8   Management of Suspected or Confirmed Hypertensive Heart Disease

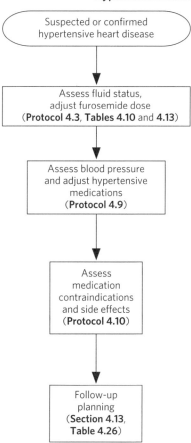

4.9.1   Vital Sign Assessment

As with all types of heart failure, management of hypertensive heart disease begins with an assessment of the patient's vital signs and overall condition. Decompensation in patients with hypertensive heart disease is often caused by uncontrolled, very high blood pressure (SBP ≥ 180 mmHg), resulting in stiffening of the heart. As described in **CHAPTER 8**, the approach in this situation is to lower the blood pressure gradually— by approximately 25% in the first 2 to 4 hours.

4.9.2   Fluid Status Assessment

The next step in the management of hypertensive heart disease is the evaluation of fluid status and titration of diuretics. See **SECTION 4.7**, **TABLE 4.10**, and **PROTOCOL 4.3**. All patients should have a creatinine checked regularly to assess renal function. Renal failure is common in patients who have had long-standing, severe hypertension.

4.9.3 Titration of Antihypertensives

In order to prevent worsening heart failure symptoms, antihypertensives should be titrated to achieve a blood pressure goal of ≤ 130/80 mmHg. See **PROTOCOL 4.9**, **PROTOCOL 4.10**, and **TABLE 4.19**. In general, an ACE inhibitor is first-line therapy for these patients unless contraindications exist (creatinine ≥ 200 μmol/L or pregnant/breastfeeding). If the blood pressure is not controlled or if ACE inhibitors are not appropriate for the patient, a thiazide diuretic may be started. After that, amlodipine, a peripherally acting calcium-channel blocker, should be used. Beta-blockers and hydralazine are third- and fourth-line medications, respectively.

TABLE 4.19 Antihypertensives for Hypertensive Heart Disease

First-line drug (ACE inhibitor)	Initial dose	Dose increase	Maximum dose	Side effects/cautions
Lisinopril	5 mg 1x/day	5 mg 1x/day	20 mg 1x/day	1. Birth defects (contraindicated in pregnancy)
Captopril	12.5 mg 3x/day	12.5 mg 3x/day	50 mg 3x/day	2. Chronic non-productive cough
				3. High potassium
				4. Do not use if creatinine ≥ 200 μmol/L
Second-line drug (thiazide)	**Initial dose**	**Dose increase**	**Maximum dose**	**Side effects/cautions**
Hydrochlorothiazide	12.5 mg 1x/day	12.5 mg 1x/day	25 mg 1x/day	Lowers potassium
Third-line drug (CCB)*	**Initial dose**	**Dose increase**	**Maximum dose**	**Side effects/cautions**
Amlodipine	5 mg 1x/day	5 mg 1x/day	10 mg 1x/day	Lower-extremity swelling
Nifedipine (sustained release)	20 mg 2x/day	20 mg 2x/day	40 mg 2x/day	
Fourth-line drug (beta-blocker)	**Initial dose**	**Dose increase**	**Maximum dose**	**Side effects/cautions**
Atenolol	25 mg 1x/day	25 mg 1x/day	50 mg 1x/day	1. Bradycardia
				2. Renally excreted
				3. Decrease dose for renal failure
Fifth-line drug (vasodilator)	**Initial dose**	**Dose increase**	**Maximum dose**	**Side effects/cautions**
Hydralazine	25 mg 3x/day	25 mg 3x/day	50 mg 3x/day	1. Headache
				2. Tachycardia
				3. Lower-extremity swelling

* CCB = Calcium-channel blocker

PROTOCOL 4.9 Antihypertensive Management in Hypertensive Heart Disease

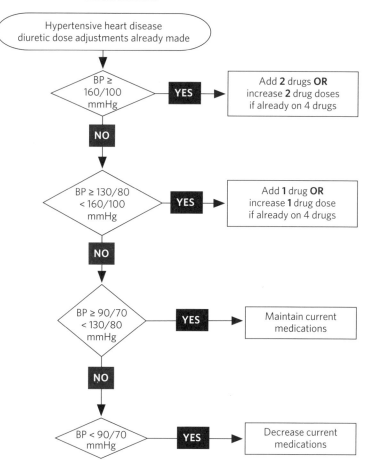

PROTOCOL 4.10 Assessment of Medication Contraindications and Side Effects in Management of Hypertensive Heart Disease

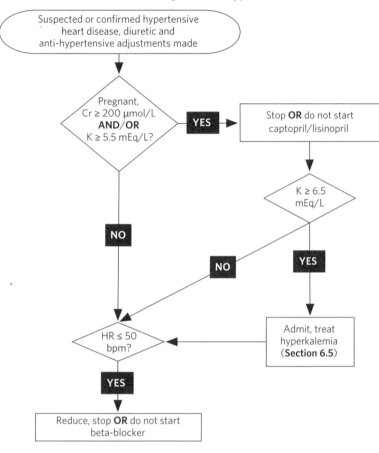

4.10 Mitral Stenosis

Mitral stenosis is a special type of valvular disease with a treatment pathway that differs from that of other valvular diseases. Untreated, mitral stenosis leads to left atrial enlargement, pulmonary hypertension, and right ventricular failure. The stretched left atrium is particularly prone to developing electrical abnormalities, leading to atrial arrhythmias. Mitral stenosis almost always results from untreated rheumatic heart disease. Mitral stenosis is most common in people between 30 and 50 years old. It may sometimes occur in younger or older patients. However, it is very rarely seen in young children. Therefore, all vital sign parameters and dosing information in this chapter refer only to adults. Often women will develop symptoms in the middle of their pregnancies. Patients with mitral stenosis are also at high risk of atrial fibrillation, which can cause rapid decompensation. Basic echocardiography can easily identify a stenotic mitral valve, which has a highly recognizable pattern in the parasternal long view.

Mitral stenosis requires a different treatment strategy than other forms of valvular heart disease. The goals of medical therapy are to manage fluid status and to minimize the negative effects of mitral stenosis on cardiac output by controlling heart rate. **PROTOCOL 4.11** outlines the steps in the medical management of mitral stenosis.

PROTOCOL 4.11 Management of Mitral Stenosis

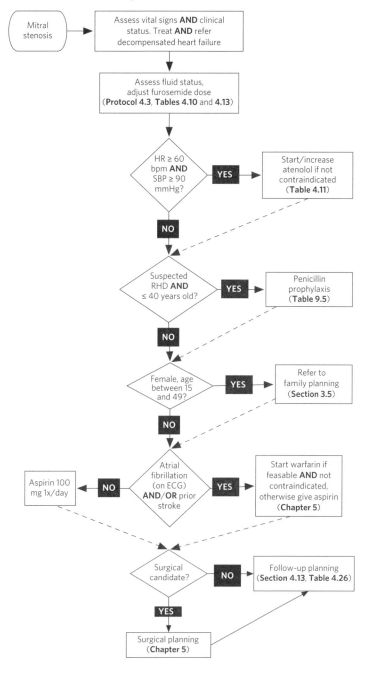

4.10.1 Vital Sign Assessment

As with all types of heart failure, mitral stenosis management begins with an assessment of the patient's vital signs and overall condition. Patients with mitral stenosis are particularly sensitive to tachycardia and will not be able to tolerate fast heart rates well.

4.10.2 Fluid Status Assessment

The next step in the management of mitral stenosis is evaluation of fluid status and titration of diuretics. The principles here are the same as in other forms of heart failure. See **SECTION 4.7**, **TABLE 4.10**, and **PROTOCOL 4.3**.

4.10.3 Control of Heart Rate

When the mitral valve doesn't open well, less blood can move from the left atrium to the left ventricle during diastole. This, in turn, decreases the amount of blood the heart can pump out with each beat. When the heart rate increases, diastole (the heart's filling time) becomes even shorter, exacerbating the problem. For this reason, it is very important to control heart rate, preferably keeping it below 60 beats per minute, if permitted by blood pressure. We recommend the use of beta-blockers for this purpose. All beta-blockers work equally well in decreasing heart rate. We suggest using atenolol because of its once-a-day dosing, low cost, and wide availability. However, any agent that slows the heart rate may be used.

Atrial fibrillation, which is common in mitral stenosis, often causes very fast heart rates. Patients with mitral stenosis are unable to tolerate these fast heart rates and will become very sick or even die if the arrhythmia is not controlled. Beta-blockers (atenolol) are the first-line therapy. However, if good heart rate control in a patient with atrial fibrillation and mitral stenosis cannot be obtained with beta-blockers alone, or if blood pressure limits the use of beta-blockers, clinicians may prescribe digoxin if the patient has a creatinine < 100 µmol/L. (See **TABLE 4.20** and **SECTION 4.16.1**.)

TABLE 4.20 Medications to Reduce Heart Rate in Mitral Stenosis

Medication	Initial dose	Dose increase	Maximum dose
Beta-blocker *(for use in sinus tachycardia or atrial fibrillation)*			
Atenolol	12.5 mg 1x/day	12.5 mg 1x/day	50 mg 1x/day
Digoxin *(only if tachycardia and atrial fibrillation and creatinine < 100 µmol/L)*			
Digoxin	0.125 mg 1x/day	0.125 mg 1x/day	0.25 mg 1x/day

4.10.4 Other Medications in Management of Mitral Stenosis

4.10.4.1 Penicillin

Rheumatic heart disease causes almost all cases of mitral stenosis in resource-poor settings. As described in **CHAPTER 9**, prevention of further attacks of rheumatic fever through penicillin prophylaxis helps slow the progression of rheumatic valvular disease. Although rheumatic fever generally affects school-aged children, we recommend penicillin prophylaxis for all patients with rheumatic valvular disease under the age of 40. See **SECTION 9.2** for specific guidelines on penicillin dosing and administration.

4.10.4.2 Birth Control

As with cardiomyopathy, mitral stenosis presents an increased danger to women during pregnancy, and for some pregnant women, it can be lethal. Not uncommonly, women will first become symptomatic from mitral stenosis in the 2nd or 3rd trimester. Women between the ages of 15 and 49 years with mitral stenosis should receive family planning counseling and be offered an acceptable form of birth control (see **CHAPTER 3**).

4.10.4.3 Anticoagulation (Aspirin and Warfarin)

All patients with mitral stenosis are at very high risk of developing clots in their dilated, stagnant left atrium. These clots have a high likelihood of embolizing to the brain and causing stroke. Atrial fibrillation further increases the chances of clot formation and stroke, and patients with mitral stenosis are at very high risk of atrial fibrillation. For this reason, all patients with mitral stenosis should receive some type of blood-thinning agent. If a patient has clear documentation of atrial fibrillation, stronger anticoagulation in the form of warfarin should be initiated if there are no contraindications to warfarin therapy (see **CHAPTER 5**). If there is no ECG-documented atrial fibrillation, then aspirin should be prescribed.

4.11   Other Valvular and Congenital Heart Disease

This category encompasses the most diverse group of heart failure patients. Most children with heart failure will fall into this diagnostic category. Unlike the previously described heart failure categories, these diseases often require advanced echocardiography skills for differentiation. Fortunately, they also share a common initial approach in management (see **PROTOCOL 4.12**). We therefore argue that at the district health center level, these patients can be safely managed as an undifferentiated group until a more advanced echocardiographer can make a definitive diagnosis.

Valvular disease (here excluding mitral stenosis) means that some insult to the heart valve (such as rheumatic fever) has caused it to either not open (stenosis) or not close (regurgitation) properly. Afflicted patients will most often have dramatic murmurs. These lesions can eventually cause dilation of the associated heart chambers, which in turn can lead to a cardiomyopathy. Valvular diseases are usually secondary to rheumatic heart disease, in which untreated streptococcal infection leads to an autoimmune response that results in valve destruction.

Congenital heart disease means that the heart was malformed at birth. Congenital disease comes in many varieties and often causes murmurs or cyanosis. It can be caused by a variety of genetic factors and/or teratogens (toxins during pregnancy).

This collection of heart failure diagnoses is both larger and more diverse than the previous categories. However, these diseases share a common pathway in their initial medical management. Moreover, differentiation among these diseases often requires a higher level of echocardiographic and other diagnostic skills than are reasonably attainable by generalist physicians or advanced nurses in resource-poor settings.

The common goals in the medical management of this group of heart failure patients include management of fluid status and reduction of the heart's workload. Definitive treatment for most congenital and valvular disease will be surgical, and thus all patients suffering this class of heart failure should be evaluated by a cardiologist, internist, or pediatrician experienced in echocardiography within 6 weeks to 6 months of preliminary diagnosis.

PROTOCOL 4.12 Valvular or Congenital Heart Disease Management (Excluding Mitral Stenosis)

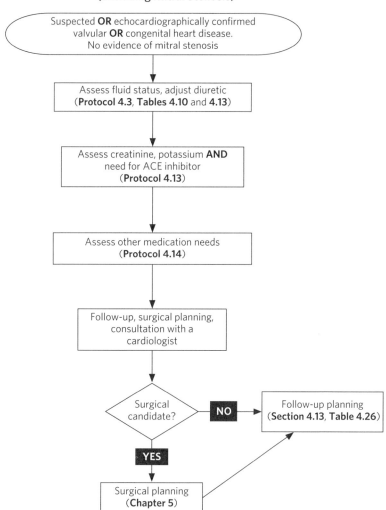

4.11.1 Vital Sign Assessment

As with all types of heart failure, management of this collection of heart failure types begins with an assessment of the patient's vital signs, weight, and overall condition.

4.11.2 Fluid Status Assessment

The next step in management is evaluation of fluid status and titration of diuretics. See **SECTION 4.7, TABLE 4.10**, and **PROTOCOL 4.3**.

4.11.3 Titration of ACE Inhibitors

In patients with valvular heart disease (excluding mitral stenosis), it is important to reduce the workload of the heart by lowering the blood pressure. The heart was designed to pump blood in only one direction. However, regurgitant lesions cause blood to flow backwards with each cardiac cycle. This results in wasted work by the heart. Lowering blood pressure helps reduce some of this extra effort by reducing the amount of force the heart needs to pump blood in the forward direction. ACE inhibitors are the preferred anti-hypertensive agent (see **TABLE 4.20**). However, if a patient has renal failure or hyperkalemia, or is pregnant, furosemide alone should be used. A cardiologist or doctor may choose to add another medication (such as isosorbide dinitrate) to reduce cardiac workload. The goal systolic blood pressure for patients with valvular heart disease is 100–120 mmHg in adults, and within normal range for age in children (see **APPENDIX E**). **PROTOCOL 4.13** outlines an approach to initiating and titrating ACE inhibitors.

PROTOCOL 4.13 **ACE-Inhibitor Titration for Valvular or Congenital Heart Disease Management (Excluding Mitral Stenosis)**

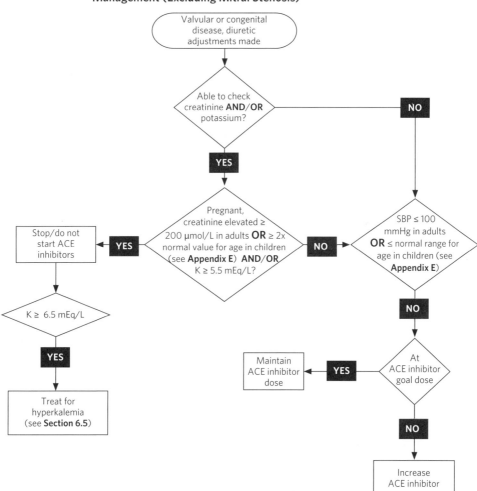

4.11.4   Other Medications

4.11.4.1   Spironolactone

Patients with disease of any of the valves on the right side of the heart can develop symptoms of right heart failure, including massive ascites. In these patients, spironolactone can be a useful adjunct to furosemide (see **TABLE 4.21** and **TABLE 4.22**). Spironolactone should only be used in patients with normal renal function (Cr ≥ 100 µmol/L or ≥ 2.3 mg/dL in adults or ≥ normal range for age if a child (see **TABLE 6.4**)), because of the risk of hyperkalemia. Concurrent use with an ACE inhibitor can also cause dangerous hyperkalemia, and these patients should have potassium monitored every six months.

4.11.4.2 Penicillin

As described in **CHAPTER 9**, penicillin prophylaxis helps slow the progression of rheumatic valvular disease by preventing further attacks of rheumatic fever. Although rheumatic fever generally affects school-aged children, we recommend penicillin prophylaxis for all patients with rheumatic valvular disease under the age of 40. See **SECTION 9.2** for specific guidelines on penicillin dosing and administration.

TABLE 4.21 Medications for Valvular/Congenital Heart Disease

	Initial dose	Dose adjustment	Maximum dose
ACE inhibitor			
Lisinopril	5 mg 1x/day	5 mg 1x/day	20 mg 1x/day
Captopril	12.5 mg 3x/day	12.5 mg 3x/day	50 mg 3x/day
Potassium-sparing diuretic			
Spironolactone	12.5–25 mg 1x/day	12.5 mg 1x/day	25 mg 1x/day

TABLE 4.22 Medications for Valvular/Congenital Heart Disease in Children (≤ 40 kg)

ACE Inhibitors					
Starting doses	< 10 kg	10 kg	15 kg	20 kg	30 kg
Lisinopril 10 mg tablet	See mg/kg dosing*	See mg/kg dosing*	See mg/kg dosing*	See mg/kg dosing*	2.5 mg ½ tab 1x/day
Initial dose: 0.07 mg/kg/day as one daily dose.					
Maximum dose: 0.6 mg/kg/day or 20 mg as one daily dose.					
Notes: Do not use in children with a creatinine ≥ 2x the normal value for age (see **APPENDIX E** for normal ranges). Not safe for use in pregnancy.					
Captopril 25 mg tablet	See mg/kg dosing*	6.25 mg ¼ tab 2x/day	6.25 mg ¼ tab 2x/day	6.25–12.5 mg ¼–½ tab 2x/day	12.5 mg ½ tab 2x/day
Initial dose: 0.3–0.5 mg/kg/dose 2–3x/day.					
Maximum dose: 2 mg/kg/dose 2–3x/day.					
Notes: Do not use in children with a creatinine ≥ 2x the normal value for age (see **APPENDIX E** for normal ranges). Not safe for use in pregnancy.					
Potassium-Sparing Diuretic					
Starting doses	< 10 kg	10 kg	15 kg	20 kg	30 kg
Spironolactone 25 mg tablet	See mg/kg dosing*	12.5 mg ½ tab	12.5 mg ½ tab	25 mg 1 tab	25 mg 1 tab
Initial dose: 1 mg/kg as one daily dose.					
Maximum dose: 3 mg/kg/dose or 50 mg as one daily dose.					
Notes: Do not use in children with a creatinine > the normal value for age (see **APPENDIX E** for normal ranges). Consider cutting the dose by half if patient is also on furosemide.					

* Note that dosing medications for small children may require crushing pills and diluting. This should only be done under the supervision of an experienced clinician.

PROTOCOL 4.14 Other Medications for Valvular or Congenital Heart Disease Management (Excluding Mitral Stenosis)

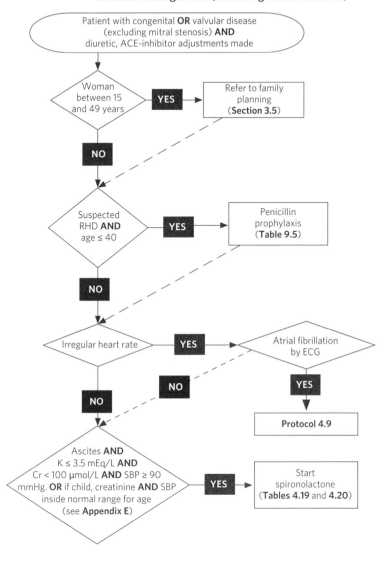

4.11.5 Cardiac Surgery Evaluation

Definitive treatment for most valvular and congenital heart disease will be surgical, and thus all patients in this class of heart failure should be evaluated by a cardiologist or experienced internist within 6 weeks to 6 months of intake. Although advanced echocardiography is not needed to guide medical management of the patient, it is necessary to evaluate the specific type of surgery that is needed. Even patients who appear well-compensated may be candidates for surgical intervention before they begin to decompensate. At times, these are the best surgical candidates. See **CHAPTER 5** for more detail on cardiac surgery evaluation.

4.12 Isolated Right-Sided Heart Failure Etiology and Diagnosis

The terms right- and left-sided heart failure are often used to describe a patient's presenting symptoms. Most etiologies of heart failure can result from left-sided heart failure symptoms (such as shortness of breath and orthopnea), and patients with signs of left-sided heart failure will often have signs of right-sided heart failure. However, patients with isolated symptoms of right-sided heart failure (ascites, hepatomegaly, elevated jugular venous pressure [JVP], lower extremity edema) fall into a distinct category of diagnoses. (See **TABLE 4.23**.)

In resource-poor settings such as Rwanda, isolated right-sided heart failure most often results from chronic diseases of the lungs that have led to pulmonary hypertension or from diseases of the pericardium (see **TABLE 4.24**). Tuberculosis is by far the most common reason for constrictive pericardial disease in most of rural sub-Saharan Africa, and as such represents a treatable cause of heart failure.

TABLE 4.23 Clinical Presentation of Right-Sided Heart Failure

Symptoms	Physical exam findings
Weight gain	Elevated JVP
Abdominal swelling	Cardiac murmur (depending on cause)
Lower-extremity edema	Enlarged or pulsatile liver
Decreased appetite	Ascites
Right-upper-quadrant pain	Lower-extremity pitting edema

Our protocols ask practitioners to first exclude left-sided heart failure (such as cardiomyopathy, hypertensive heart disease, mitral stenosis, and other valvular disease) before considering pure right-sided heart failure as a diagnosis. As with other categories of heart failure, the precise diagnosis is neither easy nor essential to the initial management of the patient. Our protocol for right-sided heart failure therefore focuses on excluding non-cardiac causes of the presenting symptoms of edema and ascites, and on identifying those patients most likely to benefit from empiric tuberculosis treatment.

Patients with ascites caused by liver failure or renal failure can resemble patients with right-sided heart failure. It is clinically very difficult to distinguish between these patients. Echocardiography is essential in differentiating patients with right-sided heart failure from those with other etiologies of edema and ascites. In particular, echocardiography can be helpful as a way to exclude heart failure as a cause of ascites. If the patient has no murmurs and has an entirely normal-appearing basic echocardiogram (including a normal inferior vena cava and right ventricle), they are unlikely to have a cardiac cause of their presenting symptoms (see **FIGURE 4.5** and **FIGURE 4.8**).

TABLE 4.24 Causes of Right-Sided Heart Failure

Cause	Notes
Left-sided heart failure	Left-sided heart failure is the most common cause of right-sided heart failure. Some common causes include cardiomyopathy, mitral stenosis, and mitral regurgitation
Tricuspid valve abnormalities	Tricuspid valve stenosis, tricuspid regurgitation, congenital heart disease
Pulmonary disease	Pulmonary TB, severe COPD
Pulmonary hypertension	HIV, congenital heart disease (commonly VSD, ASD), other
Constrictive pericarditis	Most commonly caused by TB
Endomyocardial fibrosis	Cause unknown

Treatment for patients with right-sided heart failure focuses first on identifying those patients who are likely to have disease caused by active tuberculosis. Patients with other types of right ventricular failure (usually due to pulmonary hypertension or endomyocardial fibrosis) will be mainly palliative and will mirror the approach to medical management of patients with valvular and other congenital heart disease.

PROTOCOL 4.15 outlines an approach to patients with isolated right-sided heart failure.

PROTOCOL 4.15 Management of Isolated Right-Sided Heart Failure

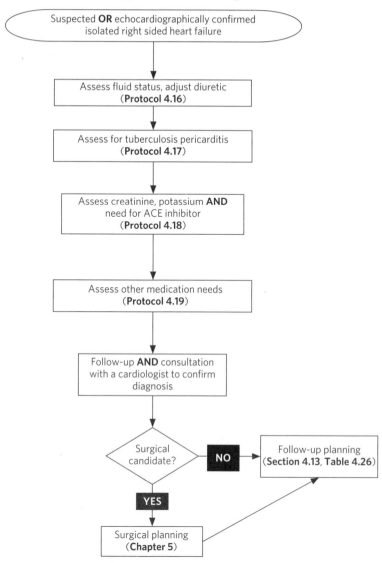

4.12.1 Vital Sign Assessment

As with all types of heart failure, management of suspected right-sided heart failure begins with an assessment of the patient's vital signs and overall condition. Patients with an effusion and hypotension should be presumed to have tamponade and should be referred to the district hospital for emergent pericardiocentesis. Likewise, patients with massive ascites that is causing respiratory distress should also be referred to the district hospital for paracentesis.

4.12.2 Fluid Status Assessment

The next step in the management of right-sided heart failure is evaluation of fluid status and titration of diuretics. These patients tend to have profound leg edema and ascites. In most cases, these patients will never reach euvolemia, and attempting to diurese them down to a dry weight will result in intravascular hypovolemia, causing renal failure, hypotension, and electrolyte imbalances. The goal should be to minimize the patient's discomfort from edema and abdominal distension.

As with other types of heart failure, furosemide is the main tool for controlling the patient's fluid status. See **SECTION 4.7.2**.

Spironolactone should be added to assist in diuresis of patients with normal renal function. In patients with severe discomfort or respiratory distress from ascites, paracentesis may be performed (see **SECTION 4.12.4**).

PROTOCOL 4.16 Fluid Status Management in Right-Sided Heart Failure

(1) Hypovolemia: Rising creatinine, low blood pressure; may still have significant edema or ascites
(2) Euvolemia: Comfortable, able to perform daily activities
(3) Hypervolemia, Moderate: Increasing ascites or edema, uncomfortable but able to do basic activities
(4) Hypervolemia, Severe: Rapid breathing, unable to walk

4.12.3 Pericardial Disease

Diseases of the pericardium fall into two main categories: (1) pericardial effusions; and (2) constrictive pericardial disease.[47] Both of these conditions can lead to heart failure by causing external compression on the heart, and by not allowing the heart to fill properly with blood.

4.12.3.1 Pericardial Effusions

Pericardial effusions are fluid collections around the heart. Small effusions (less than 1 cm in diastole) are common incidental findings in all forms of heart failure. However, large pericardial effusions without another cardiac finding are most often due to either tuberculosis (TB), cancers, or viral infections. TB is the cause of large pericardial effusions in about 90% of those infected with HIV, and in about half of those not infected with HIV.[47] On chest x-ray (CXR), the heart often appears large or globular. On an echocardiogram, the heart is surrounded by fluid (see **FIGURE 4.9**). If large enough, a pericardial effusion can cause life-threatening hypotension, which is known as cardiac tamponade. The treatment for this condition is drainage of the fluid with a needle (pericardiocentesis).

4.12.3.2 Constrictive Pericarditis

The diseases that cause a pericardial effusion can also lead to scarring and stiffening of the pericardium. This is known as constrictive pericarditis. The diagnosis of constrictive pericarditis can be difficult to make. Most patients will present with symptoms of right-sided heart failure, including ascites. Calcification around the heart on CXR is diagnostic for constrictive pericarditis, but is actually rare. Constrictive pericardial disease should be suspected in patients with signs of right-sided heart failure; a dilated, non-collapsing IVC; and no other obvious cardiac findings on echocardiography or physical examination.

Most constrictive pericardial disease in rural sub-Saharan Africa is probably due to TB. Echocardiography is helpful in the diagnosis of a pericardial effusion or constriction. However, evidence of TB infection is often subtle or nonexistent, making a definitive diagnosis unlikely in most cases. CXR demonstrates signs of pulmonary TB in only one-third of cases, and sputum smear for acid-fast bacilli is often negative.[47] Drainage or biopsy of the pericardium is difficult, expensive, and not usually available in community-based settings. Diagnosis must therefore be based on clinical presentation in the context of risk factors for TB and HIV.

4.12.3.3 Diagnosis and Treatment of Tuberculosis Pericarditis

Prompt initiation of anti-mycobacteria treatment can be lifesaving in cases of TB pericarditis. We therefore suggest that TB is the presumed diagnosis in cases of suspected constrictive pericardial disease. We recommend starting empiric therapy in these cases. All patients started on TB treatment should have three sets of sputum collected. All patients started on treatment should also be seen by a cardiologist who will decide, in conjunction with the infectious disease clinic, whether to continue or stop the anti-tuberculosis medications.

Treatment of pericardial TB is the same as for pulmonary TB and consists of a 4-drug regimen given over 6 months: 2 months of daily isoniazid, rifampin, pyrazinamide, and ethambutol, followed by 4 months of daily isoniazid and rifampin. There is no need to prolong the course of treatment. The use of corticosteroids is controversial, but in several studies, the concomitant use of prednisone with anti-TB therapy has been shown to reduce mortality and the need for surgical interventions.[48,49] We therefore recommend prescribing a steroid taper for patients treated for suspected tuberculosis pericarditis (see **TABLE 4.25**). Because rifampin increases the metabolism of steroids, prednisolone is given at relatively high doses (around 1.5 mg/kg per day in adults).

TABLE 4.25 Treatment of Tuberculous Pericarditis

Medication	Adult Dose	Pediatric dose (< 40 kg)	Schedule
Isoniazid	5 mg/kg once daily **Maximum dose:** 300 mg daily	10-15 mg/kg once daily **Maximum dose:** 300 mg once daily	26 weeks
Rifampin	10 mg/kg once daily **Maximum dose:** 600 mg once daily	10-20 mg/kg once daily **Maximum dose:** 600 mg once daily	26 weeks
Pyrazinamide	20-25 mg/kg once daily **Maximum dose:** 2 g once daily		8 weeks
Ethambutol	15-20 mg/kg once daily **Maximum dose:** 2.5 g once daily	15-25 mg/kg once daily **Maximum dose:** 2.5 g once daily	8 weeks
Prednisone	40 mg twice per day	1 mg/kg 1x/day	4 weeks, followed by
	20 mg twice per day	0.5 mg/kg 1x/day	4 weeks, followed by
	10 mg twice per day	0.25 mg/kg 1x/day	2 weeks, followed by
	5 mg once daily	0.125 mg/kg 1x/day	1 week

PROTOCOL 4.17 Diagnosis and Treatment of Tuberculosis Pericarditis

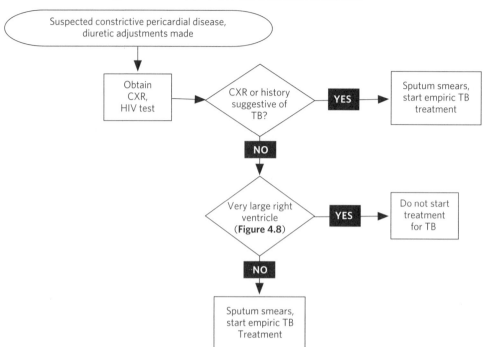

4.12.4 Titration of ACE Inhibitors and Spironolactone and Paracentesis

As described in **SECTION 4.11.4.1**, spironolactone can be used in addition to furosemide for patients with ascites. However, it should only be used in patients with normal renal function (creatinine < 100 μmol/L or < 1.1 mg/dL in adults or within normal range for age in children (see **APPENDIX E**)). When spironolactone is prescribed along with lisinopril, the patient should be monitored for hyperkalemia at least every 6 months. Spironolactone may be a useful adjunct in patients with chronically low potassium secondary to furosemide or hydrochlorothiazide use.

Patients with tense ascites may need periodic paracentesis to relieve abdominal discomfort or respiratory distress. However, without correction of the underlying cause, reaccumulation of ascitic fluid will occur. Moreover, frequent paracentesis puts patients at risk for peritoneal infections and loss of protein, which can in turn worsen the ascites.

After adding spironolactone, an ACE inhibitor may be added to the patient's regimen, if renal function and blood pressure permit. As in other types of heart failure, the ACE inhibitor can help reduce the heart's workload. In addition, patients with right-sided heart failure tend to have high levels of aldosterone, and the ACE inhibitor, like spironolactone, can counteract this.

**PROTOCOL 4.18   ACE-Inhibitor and Spironolactone Titration and
Paracentesis for Isolated Right-Sided Heart Failure**

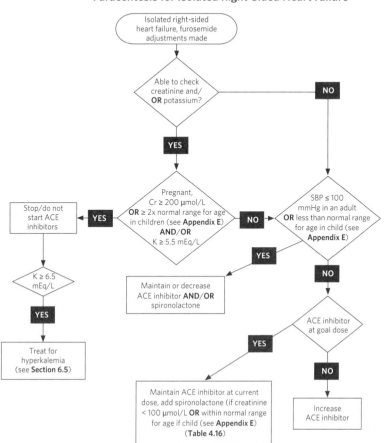

4.12.5 Other Medication Needs

Patients with isolated right-sided heart failure may suffer from various
comorbid conditions, some of which may be related to or worsen their
heart failure. For instance, patients with HIV may develop pulmonary
hypertension, which can cause right-sided heart failure. Women with
right-sided heart failure should avoid becoming pregnant, as pregnancy
may worsen their symptoms. Patients with evidence of atrial fibrillation
should be rate-controlled and anticoagulated.

PROTOCOL 4.19 Other Medication Needs in Isolated Right-Sided Heart Failure

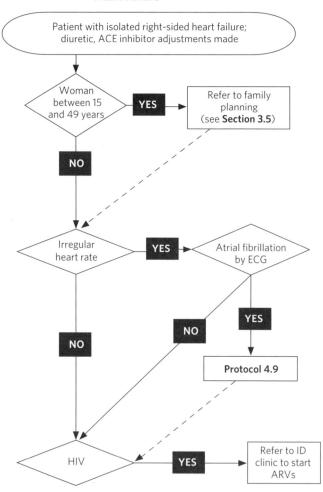

4.13 Heart Failure Patient Follow-Up

No heart failure intervention will be successful without good patient retention and follow-up. **CHAPTER 3** outlines the important role community health workers play in this effort. In addition, frequent medication adjustments require frequent clinic visits. Frequency of visits should be flexible and depend on the patient's condition. **TABLE 4.26** provides the guide used by NCD clinicians in determining how often to see patients in the clinic. Obviously, clinicians must rely on their own clinical judgment when determining how frequently a patient should be seen. In general, we encourage clinicians to see patients more frequently if they have any questions or concerns about a patient's condition or management. This allows for smaller, more frequent titration of medications and faster recognition of a deteriorating condition. Children may need to be seen more frequently given that they may quickly grow out of their medication dose.

TABLE 4.26 Clinic Follow-Up Schedule for Heart Failure Patients

	Class I or Class II heart failure, euvolemic	Class III or Class IV symptoms, new renal failure, hypervolemic or any other clinical concern
Medication change	Return in 2 weeks–1 month	Return in 1–2 weeks
No medication change	Return in 1–2 months	Return in 2 weeks–1 month

In rural, resource-poor settings such as Rwanda, travel to a clinic can pose significant hardship to patients, especially those too ill to walk long distances. As a temporary measure, we have reduced barriers to clinic attendance by providing travel reimbursement for patients traveling long distances.

4.14 Potassium Management

Many of the medications used in heart failure management can affect potassium. For instance, potassium levels may decrease over the course of diuresis. Conversely, if patients have baseline renal dysfunction, potassium may rise to dangerous levels if renal function worsens. Potassium is an essential electrolyte that, when in imbalance, can cause significant cardiac arrhythmias and even death.

In general, potassium levels will not become dangerously high as long as creatinine is normal. Many facilities are able to check creatinine but not potassium. Accordingly, we have based our algorithms on creatinine alone. See **SECTION 6.5** for discussion of management of hyperkalemia.

4.15 Arrhythmia Diagnosis and Management

Patients with heart failure of any type are at increased risk of having abnormal heart rhythms. The field of arrhythmia diagnosis and management is vast and complex, and beyond the scope of this handbook. Here we aim to provide a basic guide for district-level clinicians in recognition and management of common arrhythmias.

4.16 Role of Electrocardiography in Rural Rwanda

Electrocardiogram (ECG) use is limited at rural district hospitals in Rwanda. Many district hospitals do not have an electrocardiogram machine, and few district hospital clinicians feel comfortable in the use or interpretation of ECGs. The goal in Rwanda is to have an ECG machine at each district hospital and to provide basic training in ECG interpretation.

The main utility of an ECG in rural Rwanda is to detect arrhythmias. In this setting, few patients have coronary artery disease, and the ability to detect myocardial infarction on ECG is a less useful skill.

Almost all arrhythmias occur among patients with heart failure, particularly among those with a reduced EF or mitral stenosis and among those who have had cardiac surgery. Atrial fibrillation is likely the most common arrhythmia in this setting. NCD clinicians with no prior ECG training can easily learn to identify its characteristic ECG pattern. Other arrhythmias are less common, harder to diagnose, and more difficult to treat. Unfortunately, many patients with ventricular arrhythmias never make it to the hospital. Patients with cardiomyopathy are at high risk for these types of rhythms, and beta-blocker use following the cardiomyopathy protocols will help reduce this risk. For these reasons, we focus our ECG teaching on the detection of atrial fibrillation among patients with established heart failure.

Identification of complete heart block is a second skill that can be useful. Heart block is relatively rare but potentially deadly, and it is treatable with pacemaker implantation.

All district hospitals should have an ECG machine. However, we have found that these are often cumbersome to use. Recently, some portable, one-lead ECG machines have come onto the market and may be easier to use.

4.16.1   Atrial Fibrillation Diagnosis and Management

Our protocol for atrial fibrillation diagnosis and treatment suggests that clinicians obtain an ECG on any patient with an irregular pulse or a very rapid heart rate (≥ 120 beats per minute in an adult). The NCD nurse may perform the ECG in the clinic or accompany the patient to the inpatient ward to have the ECG performed. NCD nurses should receive basic training in ECG interpretation. However, a district hospital physician should be available to help with interpretation if there are questions. The key ECG findings suggestive of atrial fibrillation are (1) absence of P waves; and (2) irregularly spaced QRS waves (see **FIGURE 4.10**).

FIGURE 4.10 ECG of Normal Rhythm (top) and Atrial Fibrillation (bottom)

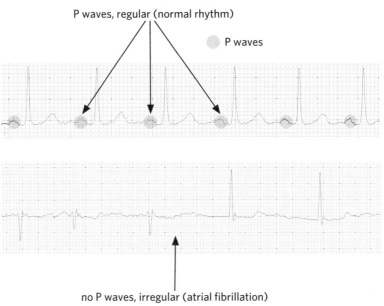

Patients with signs of decompensated heart failure should be admitted to the hospital. Patients with atrial fibrillation at a very rapid heart rate, even if it is asymptomatic, should also stay in the hospital until the rate is controlled. Adult patients with a heart rate ≥ 120 beats per minute should have their heart rate lowered if possible. Lowering the heart rate increases the time the heart has to fill and can therefore increase cardiac output. As a general rule, patients with a tachycardia (≥ 100 beats per minute in an adult) should receive a trial of beta-blocker treatment. Digoxin may also be given to help slow the heart rate and is a better choice in patients with borderline blood pressures and/or signs of decompensated heart failure. Digoxin generally takes up to a day to take effect. See **TABLE 4.18** for digoxin dosing.

Patients with decompensated heart failure, a low systolic blood pressure, and rapid atrial fibrillation may benefit from electrical cardioversion. Cardioversion machines should be available at all district hospitals.

Many of the patients who present with atrial fibrillation will have structural heart disease. Therefore, all patients found to have atrial fibrillation should have an echocardiogram.

Heart failure patients with atrial fibrillation who are rate-controlled and asymptomatic are still at high risk of stroke and should be anticoagulated. **CHAPTER 5** outlines initiation of warfarin therapy. Unlike patients who already have clots, these patients do not need to bridged with heparin therapy until they reach a therapeutic INR.

PROTOCOL 4.20 Diagnosis and Management of Atrial Fibrillation in Adults

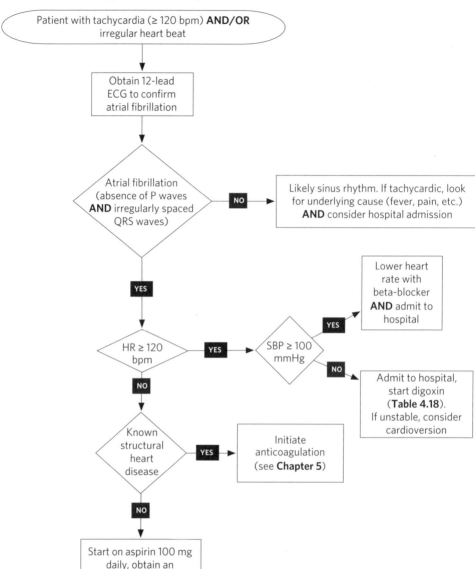

4.17 Cardioversion

The main indication for cardioversion is cardiogenic shock in the setting of rapid atrial fibrillation. This most often occurs with mitral stenosis. Every district hospital should have a cardioversion machine. Patients who are potentially in need of cardioversion should be admitted to the hospital and managed by the inpatient physician.

4.18 Palpitations and Somatization

In Rwanda, many otherwise healthy patients seek medical care for palpitations. The vast majority of these patients have normal vital signs, physical exams, and echocardiograms. When asked in greater detail about their symptoms, many patients report that the palpitations began after the 1994 Rwanda genocide. Anecdotally, palpitations (like shortness of breath) seem to be common as a somatized expression of depression, grief, and stress.

We have developed a protocol for managing palpitations in conjunction with our mental health team (see **PROTOCOL 4.21**). If history and physical exam reveal no signs of heart failure or murmurs, and the patient has a regular heart rate and rhythm, arrhythmia is unlikely. The clinician reassures the patient and explains that there doesn't seem to be anything wrong with the heart. These patients should be asked about stressors and should be told that it is common for people to experience sadness or stress as physical complaints. These patients should be offered an appointment with the mental health team.

PROTOCOL 4.21 Palpitations in Adults

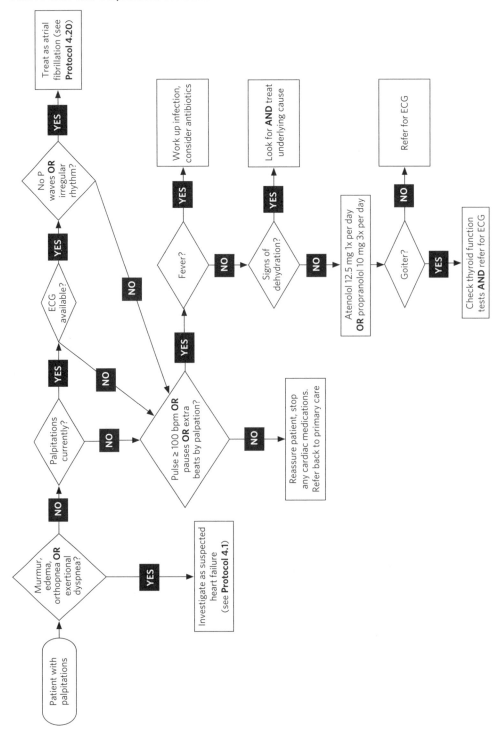

4.19 Palliative Care for Patients with Heart Failure

Palliative care is an essential part of heart failure treatment. A study comparing patients with symptomatic heart failure to patients with advanced cancers found that the two groups had similar numbers of physical symptoms and similar depression scores.[50] A study of patients dying of heart failure found that 63% experienced severe dyspnea.[51] A review of studies reporting symptoms in patients with end-stage heart disease, cancer, AIDS, chronic obstructive lung disease, and renal disease found that three symptoms—pain, dyspnea, and fatigue—had a prevalence of more than 50% in patients with each of the five diseases.[52] These physical symptoms often make it impossible for heart failure patients to work or even to be independent in self-care. Thus, symptom relief and psychosocial supports are as important for heart failure patients as they are for cancer patients.

Because heart failure typically has a relapsing and remitting course, recurrences of dyspnea and other symptoms should be anticipated and plans made—during an NCD clinic visit or prior to hospital discharge—to relieve them quickly wherever the patient might be, including in the home. When dyspnea occurs despite standard disease-modifying treatment, opioid therapy can be beneficial.[53] Morphine may improve exercise tolerance for patients with NYHA Class III disease and also can make comfortable patients with Class IV disease (see **CHAPTER 2, SECTION 2.2.4**). The usual starting doses can be used for opioid-naïve patients: 5 mg orally or in adults or 0.2–0.4 mg/kg/dose orally in children every 4 hours as needed or every four hours (see **CHAPTER 2, SECTION 2.2.3**). Because of its venodilating effect, morphine also is an effective treatment along with furosemide for acute exacerbations of pulmonary edema due to heart failure when the blood pressure is normal or elevated. In hypotensive or hypovolemic patients, however, it can cause a dangerous drop in blood pressure and thus should be used cautiously unless the only goal of care is comfort. When there is concern about side effects, morphine can be started at half the usual starting doses: 2.5 mg orally or 1 mg IV/SC in adults or 0.1–0.2 mg/kg/dose in children every 4 hours as needed.

Patients actively dying of heart failure sometimes have hours or days of dyspnea and other symptoms and require careful titration of morphine given around-the-clock to assure comfort. In some cases, health center nurses and community health workers may be able to provide this care in patients' homes once appropriate prescriptions have been written by a district-level physician. Patients with severe or complex symptoms may require end-of-life care at the health center or district level.

Patients with heart failure also may have sudden cardiac death. It may be appropriate to inform some families and patients of this possibility. Care should be taken whenever giving bad news to minimize emotional distress for the patient and family. This can be done in several ways: 1) by suggesting that support persons such as family members or friends be present when bad news will be discussed; 2) by taking the time to sit down with the patient or family and give them a chance to absorb the news; 3) by first exploring the patient's or family's understanding of the disease and gently correcting misconceptions; 4) by being prepared for strong reactions, such as anger or grief; 5) by offering to see the patient or family again soon to answer questions and provide emotional support.

Chapter 4 References

· ·

1   Beet EA. Rheumatic heart disease in Northern Nigeria. Trans R Soc Trop Med Hyg 1956;50:587-92.

2   D'Arbela PG, Kanyerezi RB, Tulloch JA. A study of heart disease in the Mulago hospital, Kampala, Uganda. Trans R Soc Trop Med Hyg 1966;60:782-90.

3   Nhonoli AM. Heart disease in Dar es Salaam. East Afr Med J 1968;45:118-21.

4   Baldachin BJ. Cardiovascular disease in the African in Matabeleland. Cent Afr J Med 1963;28:463-9.

5   Obineche EN. Pattern of cardiovascular disease in Lusaka. A review. East Afr Med J 1976;53:435-9.

6   Bukhman G, Kidder A. Cardiovascular disease and global health equity: lessons from tuberculosis control then and now. Am J Public Health 2008;98:44-54.

7   Miller DC, Spencer SS, White PD. Survey of cardiovascular disease among Africans in the vicinity of the Albert Schweitzer Hospital in 1960. Am J Cardiol 1962;10:432-46.

8   White PD. Notes on cardiovascular disease in Africa as encountered by an American physician on a brief visit to that continent in March and April, 1959. Am Heart J 1961;61:133-4.

9   Freers J, Mayanja-Kizza H, Ziegler JL, Rutakingirwa M. Echocardiographic diagnosis of heart disease in Uganda. Trop Doct 1996;26:125-8.

10 Sliwa K, Wilkinson D, Hansen C, et al. Spectrum of heart disease and risk factors in a black urban population in South Africa (the Heart of Soweto Study): a cohort study. Lancet 2008;371:915-22.

11 Commerford P, Mayosi B. An appropriate research agenda for heart disease in Africa. Lancet 2006;367:1884-6.

12 Damasceno A, Cotter G, Dzudie A, Sliwa K, Mayosi BM. Heart failure in sub-saharan Africa: time for action. J Am Coll Cardiol 2007;50:1688-93.

13 Mocumbi AO, Ferreira MB. Neglected cardiovascular diseases in Africa: challenges and opportunities. J Am Coll Cardiol 2010;55:680-7.

14 Mayosi BM. Contemporary trends in the epidemiology and management of cardiomyopathy and pericarditis in sub-Saharan Africa. Heart 2007;93:1176-83.

15 Mayosi B, Robertson K, Volmink J, et al. The Drakensberg declaration on the control of rheumatic fever and rheumatic heart disease in Africa. S Afr Med J 2006;96:246.

16 Sliwa K, Damasceno A, Mayosi BM. Epidemiology and etiology of cardiomy-opathy in Africa. Circulation 2005;112:3577-83.

17 Bukhman G, Ziegler JL, Parry EH. Endomyocardial fibrosis: still a mystery after 60 years. In: PLoS Neglected Trop Dis; 2008:e97.

18 Mocumbi AO, Ferreira MB, Sidi D, Yacoub MH. A population study of endomyocardial fibrosis in a rural area of Mozambique. N Engl J Med 2008;359:43-9.

19 Amoah AG, Kallen C. Aetiology of heart failure as seen from a National Cardiac Referral Centre in Africa. Cardiology 2000;93:11-8.

20 Kingue S, Dzudie A, Menanga A, Akono M, Ouankou M, Muna W. A new look at adult chronic heart failure in Africa in the age of the Doppler echocardiog-raphy: experience of the medicine department at Yaunde General Hospital. Ann Cardiol Angeiol (Paris) 2005;54:276-83.

21   Thiam M. L'insuffisance cardiaque en milieu cardiologique africain. Bull Soc
      Pathol Exot 2002;96:217-18.

22   Quinones MA, Douglas PS, Foster E, et al. American College of Cardiology/
      American Heart Association clinical competence statement on echocardiog-
      raphy: a report of the American College of Cardiology/American Heart
      Association/American College of Physicians—American Society of Internal
      Medicine Task Force on Clinical Competence. Circulation 2003;107:1068-89.

23   Shah S, Noble VE, Umulisa I, et al. Development of an ultrasound training
      curriculum in a limited resource international setting: successes and
      challenges of ultrasound training in rural Rwanda. Int J Emerg Med
      2008;1:193-6.

24   Shah S, Price D, Bukhman G, Shah S, Wroe E, eds. The Partners In Health
      Manual of Ultrasound for Resource-Limited Settings. Boston: Partners In
      Health; 2011.

25   Shah SP, Epino H, Bukhman G, et al. Impact of the introduction of ultrasound
      services in a limited resource setting: rural Rwanda 2008. BMC Int Health
      Hum Rights 2009;9:4.

26   McMurray JJ, Pfeffer MA. Heart failure. Lancet 2005;365:1877-89.

27   Effect of metoprolol CR/XL in chronic heart failure: Metoprolol CR/XL
      Randomised Intervention Trial in Congestive Heart Failure (MERIT-HF).
      Lancet 1999;353:2001-7.

28   Packer M, Bristow MR, Cohn JN, et al. The effect of carvedilol on morbidity
      and mortality in patients with chronic heart failure. U.S. Carvedilol Heart
      Failure Study Group. N Engl J Med 1996;334:1349-55.

29   Packer M, Coats AJ, Fowler MB, et al. Effect of carvedilol on survival in severe
      chronic heart failure. N Engl J Med 2001;344:1651-8.

30   Waagstein F, Bristow MR, Swedberg K, et al. Beneficial effects of metoprolol
      in idiopathic dilated cardiomyopathy. Metoprolol in Dilated Cardiomyopathy
      (MDC) Trial Study Group. Lancet 1993;342:1441-6.

31   The Cardiac Insufficiency Bisoprolol Study II (CIBIS-II): a randomised trial.
      Lancet 1999;353:9-13.

32   WHO Model Formulary 2008. Geneva: World Health Organization; 2009.

33   Go AS, Yang J, Gurwitz JH, Hsu J, Lane K, Platt R. Comparative effectiveness
      of beta-adrenergic antagonists (atenolol, metoprolol tartrate, carvedilol)
      on the risk of rehospitalization in adults with heart failure. Am J Cardiol
      2007;100:690-6.

34   Effect of enalapril on survival in patients with reduced left ventricular
      ejection fractions and congestive heart failure. The SOLVD Investigators.
      N Engl J Med 1991;325:293-302.

35   Jong P, Yusuf S, Rousseau MF, Ahn SA, Bangdiwala SI. Effect of enalapril on
      12-year survival and life expectancy in patients with left ventricular systolic
      dysfunction: a follow-up study. Lancet 2003;361:1843-8.

36   Pfeffer MA, Braunwald E, Moye LA, et al. Effect of captopril on mortality and
      morbidity in patients with left ventricular dysfunction after myocardial
      infarction. Results of the survival and ventricular enlargement trial. The
      SAVE Investigators. N Engl J Med 1992;327:669-77.

37   Packer M, Poole-Wilson PA, Armstrong PW, et al. Comparative effects of low
      and high doses of the angiotensin-converting enzyme inhibitor, lisinopril, on
      morbidity and mortality in chronic heart failure. ATLAS Study Group.
      Circulation 1999;100:2312-8.

38   Taylor AL, Ziesche S, Yancy C, et al. Combination of isosorbide dinitrate and
      hydralazine in blacks with heart failure. N Engl J Med 2004;351:2049-57.

39 Cohn JN, Johnson G, Ziesche S, et al. A comparison of enalapril with hydralazine-isosorbide dinitrate in the treatment of chronic congestive heart failure. N Engl J Med 1991;325:303-10.

40 Cohn JN, Archibald DG, Ziesche S, et al. Effect of vasodilator therapy on mortality in chronic congestive heart failure. Results of a Veterans Administration Cooperative Study. N Engl J Med 1986;314:1547-52.

41 Pitt B, Remme W, Zannad F, et al. Eplerenone, a selective aldosterone blocker, in patients with left ventricular dysfunction after myocardial infarction. N Engl J Med 2003;348:1309-21.

42 Pitt B, Zannad F, Remme WJ, et al. The effect of spironolactone on morbidity and mortality in patients with severe heart failure. Randomized Aldactone Evaluation Study Investigators. N Engl J Med 1999;341:709-17.

43 The effect of digoxin on mortality and morbidity in patients with heart failure. The Digitalis Investigation Group. N Engl J Med 1997;336:525-33.

44 Rathore SS, Wang Y, Krumholz HM. Sex-based differences in the effect of digoxin for the treatment of heart failure. N Engl J Med 2002;347:1403-11.

45 Twagirumukiza M, Nkeramihigo E, Seminega B, Gasakure E, Boccara F, Barbaro G. Prevalence of dilated cardiomyopathy in HIV-infected African patients not receiving HAART: a multicenter, observational, prospective, cohort study in Rwanda. Curr HIV Res 2007;5:129-37.

46 Barbaro G, Di Lorenzo G, Grisorio B, Barbarini G. The Gruppo Italiano per lo Studio Cardiologico dei Pazienti Affetti da A. Incidence of Dilated Cardiomyopathy and Detection of HIV in Myocardial Cells of HIV-Positive Patients. N Engl J Med 1998;339:1093-9.

47 Syed FF, Mayosi BM. A modern approach to tuberculous pericarditis. Prog Cardiovasc Dis 2007;50:218-36.

48 Strang JI, Kakaza HH, Gibson DG, Girling DJ, Nunn AJ, Fox W. Controlled trial of prednisolone as adjuvant in treatment of tuberculous constrictive pericarditis in Transkei. Lancet 1987;2:1418-22.

49 Mayosi BM, Ntsekhe M, Volmink JA, Commerford PJ. Interventions for treating tuberculous pericarditis. Cochrane Database Syst Rev 2002:CD000526.

50 Bekelman DB, Rumsfeld JS, Havranek EP, et al. Symptom burden, depression, and spiritual well-being: a comparison of heart failure and advanced cancer patients. J Gen Intern Med 2009;24:592-8.

51 Levenson JW, McCarthy EP, Lynn J, et al. The last six months of life for patients with congestive heart failure. J Am Geriatr Soc 2000;48(suppl 5):S101-S109.

52 Solano JP, Gomes B, Higginson IJ. A comparison of symptom prevalence in far advanced cancer, AIDS, heart disease, chronic onstructive pulmonary disease and renal disease. J Pain Symptom Manage 2006;31:58-69.

53 Pantilat SZ, Steimle AE. Palliative care for patients with heart failure. JAMA 2004;291:2476-82.

CHAPTER 5

Cardiac Surgery Screening, Referral, Anticoagulation, and Postoperative Management

As mentioned in **CHAPTER 4**, about a third of patients identified through district NCD clinics in Rwanda have valvular or congenital lesions amenable to surgical intervention. A much smaller number may benefit from surgical repair of pericardial lesions. The goal is to find these patients before they develop irreversible cardiomyopathies, severe pulmonary hypertension, or renal failure as a result of their disease, all of which would make them poorer surgical candidates later in life.

Cardiac surgery for children and young adults with congenital, valvular, or pericardial disease can be an excellent public health investment (see **APPENDIX B**). NCD clinics at district hospitals, working in conjunction with specialists from tertiary centers, can be the key to timely referral for possible surgical candidates. At the same time, good long-term outcomes for patients after cardiac surgery require strong chronic care infrastructure. In this way, cardiac surgery and chronic care integration are synergistic strategies for health-system strengthening.

This chapter discusses some of the issues specific to referral and follow-up of cardiac surgical patients, as well as issues around anticoagulation more broadly.

5.1 History of Cardiac Surgery in Rwanda

The history of cardiac surgery in Rwanda prior to 1994 is not well known. Between 1994 and about 2006, cardiac surgery was largely unavailable, even to relatively wealthy citizens. Since that time, a Rwandan pediatric cardiologist has returned from training in Belgium and has collaborated with the Rwandan Medical Referral Board and the King Faisal Hospital in Kigali to arrange for more patients to be sent out of country for cardiac surgery and to attract visiting cardiac surgical teams. The goal has been to ultimately establish a Rwandan cardiac surgical program. Between 2006 and 2011, there have been more than 200 cardiac surgical operations in Rwanda, with only 6 deaths. **FIGURE 5.1** and **FIGURE 5.2** show the distribution of indications and sources of surgery for Rwandan patients who received cardiac surgery between November 2007 and February 2010.

FIGURE 5.1 Indication for Cardiac Surgery between Nov. 2007 and Feb. 2010 (%)

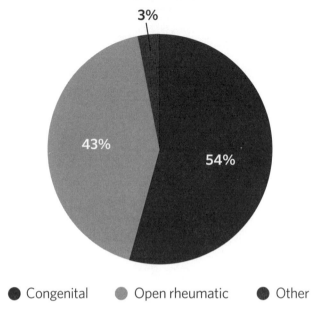

● Congenital   ● Open rheumatic   ● Other

FIGURE 5.2 Source of Cardiac Surgery in Rwanda between Nov. 2007 and Feb. 2010 (n)

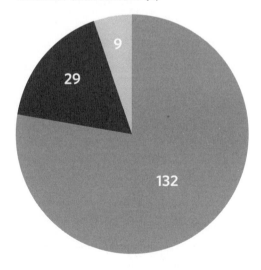

● Visting cardiac surgical team
● External referral
● Closed cardiac surgery by local thoracic surgeon

5.1.1 Out-of-Country Referral to External Cardiac Surgical Centers

Referral to external cardiac surgical centers is the main source of cardiac surgery for many countries in sub-Saharan Africa. External referral plays an important role, even as African countries work to establish their own cardiac surgical programs. Visiting cardiac surgical teams are not available for emergency cases. Furthermore, external centers are often best equipped to manage complex cases requiring intense and prolonged post-operative care. However, in our experience, raising funds for external referral is challenging (see **FIGURE 5.2**).

There are two kinds of external centers: those that raise money themselves to provide surgery free of charge (philanthropic centers), and those that ask the referring organization to raise the required funds (fee-for-service centers). Both kinds of centers play an important role for increasing access to cardiac surgery.

5.1.1.1 Philanthropic Centers

Many centers in the United States and Europe will occasionally perform cardiac surgery on a philanthropic basis. These centers must raise funds to cover the real costs of these procedures and often look to regional donors for support. However, the cost of care at these centers is high, regardless of who is paying for it. On the other hand, patients flown from Africa often raise awareness and lead to increased engagement from institutions in wealthy countries. These effects have value above and beyond the value of life-saving surgery itself. In the longer run, however, we feel that money raised for philanthropic cardiac surgery could be better directed toward supporting lower-cost care through regional centers in middle-income countries and in Africa itself.

A very important regional center for Central and Eastern Africa is the Salam Heart Center in Khartoum, Sudan.[1] This center is operated by the Italian non-governmental organization Emergency. Emergency raises the funds for the surgeries and hospitalization costs, but needs referring organizations to pay the cost of plane tickets. Emergency has estimated that their real cost per surgery is around $14,000. Since 2007, this center has performed more than 3000 surgical operations.

The Walter Sisulu Heart Center in Johannesburg, South Africa, is another important site that performs a limited number of surgeries for pediatric patients.[2] Although these surgeries are provided free of charge to the referring organization, the real costs of these procedures are probably relatively high in South Africa.

Save A Child's Heart is an Israeli organization that both provides cardiac surgery for children from Africa, and trains African professionals.[3,4] The funding for this organization is limited, and increasingly their center in Holon, Israel, is asking for a financial contribution from referring organizations.

5.1.1.2   Fee-for-Service Centers

International fee-for-service centers are an important resource for African countries. There are many centers in India that provide excellent care through impressively high-volume, low-cost models. By one estimate, more than 60,000 open-heart surgeries are performed in India each year—around 600 for every 10 million people.[5] The experience in Rwanda has been primarily with the Miot center in Chennai.[1] Results from this center have been good, even with complex cases. The total charges per patient, including air transportation and housing, have been between $10,000 and $15,000.

5.1.2   Visiting Cardiac Surgical Teams

Visiting cardiac surgical teams have played a critical role in development of cardiac surgical capacity in Rwanda. The real costs of surgeries performed by these teams may well be higher than the cost of transfer to external centers. We believe this cost is worth it as long as skills continue to be transferred to local professionals with each trip. In the end, the goal of the visiting cardiac surgical teams is to support self-sufficient local teams of surgeons, anesthesiologists, and nurses.

Visiting teams are, of necessity, large, and require substantial funds for travel, food, and lodging (see below). These costs are particularly high in Rwanda compared with other low-income countries. Moreover, up until the present, visiting teams have needed to ship large quantities of medication and equipment from abroad.

Cardiac surgical teams visiting Rwanda have raised money for equipment, supplies, and travel. Heath providers have also donated their vacation time. These teams meticulously procure, label, pack, and ship nearly every single item needed for the performance of complex cardiac surgical procedures. These items include, but are not limited to, heart-lung machines, ultrasound equipment, and surgical instruments, as well as consumables such as perfusion supplies, medications, intravenous fluids, surgical masks, globes, and prosthetic heart valves and rings. Some teams have also supported the cost of patient follow-up and social support (e.g., school fees, housing).

The Rwandan Ministry of Health (MOH) has made an equally important contribution. The MOH has paid for lodging costs for essential members of visiting teams. The MOH has also absorbed the hospitalization costs at the hosting institution, the King Faisal Hospital.

The first cardiac surgical team to operate in Rwanda was Operation Open Heart (OOH) in April 2006.[6,7] This Australian group already had several decades of experience supporting a cardiac program in Papua New Guinea and other Asian and Pacific island countries.[8,9] Since that time, OOH has operated in Rwanda every November. This surgical group performs adult and pediatric surgeries, and has paved the way for other visiting teams.

In April 2008, Team Heart became the second cardiac surgical group to operate in Rwanda.[10] Team Heart is a Boston-based cardiac surgical group affiliated with the Brigham and Women's Hospital. Team Heart has focused on surgery for teenagers and young adults with rheumatic valvular disease. This surgical group has completed an annual surgical mission for four consecutive years, most recently in February of 2011. Team Heart has also been an important advocate for strategies to prevent rheumatic heart disease and rheumatic fever, including school-based screening.

In February 2010, Healing Hearts Northwest (HHNW) joined the group of cardiac surgical teams supporting Rwanda through annual missions.[11] HHNW performs both adult and pediatric surgeries.

Chain of Hope Belgium has also brought pediatric interventional teams to Rwanda. Although there is no cardiac catheterization laboratory in Rwanda at present, Chain of Hope has been able to operate using echocardiographic and fluoroscopic guidance.[12] The Chain of Hope team has also been instrumental in training another Rwandan pediatric cardiologist, who recently returned from Belgium and joined the public sector.

5.2   Building a National Cardiac Surgery Program

There are very few national cardiac surgical programs in Africa.[13-18] The challenges of establishing such centers and achieving good surgical outcomes are significant. At the same time, countries with populations of 10 million or more people can easily justify the need for at least one local center to perform 300 or more surgeries per year. We have estimated that such centers could provide valvular replacements for under $5000 per case (see **APPENDIX B**). Programs that operate on 300 or more cases per year must be able to rely on a strong system of chronic care capable of anticoagulation monitoring at district-hospital level. The following sections describe strategies for case finding and follow-up.

5.2.1   Cardiac Surgical Referral

Cardiac surgical programs need to have access to a large and nationally inclusive set of potential cardiac surgical candidates. One challenge for cardiac surgical programs is ensuring that the poor living in rural communities, located far from the capital, have equal access to referral for cardiac surgery. Traditionally in Rwanda, as in many countries, cardiac surgery programs have relied upon a combination of existing referral systems and intermittent cardiac surgical screening camps. National scale-up of NCD clinics at district hospitals will play a crucial role in expanding and enriching the pool of possible cardiac surgical candidates available for evaluation by specialists at the University Teaching Hospitals (CHUK and CHUB) and King Faisal Hospital. Here we briefly describe how NCD clinics feed into the cardiac surgical selection system.

Once a district NCD clinic system is in place, heart failure cases are evaluated first at district-hospital level by the NCD nurse (see **CHAPTER 4**). Once the NCD nurse has confirmed probable heart failure and excluded a cardiomyopathy or hypertensive heart disease, the patient is referred to a cardiologist for complete evaluation and advanced echocardiography. Heart failure clinics are held on the same day each week and patients are divided into groups. This kind of organization allows both cardiologists from visiting teams and those working in the referral centers to do efficient outreach to district hospitals around the country.

Once the cardiologist determines that a patient is a suitable surgical candidate, he or she adds them to a national cardiac surgical waiting list. Prior to each cardiac surgical mission, visiting teams can review this list as part of their initial patient case selection.

TABLE 5.1 shows the typical evaluations requested by cardiac surgical teams prior to surgery.

TABLE 5.1   Typical Preoperative Evaluation for Cardiac Surgery

History
• Heart failure symptom class
• Careful examination for possible tuberculosis
• Social evaluation (including housing, education, and employment needs)
• Reproductive history
Physical examination
• Evaluation for obvious comorbidities
• Careful evaluation of the liver
• Evaluation for malnutrition
• Dental evaluation
Laboratory studies
• Complete blood cell count with differential
• HIV
• Hepatitis C
• Liver function tests
• Creatinine, glucose, electrolytes
• Urinalysis
• Blood smear for malaria
Imaging
• Chest x-ray
• Echocardiogram (within 1 month)

5.2.2   Principles of Case Selection

It has been the observation of visiting adult cardiac surgical teams in Rwanda that patients with rheumatic valvular disease, and particularly the poorest and those from rural areas, present late in their clinical course. By this time, these patients are already experiencing NYHA Class III and IV heart failure symptoms, with involvement of two, and sometimes three, cardiac valves.

Thus, while it is desirable that local cardiac surgery programs in Africa initially focus on lower-risk surgical candidates, systematically excluding salvageable patients with advanced disease is not a good option. This, among numerous additional factors, will impact the pace with which local, independent cardiac surgery programs can develop, and will continue to mandate involvement of visiting programs to perform surgeries, while training local personnel to assume direction of the programs.

In Rwanda, cardiac surgical case selection is coordinated nationally by the cardiac surgery program director with input from all cardiologists. Here we describe some principles of case selection in a setting where available options for cardiac surgery include (1) limited numbers of visiting teams and, to a lesser degree, (2) external referral. The total number of available surgical slots has been around 60 per year, although this continues to grow.

First, given very limited access to cardiac surgery in Rwanda, patients under age 40 are prioritized.

Second, many patients unfortunately have disease that is so advanced that they are unlikely to have a good outcome even with surgery.

Third, some patients would require multiple staged surgeries to achieve a full repair (e.g., congenitally single ventricles). These patients are currently considered too complex to fix. For these patients, a palliative shunt is the best available option.

Fourth, most visiting cardiac surgical teams do not feel that it is safe to operate on more than one highly complex case per day. Visiting teams must balance the sometimes competing demands of patient acuity and complexity with the realities of postoperative care availability. Despite these resource limitations, more adult patients have received multiple, rather than single, valve procedures for the past 3 years. Over the past 4 years, multiple valve operations have become the norm for patients with rheumatic valvular disease, including several triple valve surgeries.

Fifth, out-of-country referral is used to make surgery available for emergent cases and reasonable candidates who are unlikely to survive for evaluation by the next visiting team.

As of December 2010, there were more than 100 patients awaiting cardiac surgery in Rwanda.

5.3   Common Procedures for Cardiac Valves

NCD nurses and generalist physicians working at district hospitals need to understand some of the basics of cardiac valvular surgery.[19] The follow-up issues for patients following cardiac surgery depend, in part, on the nature of the surgery they have undergone.

There are two basic types of valvular surgeries: valve repair and valve replacement. Mitral valves and tricuspid valves can sometimes be repaired. Valve repair has the advantage of preserving more of the normal function of the valve. On the other hand, patients with a valve repair often require a second operation later in life.

Access to heart surgery in Rwanda and surrounding countries is limited. Given the fact that reoperative heart surgery is not likely to be a priority in the near future, experienced visiting teams are opting more often for valve replacement therapy for patients with rheumatic heart disease.

The decision of mechanical versus tissue prostheses is often challenging, and must incorporate both medical as well as cultural factors. One of the common situations encountered is operating on a female of child-bearing age who may wish to have children. Mechanical valves require patients to take teratogenic anticoagulants. Even though tissue valves do not last as long in young individuals, in this circumstance, we choose to honor the patient's wishes, and give her tissue prostheses. Another not-uncommon situation is a patient who may be from such a remote part of the country that warfarin follow-up is not feasible. In this case, tissue valves would also be the safer option, though perhaps not the most durable. In most cases, mechanical valves are preferred, provided warfarin follow-up is available.

The sections below discuss the considerations involved with each type of surgery.

5.3.1 Mitral or Tricuspid Valve Repair

Some valvular damage is mild enough to be repaired. The main advantage of a valve repair is that it leaves the part of the valve below the leaflets intact. This contributes to better function of the associated ventricle. The risk of reoperation due to failure of the repair probably falls somewhere between the risks of failure in bioprosthetic and mechanical valves.[20]

For patients with mitral stenosis due to fusion of the anterior and posterior leaflets, successful surgery involves separating the two leaflets. This is called a *commissurotomy* (see **TABLE 5.2**). In patients with regurgitant mitral valve disease, a metal ring can be used to slightly narrow the valve. The ring is placed around the outer edge of the valve (also called the annulus). This procedure is called a *ring annuloplasty*. In addition, some patients may also need to have part of their valve cut away, or augmented with pericardium, to fix the regurgitation.

TABLE 5.2   Types of Valve Repairs

	Ring annuloplasty	Commissurotomy
Indication	Mitral or tricuspid regurgitation	Mitral or tricuspid stenosis
Anticoagulation	Yes, with aspirin	Yes, with aspirin

5.3.2 Percutaneous Procedures

A minimally invasive procedure can open up stenotic valves and can close certain congenital heart lesions. A small catheter is placed through the groin (into the femoral artery or vein) and is passed upward toward the heart. Small corrective devices can be passed through these catheters to repair the defect. If this type of procedure can be done, it is preferred, since it carries the smallest risk.

Rwanda currently does not have a cardiac catheterization laboratory, but it is possible to perform some congenital procedures with echocardiographic and fluoroscopic guidance alone.

There are two issues with balloon valvuloplasty for mitral and tricuspid stenosis at this point. First, we have very few patients in our surgical series with pure mitral or tricuspid stenosis amenable to valvuloplasty. In order to maintain skills in this procedure, a certain volume is required, and it may be that this will only be possible at a later stage of health service development, when patients are diagnosed at an earlier stage of disease progression. Secondly, due to the risks of balloon valvuloplasty, there must be a cardiac surgical team available on site at the time of the procedure as back-up.

We feel that the main justifications for a cardiac catheterization laboratory early in the development of a cardiac surgical program are (1) the need for diagnostic catheterization, and (2) delivery of low-risk procedures for congenital heart disease.

5.3.3 Mechanical Valves

Mechanical valves are made out of an artificial material and are very durable. Once these valves are in place, the patient may never need another heart surgery. This is the great advantage of these valves, especially in settings where access to repeat cardiac surgery is very limited. The disadvantage of these kinds of valves is that they are all susceptible to forming clots on their surface. (See **TABLE 5.3.**) For this reason, patients with mechanical valves need to be continuously anticoagulated with warfarin to prevent stroke, valve thrombosis, and other complications. Warfarin is a drug with unpredictable effects and needs to be monitored closely (see **SECTION 5.8**).

Outcomes in general for patients with mechanical valves have been poor in Africa because of weak chronic care infrastructure.[21] We believe that use of community health workers to support adherence with therapy can improve these outcomes as they have in the case of HIV and tuberculosis.

In general, we prefer mechanical valves because of their durability. The following section describes types of patients for whom mechanical valves are not a good option.

5.3.4 Bioprosthetic Valves

Bioprosthetic valves are made from living tissue (from a cow, pig, or human) and are shaped to resemble a normal heart valve. Since they are made of living tissue, the risk of thrombosis is greatly reduced, and only aspirin (100 mg, 1x/day) is needed. However, normal heart function can damage these valves. They rarely last more than 10 years, and some-times much less.[22] (See **TABLE 5.3**.)

Bioprosthetic valves are good for the following types of patients:

1. **Young children.** Young children are likely to need a second operation at some point because they will outgrow their valve; a mechanical valve would expose them to extra risks without much benefit over a repair or replacement.

2. **Women of child-bearing age who want to have children.** Warfarin causes birth defects in pregnancy and increases the risk of miscarriage. There is no ideal strategy for managing women who are pregnant and have a mechanical valve.[23,24] For all women of child-bearing age with a mechanical valve, contraception will be very important.

3. **Patients that live in districts without chronic care infrastructure.** Mechanical valves can be dangerous if there is not a good system of follow-up close to the patient's home. In this scenario, a bioprosthetic valve may be a less risky option.

TABLE 5.3 Types of Replacement Heart Valves

	Bioprosthetic	Mechanical
Anticoagulation	Aspirin	Warfarin
Longevity	~10 years, probably less	~20 years, potentially life-long
Endocarditis risk	Increased	Increased
Used in	• children • women of child-bearing age who desire future pregnancies	• men • women of child-bearing age who do not desire more children • women not of child-bearing age

5.4 Early Post-Operative Evaluation (First 3 Months)

In addition to their regular visits to a chronic care clinic, post-cardiac surgery patients should be seen by a cardiologist at least 4 times in the first year (1 month, 3 months, 6 months, and 12 months following their operations).[25] Careful records should be kept for these patients on a post-cardiac surgery follow-up chart. In our system, patients who go to referral hospitals to follow up are asked to bring this chart. Information from each visit should also be recorded in a central electronic medical record. Ideally, a national cardiac surgery coordinator will oversee this process. Any concern about these patients should be communicated immediately to the larger cardiac surgery network.

At each post-operative visit, the patient should be physically examined (including auscultation) with special attention to crisp valve clicks (in the case of mechanical valves), and to the absence of new heart murmurs. Patients should have their vital signs measured (including weight, height, blood pressure, pulse, and respiratory rate if in any respiratory distress). They should then have their volume status assessed in the same manner as with preoperative heart failure patients (see **SECTION 4.7**). Patients should be asked about medication adherence. Women less than 49 years of age should be asked about birth control measures and referred accordingly (see **SECTION 3.5**). All patients should have a creatinine drawn if they are on any heart failure medications. Patients on anticoagulation should also have an INR drawn.

Certain complications, described below, are most common in the first 3 months after surgery.

5.4.1   Heart Failure
Great shifts of fluid occur during heart surgery. The heart muscle can also be damaged. After 3 to 6 months, patients will often stabilize. During the early post-operative period in particular, careful attention must be paid to the patient's weight, and furosemide must be adjusted to prevent decompensation from fluid overload. Patients with persistently depressed left ventricular function after cardiac surgery should be treated for heart failure according to the cardiomyopathy protocol (see **PROTOCOL 4.4**). Patients with normal right and left heart function should ultimately not require any furosemide.

Continued heart failure—especially a change in the patient's status— can signify a new problem with a valve (such as endocarditis, thrombosis, or valve dehiscence/detachment). It can also signify pericardial tamponade (see below), or an arrhythmia (such as atrial fibrillation). For this reason, scheduled echocardiograms performed by a specialist are important shortly after surgery.

5.4.2   Sternal Wound Infection and Dehiscence
To access the heart for surgery, the sternum must be cut. At the end of the procedure, the sternum is repaired using wires. On occasion, some

of these wires may separate, causing dehiscence and instability of the sternum. If this occurs, patients are at risk for infections of the wound and of the deeper structures of the heart. This is an emergency; patients need immediate treatment with antibiotics. At each of the early visits following surgery, the sternum should be checked for stability. A practitioner can check for instability by placing the palm of the hand on the sternum and rocking it back and forth. If there is instability, a click will be felt. Some post-operative sternal pain is normal, and usually resolves with time. But a sternum that moves significantly with gentle pushing is a concern and should quickly be brought to the attention of the cardiac surgery team.

5.4.3   Pericardial Tamponade

During cardiac surgery, the pericardium is opened. Most patients will have a small pericardial effusion that resolves after 3 to 6 months. In some patients, however, the fluid collection grows and eventually interferes with the heart's function (tamponade). This condition can kill the patient if the fluid is left undrained. A large effusion can be seen easily on a preliminary echocardiogram (see **FIGURE 4.9**), which should be attempted at each of the early follow-up visits. If there is a concern, the cardiac surgery team should be contacted immediately, and echocardiographic images should be transmitted by email if possible. In the event of cardiovascular collapse, bedside drainage of the effusion should be attempted if a clinician experienced in the procedure is available. Sometimes, there are fluid collections localized around just one part of the heart. These can cause problems and may only be noticed by a specialist. Clinicians should suspect pericardial tamponade if a post-operative patient presents with hypotension.

5.4.4   Endocarditis

Infection of a prosthetic heart valve can be aggressive. Although such infections can occur any time after surgery, they are particularly common in the first 6 months. On physical examination, new signs of heart failure or new murmurs can be suggestive of endocarditis. Most important, the patient's temperature should be checked at every visit.

Antibiotic prophylaxis is recommended prior to any dental procedure.[26] Amoxicillin should be given 60 minutes prior to the procedure in a single dose of 2 gm (adult) and 50 mg/kg (children ≤ 40 kg). Clindamycin is an alternative in those with a penicillin allergy: 600 mg in adults, 20 mg/kg in children (maximum 600 mg).

5.4.5   Atrial Arrhythmias

After cardiac surgery, patients are at high risk for developing atrial fibrillation. The use of beta-blockers in the post-operative setting helps to reduce the risk of atrial fibrillation. Post-operative patients should be treated with a beta-blocker (generally atenolol) for the first 6 weeks after surgery. After that, the atenolol should be gradually reduced and eventually stopped.

5.5   Ongoing Monitoring of the Post-Operative Patient

After the early post-operative period, most patients should be able to be followed primarily at district level, in NCD clinics. Referral to a cardiologist or to referral centers should be on an as-needed basis. However, information about the patients should still be communicated to a central coordinator to aid with monitoring and evaluation of the national referral system.

Patients continue to be at risk for certain complications. NCD clinicians should evaluate for these at each follow-up visit. Any complication should be recorded in the patient chart and communicated to the national cardiac surgery coordinator.

5.5.1   Fever in Patients with Prosthetic Heart Valves

Patients with any type of prosthetic heart valve remain at risk for valve infections (endocarditis). The patient's temperature should be checked at each follow-up visit and the patient should be asked about subjective fevers. If a fever ≥ 38°C (≥ 100.4°F) is found, the practitioner should be concerned about endocarditis and involve the district hospital physician on call immediately. In Rwanda, the clinician sends an email message to the cardiac surgery network.

Methicillin-resistant Staphylococcus aureus has been identified as a cause of prosthetic valve endocarditis in Rwanda. An emergency stock of vancomycin should be made available to all district hospitals that are following patients after valvular heart surgery.

If a patient with a fever has a blood pressure ≤ 80/40 mmHg, signs of sepsis (tachycardia, labored breathing), or a new murmur, the patient should be immediately transferred to the inpatient district hospital ward. Two sets of blood should be drawn for cultures (each from a separate intravenous puncture). Blood cultures are generally positive in cases of endocarditis and are essential for the choice of long-term antibiotics. Blood is sent to the referral center lab in the capital, since district hospitals are currently unable to process blood cultures.

The patient should be stabilized at the district hospital (with fluids and peripheral vasopressors such as dopamine if needed) and then transferred to the capital for referral center–level care. Such transfers should be communicated promptly to the national cardiac surgery coordinator and to the cardiologist following the patient.

After blood cultures are drawn, empiric antibiotics should be started. Intravenous vancomycin is the preferred empiric treatment, but if this drug is not available, then the combination of cloxacillin and ceftriaxone is an alternative (see **TABLE 5.4**).

TABLE 5.4   Empiric Antibiotic Treatments for Endocarditis

Antibiotic	Indication	Adult dose	Pediatrics dose	Effect on warfarin
Vancomycin	Empiric endocarditis therapy, methicillin-resistant *Staphylococcus aureus, Staphylococcus epidermidis*, enterococcus	1 gm/dose 2x/d	10 mg/kg/dose 4x/d (maximum 1 gram per dose)	No effect
OR (Combination therapy with cloxacillin + ceftriaxone or penicillin G)				
Cloxacillin	Empiric endocarditis therapy, methicillin-sensitive *Staphylococcus aureus,* empiric treatment of cellulitis in patients with prosthetic heart valves	2 gm/dose every 4 hours IV	50 mg/kg/dose every 4 hours IV	No effect
Ceftriaxone	Empiric endocarditis therapy, *Streptococcus viridans,* empiric treatment of urinary tract infection, pneumonia in patients with prosthetic heart valve	2 gm daily IV **OR** IM	100 mg/kg/daily IV **OR** IM (maximum 2 gm)	Decreases warfarin effect
Penicillin G	Empiric endocarditis therapy, *Streptococcus viridans*	4.5 million units/dose IV 4x/d	50,000 units/ kg/dose IV 4x/d (maximum 24 million units/day)	No effect

Patients who have a fever but none of the other warning signs can be evaluated for other common infections, such as malaria, urinary tract infections, pneumonia, or cellulitis. Blood cultures should be drawn and sent to the referral hospital before starting empiric antibiotics. Patients should be hospitalized while awaiting blood culture results. If there is no improvement in a patient's status within 24 hours, transfer to the referral center should be arranged. (See **PROTOCOL 5.1**.)

PROTOCOL 5.1   Management of Fever in Patients with Prosthetic Heart Valves

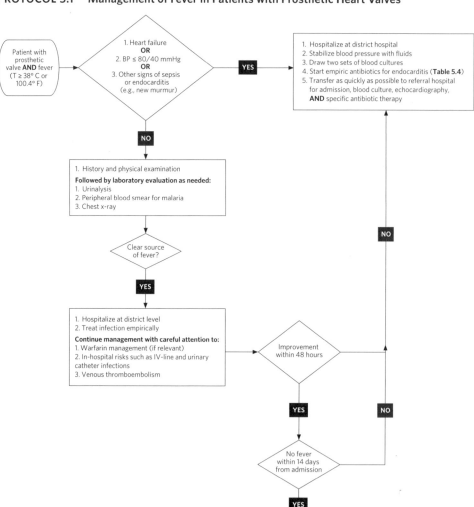

We do not address the long-term treatment of endocarditis in this guide. One major issue in the treatment of prosthetic-valve endocarditis is that it usually involves intravenous antibiotics for at least 6 weeks (see **TABLE 5.5**). Oral antibiotics alone are not an acceptable alternative to intravenous treatment, and the need to frequently change peripheral intravenous catheters can be a problem. Efforts should be made to introduce skills in midline intravenous catheter placement and care at the district hospital level.

An additional consideration is that many antibiotics modify the effect of warfarin (see **TABLE 5.6**). In patients taking warfarin, the international normalized ratio (INR) should also be followed closely during antibiotic treatment.

Finally, *Staphylococcus aureus* endocarditis is particularly aggressive in prosthetic heart valves and may even require reoperation. All endocarditis cases should be managed very closely with the director of the national cardiac surgical program in discussion with the national cardiac surgical community.

TABLE 5.5   Some Organism-Specific Treatments for Prosthetic Valve Endocarditis

Antibiotic	Duration of therapy	Adult dose	Pediatrics dose	Effect on warfarin
Staphylococcus aureus (methicillin-resistant): combination therapy				
Vancomycin	6 weeks	1 gm/dose 2x/d	15 mg/kg/dose 4x/day (maximum 1 gram per dose)	No effect
Gentamicin	2 weeks	1 mg/kg/dose IV **OR** IM 3x/d	1 mg/kg/dose IV **OR** IM 3x/day	No effect
Rifampin	6 weeks	300 mg orally 3x/day	7 mg/kg/dose orally 3x/d	Markedly decreases warfarin effect
Staphylococcus aureus (methicillin-sensitive): combination therapy				
Cloxacillin	6 weeks	2 gm daily IV	50 mg/kg/dose every 6 hours IV	No effect
Gentamicin	2 weeks	1 mg/kg IV **OR** IM 3x/d	1 mg/kg/dose IV **OR** IM 3x/day	No effect
Rifampin	6 weeks	300 mg orally 3x/day	7 mg/kg/dose orally 3x/d	Markedly decreases warfarin effect
Streptococcus viridans (ceftriaxone or penicillin G)				
Ceftriaxone	6 weeks	2 grams daily IV **OR** IM	100 mg/kg/daily IV **OR** IM (maximum 2 gm)	Decreases warfarin effect
Penicillin G	6 weeks	4.5 million units/dose IV 4x/d	50,000 U/kg IV 4x/d (maximum 2.4 units/d)	No effect

5.5.2   Valve Thrombosis

All patients with mechanical heart valves should be on lifelong anticoagulation therapy with warfarin to prevent blood clots in the heart and strokes. If the level of anticoagulation drops below the goal range, patients will be at increased risk for the formation of blood clots on the valves (thrombosis). The risk of thrombosis varies with type and position of the valve. Mechanical tricuspid valves are at the highest risk, followed by mitral and aortic valves.

If thrombosis occurs in a patient with a mechanical valve, the heart valve will lose its usual crisp closing sound. Cardiac auscultation should be performed in all post-cardiac surgery patients with mechanical valves. Appreciating the difference between a normal mechanical heart valve and one without a crisp sound can be difficult. This skill is usually acquired after listening to many normal mechanical valves. If there is a concern for valve thrombosis, the patient should be referred to the patient's cardiologist immediately. While preparing for transfer, these patients should have an INR checked and, if it is below goal range, should be given heparin subcutaneously to reduce the chance of further clot propagation.

5.5.3 Valve Dehiscence

When a valve is repaired or replaced, new components are generally attached to the heart's structure with sutures. In rare cases, these sutures may loosen, opening defects near the margin of the heart valve. Blood may then regurgitate through these defects, generating a new murmur. If a new murmur is noted during auscultation of a post-cardiac surgery patient's heart, the practitioner should suspect dehiscence or endocarditis and should refer the patient to the patient's cardiologist.

5.6 Penicillin Prophylaxis for Patients with Surgically Corrected Rheumatic Valvular Disease

Patients with rheumatic valvular disease should be treated with penicillin to prevent further streptococcal throat infections and recurrent rheumatic fever. In patients who have surgically repaired or replaced valves for rheumatic heart disease, penicillin prophylaxis should be continued. Repeat infections can result in damage to other heart valves, which may also require surgery. These outcomes can be avoided with the appropriate use of penicillin. See **TABLE 9.5** for details on the use of penicillin for prophylaxis.

5.7 Methods of Anticoagulation and Indications

Anticoagulation can be lifesaving for many patients. It is essential for post–cardiac surgery patients with mechanical valves. However, using anticoagulants safely in resource-poor settings has often been seen as unachievable. Here we detail our approach to this problem.

Anticoagulation can be achieved by several means. In Rwanda, the main options are aspirin, subcutaneous enoxaparin (Clexane), subcutaneous unfractionated heparin, and oral warfarin.

Aspirin is a safe, effective, and inexpensive option for patients who have an increased, but still relatively low, risk of thrombosis. These include patients with mitral stenosis in sinus rhythm and stable peripartum cardiomyopathies, as well as those who have bioprosthetic valves.

However, patients at higher risk of stroke, such as those with a known thrombus or a mechanical heart valve, require a greater degree of anticoagulation. This is achieved with warfarin, which inhibits synthesis of several blood coagulation proteins. Warfarin is a tricky drug. Metabolism varies greatly from person to person and within the same patient from day to day, and even hour to hour, depending on interactions with food and medications. **TABLE 5.6** lists some of the common medications that interact with warfarin.

TABLE 5.6   Common Drug Interactions with Warfarin

Drug	Effect on INR
Co-trimoxazole	Increase
Metronidazole	Increase
Ciprofloxacin	Increase
Cimetidine	Increase
Rifampin	Decrease
Antiretroviral drugs	Increase or decrease
Alcohol	Increase or decrease

Moreover, warfarin takes several days to achieve a therapeutic level of anticoagulation. Subcutaneous enoxaparin (Clexane) or subcutaneous unfractionated heparin is used in patients at a very high risk of stroke who require additional anticoagulation (a "bridge") until the warfarin takes effect. District hospitals in Rwanda currently don't use IV heparin because IV pumps for drips and PTT monitoring are not available.

The international normalized ratio, or INR, is the main blood test used to measure the degree of anticoagulation in patients on warfarin. The INR is calculated from a prothrombin time, which is compared to that of a normal individual. As the blood becomes more anticoagulated (or "thinner"), the INR value will rise. A normal INR is 1.0.

Different conditions can be more or less prone to the development of thrombosis. In general, conditions in which blood is stagnant are particularly thrombogenic. For instance, patients with mechanical mitral or tricuspid valves (where blood does not move at high velocities) are more likely to develop thrombosis compared to those with mechanical aortic valves. Different INR targets are used for the different types of indications.

Common indications for anticoagulation in our clinics and district hospitals include post–cardiac surgery status, atrial fibrillation, mitral stenosis, left ventricular thrombus, atrial thrombus, deep venous thrombosis, and pulmonary embolism. Treatment aims to prevent stroke and other embolic disease while minimizing the risks of bleeding. **TABLE 5.7** lists our indications for anticoagulation and the agents we use.

TABLE 5.7   Anticoagulation Agents and Indications

Indications	Warfarin or aspirin?	Heparin bridge?	Goal INR	Duration of therapy
Heart failure and atrial fibrillation				
Peripartum cardiomyopathy	Aspirin	N/A	N/A	Lifelong
Mitral stenosis in sinus rhythm	Aspirin	N/A	N/A	Lifelong
Mitral stenosis with signs of prior stroke	Warfarin	No	2.0-2.5	Lifelong
Atrial fibrillation (without heart failure)	Aspirin	N/A	N/A	Lifelong
Atrial fibrillation (with heart failure)	Warfarin	No	2.0-2.5	Lifelong
Prosthetic valves				
Bioprosthetic tricuspid valve	Warfarin for the first 3 months, then aspirin	Yes	2.5-3.0	Lifelong
Other bioprosthetic valves (not tricuspid)	Aspirin	N/A	N/A	Lifelong
Mechanical aortic valve	Warfarin	Yes	2.5-3.0	Lifelong
Mechanical mitral valve	Warfarin	Yes	3.0-3.5	Lifelong
Mechanical tricuspid valve	Warfarin	Yes	3.0-3.5	Lifelong
Thrombus				
Ventricular thrombosis	Warfarin	Yes	2.0-2.5	6 months
Deep-vein thrombosis	Warfarin	Yes	2.0-2.5	3 months
Pulmonary embolism	Warfarin	Yes	2.0-2.5	6 months

5.8   Initiating Warfarin Therapy

Protocols in previous chapters have indicated when anticoagulation should be started in patients with heart failure and atrial fibrillation.

5.8.1   Contraindications to Warfarin Therapy

Before starting warfarin therapy, patients should be assessed for relative contraindications to warfarin therapy.

Warfarin in pregnancy can cause serious birth defects as well as fetal loss. The risks and benefits of initiating warfarin should be discussed with the woman. In some cases, such as the presence of a mechanical valve, the risk to the mother of not taking warfarin will likely outweigh the risks to the fetus. In other cases, such as atrial fibrillation, the risk of an embolic event may be deemed low enough that the woman will choose not to take warfarin during the pregnancy.

Recent, serious bleeding is another relative contraindication. Again, this should be weighed against the risk of embolic events in deciding whether or not to start warfarin.

Patients should also be assessed for signs of liver disease. A patient with a large, palpable liver on exam, ascites, or a history of heavy alcohol use should have an INR checked prior to initiating warfarin therapy. Warfarin should still be given if the INR is below the goal range, but therapy should be started at half the normal dose.

5.8.2   Monitoring Warfarin

In many low-income settings, the costs of warfarin and of monitoring devices are seen as an insurmountable barrier to anticoagulation. In our experience, investment in this intervention is cost-effective and less dangerous than generally perceived. Patients are usually very vigilant about checking their own INR. Properly trained community health workers are a great aid in helping to monitor and titrate warfarin doses.

Patients who have an indication for warfarin should first be assessed for their risk of stroke or other embolic events. Patients at low risk of embolic events include those with atrial fibrillation. These patients may have warfarin initiated in the outpatient setting with close follow-up.

TABLE 5.8 lists recommended dosing for outpatient initiation of warfarin. Note that this dosing is lower than typically used in settings with more intensive monitoring.

TABLE 5.8   Initial Outpatient Warfarin Dosing

Patient age	Initial dose
Adults	2.5 mg/day
Children (5–40 kg)	0.1 -0.2 mg/kg/day (maximum 10 mg/dose)

Patients at high risk of embolic events include those with mechanical valves and those with an active clot in the heart or the deep veins of the legs. Any patient who is at very high risk of thrombosis and who therefore requires a heparin bridge must be started on warfarin in the hospital. Unfortunately, all low-molecular-weight heparins are relatively expensive and in our experience not affordable to procure on a large scale. Therefore, in Rwanda we often use subcutaneous heparin at treatment doses as a bridging therapy. Partial thromboplastin time (PTT) is not available to monitor the level of anticoagulation. Because infusion pumps are not available at district hospitals, we use subcutaneous heparin. **TABLE 5.9** lists doses for bridging medications. Because warfarin takes 3 days to reach its full effect, the warfarin dose should not be increased more frequently than every 3 days.

If the warfarin is discontinued and therapy has to be re-initiated due to an INR below 1.5, it is best to hospitalize the patient and administer another agent until the INR rises higher than 2.0.

TABLE 5.9   Therapies For Bridging Anticoagulation

Medication	Dosing
Enoxaparin (Clexane)	1 mg/kg/dose twice per day
Heparin (subcutaneous)[27,28]	**Adult:** 15,000 units/dose 2x/d **Child:** 250 units/kg/dose 2x/d

Some patients, such as those with atrial fibrillation, can be started on warfarin on an outpatient basis without a heparin bridge. **PROTOCOL 5.2** outlines the steps involved in initiating warfarin therapy.

PROTOCOL 5.2   Initiating Warfarin Therapy

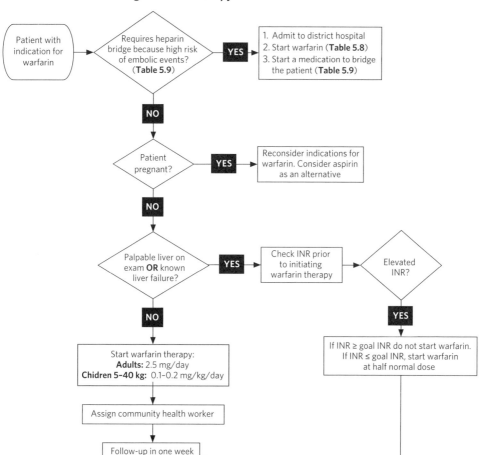

5.9   Titrating Warfarin Therapy

The main principle in adjusting warfarin is to make small, incremental changes in dosage. Warfarin is supplied in tablets of 1 mg and 5 mg. In general, dose adjustments of 0.5–1 mg (10%–20%) are appropriate. When a patient's INR is not in the therapeutic range, the clinician reviews the patient's diet, compliance with the medication, possible pharmacy or prescription errors, warfarin expiration date, and any medication changes (including herbal/traditional remedies) in detail. The clinician also reviews the recent trend in the INR relative to the recent doses of warfarin. If a patient's INR has remained in the goal range on a stable dose of warfarin for a few months, a current INR that is slightly out of range may return to the goal range in a few days without a change in dosage. Such patients may only need to follow up in a few weeks to verify that the INR has returned to the goal range. If a patient's last INR was low and then increased to above the goal on an increased dose of warfarin, the appropriate dose may lie between the first and second doses.

In general, if a patient's INR is below the therapeutic range, the dose should be increased by 10%–20% (roughly 0.5–1 mg for adults). If the INR is above the therapeutic range, the dose should be decreased by 10%–20% (roughly 0.5–1 mg for adults). However, if a patient's INR is found to be increasing rapidly (for instance, from 2.0 to 5.0), the warfarin should be stopped for 2 days before being resumed at a lower dose (decreased by 20% or roughly 1 mg for adults).

Most adult patients will require between 3 mg and 6 mg of warfarin each day, but responses can vary widely. One patient may require 20 mg each day; another may need only 2 mg. There is increasing evidence of genetic variation in warfarin metabolism.[29,30]

Despite a practitioner's best attempts to regulate a patient's warfarin, some patients may need frequent adjustments in the dose. This is especially true at the beginning of treatment. As time goes on, the patient's response to warfarin tends to stabilize. If there is ever a question about the appropriate warfarin dose for a patient, the provider should discuss the case with an experienced provider.

Because warfarin can cause birth defects, all women of childbearing age (15–49 years old) should be tested for pregnancy prior to initiating warfarin and referred to family planning.

PROTOCOL 5.3 outlines the steps involved in adjusting warfarin dosing in all patients on anticoagulation. As noted, however, individual patients will respond differently to warfarin. When in doubt, the treating clinician should consult a more senior provider. NCD nurses in Rwanda are encouraged to call or email one of the cardiologists in the capitol for guidance.

PROTOCOL 5.3   Titrating Warfarin Therapy

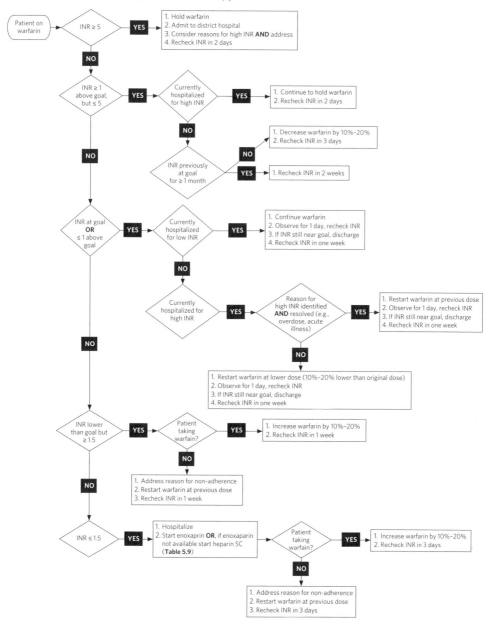

5.10   Drug Supply and Patient Monitoring

In Rwanda, aspirin is the only anticoagulant widely available at the district hospital level. PIH-supported district hospitals procure a limited supply of warfarin and heparin, and our district NCD clinics all have point-of-care INR machines to monitor patients. All patients on warfarin receive directly observed therapy administered by a community health worker. Patients who require a heparin bridge until their INR is therapeutic are hospitalized.

Rwanda's National Cardiac Surgery program has created a need for anticoagulation services beyond the catchment area of current NCD clinics. As a stopgap measure, the cardiac surgery program has started to build a closely monitored system of central distribution to districts where the affected patients reside. A clinician at a nearby health facility is identified and contracted to follow the patient. These clinicians are given an INR machine, a protocol for warfarin adjustment, and a standardized form to record the patient's dose, lab values, and quantity of drugs reserved for them. The patient is then given a supply of anticoagulation materials. The clinician keeps track of this inventory at each visit and is responsible for requesting refills from the capitol when the patient has less than a 3-month supply left. All information is transmitted on a bimonthly basis to a central database.

5.11   Dangers of Anticoagulation

Inappropriate anticoagulation can have very serious consequences. If the patient's INR is too low, thrombosis can occur, resulting in valve dysfunction or in stroke. If the patient's INR is too high, life-threatening bleeding can occur. Bleeding can be difficult to detect. Because of this, medication adherence is essential. If possible, all patients on warfarin anticoagulation should be assigned a community health worker to provide directly observed therapy.

Chapter 5 References

1   The Salam Centre for Cardiac Surgery. (Accessed at **http://salamcentre.emergency.it/**.)

2   Walter Sisulu Pediatric Cardiac Centre for Africa. (Accessed at **http://www.wspcca.org.za/**.)

3   Cohen AJ, Tamir A, Houri S, et al. Save a child's heart: We can and we should. Ann Thorac Surg 2001;71:462-8.

4   Save a Child's Heart. (Accessed at **http://www.saveachildsheart.org/**.)

5   Chaturvedi V, Talwar S, Airan B, Bhargava B. Interventional cardiology and cardiac surgery in India. Heart 2008;94:268-74.

6   Tippett B, Wilson J, Shepherd J, Cutler R, Webster P. Operation Open Heart–Rwanda. Heart Lung Circ 2008;17 Suppl 4:S82-3.

7   Operation Open Heart Rwanda. (Accessed at **http://rwanda.ooh.org.au/**.)

8   Tefuarani N, Vince J, Hawker R, et al. Operation Open Heart in PNG, 1993-2006. Heart Lung Circ 2007;16:373-7.

9   Tefuarani N, Vince J, Hawker R, Sleigh A, Williams G. The medium-to-long-term outcome of Papua New Guinean children after cardiac surgery. Ann Trop Paediatr 2004;24:65-74.

10 Team Heart. (Accessed at **http://www.teamheart.org**.)

11 Healing Hearts Northwest. (Accessed at **http://www.healingheartsnorthwest.com/**.)

12 Chain of Hope Belgium. (Accessed at **http://www.chaine-espoir.be/**.)

13 Pezzella AT. International cardiac surgery: A global perspective. Semin Thorac Cardiovasc Surg 2002;14:298-320.

14 Mocumbi AO, Lameira E, Yaksh A, Paul L, Ferreira MB, Sidi D. Challenges on the management of congenital heart disease in developing countries. Int J Cardiol 2009.

15 Khwa Otsyula BO. Cardiothoracic surgery in sub-Saharan Africa: Problems and perspectives. East Afr Med J 1993;70:129-30.

16 Yacoub MH. Establishing pediatric cardiovascular services in the developing world: A wake-up call. Circulation 2007;116:1876-8.

17 Hewitson J, Brink J, Zilla P. The challenge of pediatric cardiac services in the developing world. Semin Thorac Cardiovasc Surg 2002;14:340-5.

18 Global Efforts for Improving Pediatric Heart Health. Minneapolis, MN: Children's Heart Link; 2007.

19 Sun JC, Davidson MJ, Lamy A, Eikelboom JW. Antithrombotic management of patients with prosthetic heart valves: Current evidence and future trends. Lancet 2009;374:565-76.

20 Antunes MJ. Reoperation after repair of rheumatic mitral regurgitation. Am J Cardiol 1994;73:722-3.

21 Antunes MJ, Wessels A, Sadowski RG, et al. Medtronic Hall valve replacement in a third-world population group. A review of the performance of 1000 prostheses. J Thorac Cardiovasc Surg 1988;95:980-93.

22 Pibarot P, Dumesnil JG. Prosthetic heart valves: Selection of the optimal prosthesis and long-term management. Circulation 2009;119:1034-48.

23 Sareli P, England MJ, Berk MR, et al. Maternal and fetal sequelae of anticoagulation during pregnancy in patients with mechanical heart valve prostheses. Am J Cardiol 1989;63:1462-5.

24   Elkayam U, Bitar F. Valvular heart disease and pregnancy. Part II: Prosthetic valves. J Am Coll Cardiol 2005;46:403-10.

25   Butchart EG, Gohlke-Barwolf C, Antunes MJ, Hall RJ, eds. Heart Valve Disease: A Guide to Patient Management after Surgery. Oxon, UK: Informa Healthcare; 2006.

26   Wilson W, Taubert KA, Gewitz M, et al. Prevention of infective endocarditis: Guidelines from the American Heart Association: A guideline from the American Heart Association Rheumatic Fever, Endocarditis, and Kawasaki Disease Committee, Council on Cardiovascular Disease in the Young, and the Council on Clinical Cardiology, Council on Cardiovascular Surgery and Anesthesia, and the Quality of Care and Outcomes Research Interdisciplinary Working Group. Circulation 2007;116:1736-54.

27   Robinson AM, McLean KA, Greaves M, Channer KS. Subcutaneous versus intravenous administration of heparin in the treatment of deep vein thrombosis; which do patients prefer? A randomized cross-over study. Postgrad Med J 1993;69:115-6.

28   Prandoni P, Bagatella P, Bernardi E, et al. Use of an algorithm for administering subcutaneous heparin in the treatment of deep venous thrombosis. Ann Intern Med 1998;129:299-302.

29   Rieder MJ, Reiner AP, Gage BF, et al. Effect of VKORC1 haplotypes on transcriptional regulation and warfarin dose. N Engl J Med 2005;352: 2285-93.

30   Schwarz UI, Ritchie MD, Bradford Y, et al. Genetic determinants of response to warfarin during initial anticoagulation. N Engl J Med 2008;358:999-1008.

CHAPTER 6
Chronic Kidney Disease
. . . .

6.1   Etiology of Chronic Kidney Disease in Rural Rwanda

There are no published population-based studies of kidney disease in
Rwanda. Studies from other countries in sub-Saharan Africa suggest
that most renal failure is probably caused by infections and hypertension. The major infectious causes are probably streptococcus, malaria,
and tuberculosis (see **TABLE 6.1**).[1] Untreated urinary tract infections
can also lead to renal dysfunction. HIV nephropathy is a major cause of
kidney disease in areas with high HIV prevalence. Schistosomiasis may
cause renal failure by obstructing the ureters. Other chronic diseases
such as heart failure can also cause chronic renal failure. Toxins, such as
those from a snakebite or from traditional medications, can directly in-
jure the kidneys.[2] Patients who are seriously ill from any cause will often
develop renal failure because of poor perfusion of the kidneys. Diabetic
nephropathy is relatively rare in sub-Saharan Africa.

By contrast, the causes of acute renal failure are similar throughout the
world. They are most frequently dehydration, infection, hypotension,
and exposure to nephrotoxins.

Sub-Saharan Africa has a relatively low estimated prevalence of end-
stage renal disease: 100 cases per 1 million people, compared with 1500
cases per million in the United States and 400 cases per million in Latin
America.[2] By this measure, a country such as Rwanda, with a population
of approximately 10 million, would have about 1000 people who require
renal replacement therapy. This low prevalence reflects both the relatively high mortality associated with renal failure in sub-Saharan Africa
and also the relatively low rate of diabetes and hypertension, the major
drivers of renal failure in more developed countries.

TABLE 6.1   Causes of End-Stage Renal Disease in Sub-Saharan Africa
and the U.S.

	Glomerulonephritis or unknown	Hypertension	Diabetes	Other
Average (Nigeria and Senegal)[1]	54%	27.4%	11.9%	6.7%
USA[3]	15.4%	24.2%	37.3%	22.9%

6.2 Screening for Renal Failure in High-Risk Populations

Most patients followed for renal failure in the Rwandan NCD clinics presented with overt symptoms such as anasarca. These patients had typically been hospitalized and then referred to the clinic at discharge. Many had end-stage renal disease. Access to renal replacement therapy or renal transplantation is extremely limited in Rwanda.

ACE inhibitors given to patients early in the course of their disease can dramatically retard the progression of kidney damage. Accordingly, the International Society of Nephrology has suggested population screening for urine protein as part of an integrated, community-based, case-finding strategy.[4,5] Some sites in resource-poor settings, including sub-Saharan Africa, have begun to investigate the value of this approach.[6] In Rwanda, we have not yet pursued population screening. Instead, we have focused initially on improving the care of patients with advanced disease (including palliation) while screening for renal disease in high-risk populations.

The three populations identified as at risk for asymptomatic chronic renal disease in Rwanda are those with hypertension, diabetes, and HIV. These patients are followed in their respective continuity clinics (at health-center level). Referral to the district-hospital NCD clinics is triggered once a creatinine test is needed.

6.2.1 Hypertension

All adult patients with a persistent blood pressure greater than 160/100 mmHg are screened for proteinuria. Patients found to have greater than 2+ proteinuria in an uncontaminated specimen are referred to the district NCD clinic for confirmation of proteinuria, and to have their creatinine measured (see **SECTION 8.2** and **PROTOCOL 8.2**). In addition, adult patients younger than 40 who have stage II or greater hypertension are referred to the district NCD clinic for creatinine measurement (see **PROTOCOL 8.3** and **SECTION 8.6**). Hypertension in these patients may be secondary to another cause; advanced renal disease is one common culprit. Hypertension in children ≤ 15 years is almost always a sign of an underlying disorder, most frequently renal failure. These patients are referred to the district hospital for an inpatient evaluation, including assessment of renal function (see **SECTION 8.8**).

6.2.2 Diabetes

All patients diagnosed with diabetes should have a urine dipstick test performed twice per year and serum creatinine checked annually. Urine microalbumin testing is currently not available.

6.2.3 HIV

HIV is thought to cause renal failure primarily through damage to the glomerulus, resulting in HIV-related nephropathy (HIVAN).[7,8] Studies in sub-Saharan Africa report HIVAN prevalence that varies by population and severity of HIV disease, ranging from 6% to 45% of HIV patients. Higher rates are associated with more severe HIV disease and hospitalization at the time of survey. Most studies show an improvement in renal function with initiation of highly active antiretroviral therapy, or HAART.[7]

We recommend that all HIV patients be screened for proteinuria. Those with proteinuria should be started on an ACE inhibitor unless contraindications exist. The WHO categorizes all HIV patients with symptomatic HIV-associated nephropathy as meeting the definition of stage IV HIV disease, regardless of CD4 count. Patients with HIV and nephrotic syndrome or kidney failure should be started on antiretroviral therapy at any CD4 count. Some experts have advocated that all HIV patients with proteinuria and no other clear cause should be started on antiretrovirals, especially in places where renal replacement therapy is unavailable. This may be difficult in settings where many patients with low CD4 counts are still not on treatment because of lack of resources. Some antiretrovirals, such as tenofovir, should be dosed differently or not used in renal failure.

In screening for renal failure with a urine dipstick, it is very important to avoid false positives. **TABLE 6.2** shows the approximate relationship between urine dipstick results and 24-hour urine protein collection. Urine concentration affects dipstick results. For this reason, we have chosen a threshold of 2+ positivity. This threshold avoids false positives because it corresponds to more than 500 mg of protein in 24 hours at almost any urinary concentration. An alternative approach is to base the urine dipstick threshold on the specific gravity.[9] There is an online calculator that assists with this as well (see **http://www.metrohealthresearch. org/schelling**).

TABLE 6.2   Relationship between Urine Dipstick and 24-hour Urine Protein Results

Urine dipstick result	24-hour urine protein	Dipstick result may be suggestive of:
Trace	150 mg	Top-normal
1+	200–500 mg	Microalbuminuria*
2+	0.5–1.5 gm	Proteinuria
3+	2–5 gm	Nephrotic-range
4+	7 gm	Nephrotic-range

*Most urine dipsticks are insensitive for microalbuminuria

If initially positive, urine dipsticks should be repeated to confirm the result on at least 2 out of 3 tests. Proteinuria often accompanies urinary tract infections, but a positive test can also be caused by perineal cells contaminating the specimen. In practice, we recommend that any urine with epithelial cells, leukocytes, or nitrites not be regarded as positive for proteinuria. If there are many epithelial cells, the test should be repeated on a fresh specimen, collected using clean catch techniques. Young children may require cathertization to obtain a clean catch specimen. If there are many leukocytes (≥ 2+) but not many epithelial cells, the clinician should consider treating the patient for a urinary tract infection if there are clinical reasons to suspect one.

6.3   Classification of Renal Failure

Renal failure severity classification is traditionally based on interpretation of the serum creatinine in combination with the patient's weight, sex, and age. These factors combine to give a glomerular filtration rate (GFR), which is an estimate of how well the kidneys filter the blood. A high GFR means the kidneys are filtering the blood appropriately, while a low GFR means the kidneys have lost the ability to filter the blood very well. The formula most commonly used worldwide to estimate GFR is one developed by Donald Cockroft and Henry Gault in the 1970s in Canada (**http://www.nephron.com/cgi-bin/CGSIdefault.cgi**).[10] A report from Ghana has shown that the Cockroft-Gault equation tends to significantly overestimate the degree of kidney failure in the studied population.[11] An alternative, known as the Chronic Kidney Disease Epidemiology Collaboration (CKD-EPI) equation, estimates renal function more accurately in individuals with normal renal function and has been validated in Ghana.[12] This equation is difficult to use without an online calculator (**http://www.kidney.org/professionals/kdoqi/gfr_calculator.cfm**). Given concerns about overdiagnosis, we do not recommend using Cockroft-Gault in asymptomatic patients being screened for kidney disease.[13] There is also an online calculator available for the Schwartz equation for use in pediatric populations under age 15 (**http://www.kidney.org/professionals/kdoqi/gfr_calculatorPed. cfm** or **http://nephron.com/bedside_peds_nic.cgi**).[14]

An initial injury to the kidney can cause damage to the renal parenchyma. The kidney responds by hyperfiltration, forcing the remaining normal nephrons to work harder to maintain the same clearance of toxins from the blood. Therefore, in early chronic kidney disease, the creatinine initially does not rise. However, proteinuria may be present, suggesting some dysfunction of the nephrons that allows protein to escape from the blood to the urine. Initiation of treatment with ACE inhibitors to decrease hyperfiltration can help to protect the kidneys from further damage.

Calculating GFR for each patient in a busy clinic may be impractical. For this reason, we often give absolute cutoffs of creatinine to guide diagnosis and treatment decisions. These cutoffs are purposefully conservative to account for our patients' low average body weight and for the difficulties of closely monitoring electrolytes in our setting.

TABLE 6.3 outlines the different stages of chronic kidney disease (CKD) with corresponding ranges of GFR and creatinine for adults and children. These creatinine ranges are purposefully conservative because many of patients have low body weight. **TABLE 6.4** lists the average creatinine for age for children. The table refers to the glomerular filtration rate. CKD stages 1 and 2 refer to patients with normal GFRs ($\geq$ 60 ml/min), but with some degree of proteinuria (including microalbuminuria). Patients with CKD 3 have significant kidney impairment but are usually asymptomatic. Patients with CKD 4 and 5 have severe kidney dysfunction. These patients are likely to begin experiencing symptoms. **TABLE 6.4** gives corresponding levels of creatinine elevation for an average patient in our clinic.

TABLE 6.3 Stages of Chronic Kidney Disease

	Degree of dysfunction	Glomerular filtration rate	Approximate creatinine cutoff for adults	Approximate creatinine cutoff for children
CKD 1 and 2	Mild dysfunction	$\geq$ 60 ml/min/1.73m²	< 100 µmol/L (< 1.1 mg/dL)	Normal creatinine for age
CKD 3	Moderate dysfunction	30-59 ml/min/1.73m²	100-199 µmol/L (1.1-2.3 mg/dL)	Normal to < 2x normal creatinine for age
CKD 4 and 5	Severe dysfunction	$\leq$ 29 ml/min/1.73m²	$\geq$ 200* µmol/L (> 2.3 mg/dL)	$\geq$ 2x normal creatinine for age

* Conservative lower limit; corresponds to a GFR of about 30 ml/min in a 30-year-old, 50 kg woman.

TABLE 6.4   Normal Creatinine Ranges for Children by Age

Newborn	27–88 μmol/L (0.3–1.0 mg/dL)
Infant or pre-school-aged child (2 months–4 years)	18–35 μmol/L (0.2–0.5 mg/dL)
School-aged child (5–10 years)	27–62 μmol/L (0.3–0.7 mg/dL)
Older child or adolescent (>10 years)	44–88 μmol/L (0.5–1.0 mg/dL)

6.4   Initial Evaluation and Management of Chronic Kidney Disease (CKD)

PROTOCOL 6.1 and **PROTOCOL 6.2** outline our approach to the initial evaluation of kidney disease based on the severity of dysfunction. Most individuals are found to have CKD 1 or 2 through dipstick screening after they are already diagnosed with HIV, diabetes, or hypertension. These patients are referred to district-hospital NCD clinics to have their creatinine evaluated, since creatinine testing is not usually available at health centers. If there are signs of urinary obstruction or difficulty in breathing, patients should be hospitalized for further evaluation and treatment. All patients should have the following tests on their initial visit to the NCD clinic: blood pressure, urine dipstick, HIV test, electrolyte panel, creatinine, glucose, and hemoglobin.

PROTOCOL 6.1   Initial Evaluation of Chronic Kidney Disease Stage 1 or 2

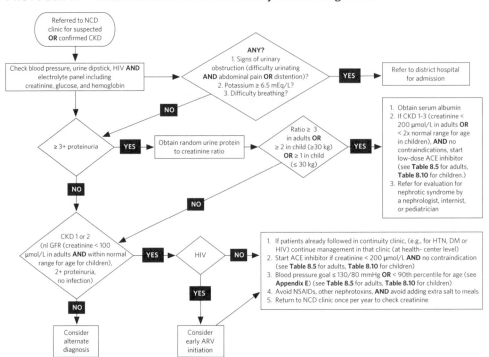

If there is evidence of 3+ or 4+ proteinuria on the urine dipstick, a spot urine protein–to-creatinine ratio should be obtained. The spot urine protein–to-creatinine ratio (mg per mg) correlates well with the number of grams of protein excreted in a 24-hour period. This will determine if there is nephrotic-range proteinuria (more than 3 gm in 24 hours in an adult or 50 mg/kg/day for children). For example, if a patient has 350 mg/dL of protein on a random urine sample and 50 mg/dL of creatinine, the urine protein–to-creatinine ratio would be 7. This corresponds to roughly 7 gm of urine protein output in 24 hours. It is important to use the same units for both protein and creatinine.

Patients with nephrotic-range proteinuria should be referred to the district or referral center level for consultation by either a nephrologist (if available), pediatrician, or internist for evaluation and initiation of steroids or other therapy if needed. It is also helpful to obtain a serum albumin test prior to further evaluation. If the patient has mild to moderate renal dysfunction (CKD 1–3, see **TABLE 6.3** and **TABLE 6.4**), it is helpful to start a low dose of an ACE inhibitor (see **TABLE 8.5** for adults, and **TABLE 8.10** and **TABLE 8.11** for children).

Once the diagnosis of CKD 1 or 2 is confirmed, patients should be followed at their usual health center clinic site. An ACE inhibitor should be initiated at a low dose (see **TABLE 8.5** for adults, and **TABLE 8.10** and **TABLE 8.11** for children) with a goal blood pressure of less than 130/80 mmHg in adults and ≤ 90th percentile for age for children (see **APPENDIX E**). Non-steroidal anti-inflammatory drugs (NSAIDs), such as ibuprofen, should be avoided along with other kidney toxins. As discussed above, HIV-positive patients should be considered for anti-retroviral therapy regardless of CD4 count to prevent progression of disease. Patients with CKD 1 or 2 should be seen once a year in a district-level NCD clinic to have their creatinine checked and their degree of CKD reassessed.

Patients with moderate to severe CKD (CKD 3, 4, or 5) should be closely evaluated for reversible causes of their disease (see **PROTOCOL 6.2**). Patients with CKD 4 or 5 will often be symptomatic and initial evaluation will take place in the hospital. Patients with CKD 3 are usually identified through screening because they have another disease (such as heart failure).

PROTOCOL 6.2   Initial Evaluation of Chronic Kidney Disease Stage 3, 4, and 5

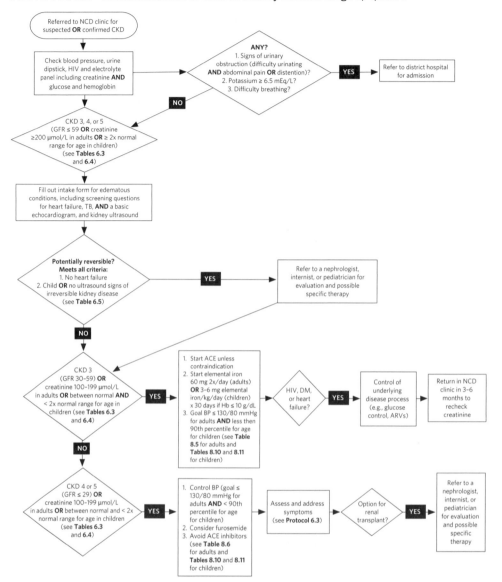

When there is no obvious cause of kidney dysfunction, the key question is whether the patient has a condition that would benefit from treatment with steroids or another immune-modifying agent. At the district hospital level, ultrasound is one simple tool that can help identify patients unlikely to benefit from specific therapies.

The *PIH Manual of Ultrasound for Resource-Limited Settings* describes how to obtain and interpret ultrasound images of the kidneys.[15] The guide is aimed at district clinicians. Assessment for kidney size and the presence of hydronephrosis should be part of the training of generalist physicians, clinical officers, and NCD nurses. Normal kidneys in an adult measure 9–13 cm in length and 4–6 cm in width. Additionally, the kidney cortex (outer portion of the organ) is usually relatively dark, compared to structures like the liver on ultrasound (see **FIGURE 6.1** and **FIGURE 6.2**). Most sources of renal disease will cause the kidneys to become smaller and brighter. Important exceptions are HIV and diabetic nephropathy (conditions that are not thought to be particularly steroid-responsive).

FIGURE 6.1   Normal Kidney Anatomy on Ultrasound *(Arrowheads show the medullary pyramids, and star shows the outer cortex)*

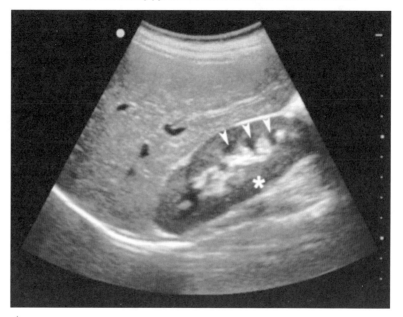

FIGURE 6.2   Ultrasound in Chronic Kidney Disease: Loss of Differentiation between Cortex and Medulla

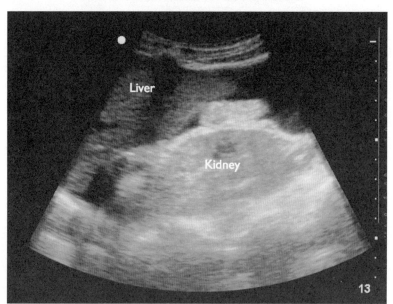

In general, kidneys that are very small and echogenic (bright on ultrasound) are likely to be affected by advanced, chronic disease that will not respond to steroids or other specific therapies. A recent study has correlated ultrasound and renal biopsy results.[16] This study found advanced, irreversible disease in 86% of patients who had both small kidneys (≤ 20 cm combined length in adults), and echogenic cortices (brighter than the liver) on ultrasound. Echogenicity alone was fairly non-specific (only 30% had advanced disease). The following combination of findings on ultrasound should preclude the need for specialist referral (see **TABLE 6.5**). Normal kidney size in children will vary by age. However, children are more likely than adults to have reversible renal failure and should always be referred to a nephrologist or pediatrician for further evaluation, regardless of ultrasound findings.

TABLE 6.5   Ultrasound Findings Specific for Severe, Irreversible Kidney Disease

1. Echogenic cortex (more than liver), plus a combined length ≤ 20 cm in adults **OR** ≤ 2 standard deviations below normal for age in children
2. Very small kidneys with a combined length less than 16 cm in adults

Obstructive nephropathy is a potentially reversible cause of renal failure that should prompt hospital admission for further evaluation (see **FIGURE 6.3**).

FIGURE 6.3 Hydronephrosis on Ultrasound

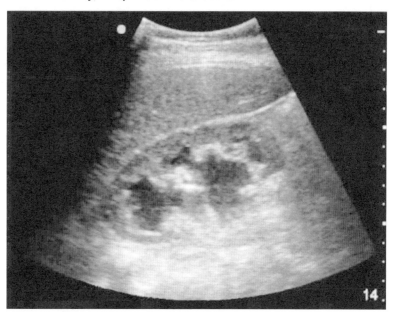

In this chapter we do not go into the details of evaluation by a nephrologist. In many settings, renal biopsy is not available. Decisions to start steroids or other therapies may have to be made with limited data. Although availability of renal replacement therapy is very limited, it may play a role in patients with acute and potentially reversible disease. Issues surrounding renal transplantation are discussed below.

The roles of the district clinician are (1) to avoid referrals for patients unlikely to be candidates for specific therapies; and (2) to direct the ongoing care and palliation of such patients.

All patients with moderate renal failure (CKD 3) should receive iron supplementation if their hemoglobin is less than 10 mg/dL. The preferred dose for adults is 60 mg twice per day of elemental iron for 30 days. The dose for children is 3–6 mg elemental iron/kg per day. Other adjuvant therapies such as phosphate binders, calcium or sodium bicarbonate are not helpful unless patients are candidates for renal replacement therapy. Additionally, blood pressures should be kept below 130/80 mmHg (for adults) and below the 90th percentile for age (for children) if possible. Patients with CKD 3 (usually with a creatinine between 100 and 200 µmol/L in adults or between normal and 2x normal range for age in children) should still be able to tolerate and will benefit from ACE-inhibition (see **TABLE 8.5** for adults, and **TABLE 8.10** and **TABLE 8.11** for children). Contraindications include a potassium greater than 5 mEq/L. Furosemide is often a helpful adjuvant therapy.

The management of patients with severe renal failure (CKD 4 or 5) without a reversible cause for their disease depends upon the availability of renal transplantation. All patients should have their blood pressure controlled if possible (see **TABLE 8.6** for adults and **TABLE 8.11** for children). ACE inhibitors should be avoided. High doses of furosemide may be required. Patients should be assessed for symptoms of their disease (see **SECTION 6.6**). These symptoms should always be addressed. When symptoms become a predominant concern and if there is no access to life-prolonging therapies such as renal replacement or transplantation, the focus should be on quality of life.

6.5 Hyperkalemia

Potassium testing has become increasingly available at district hospitals in Rwanda. All patients evaluated for CKD 3 or higher at district NCD clinics should have their potassium checked initially. If a patient is found to have hyperkalemia (≥ 5 mEq/L), ACE inhibitors, spironolactone and any potassium supplementation should be discontinued (see **PROTOCOL 6.3**). If there is an abnormally high potassium level in a patient with an estimated glomerular filtration rate of more than 60 mg/ml, in the absence of culprit medications, a false reading based on hemolysis should be suspected.

PROTOCOL 6.3   Outpatient Management of Mild Hyperkalemia

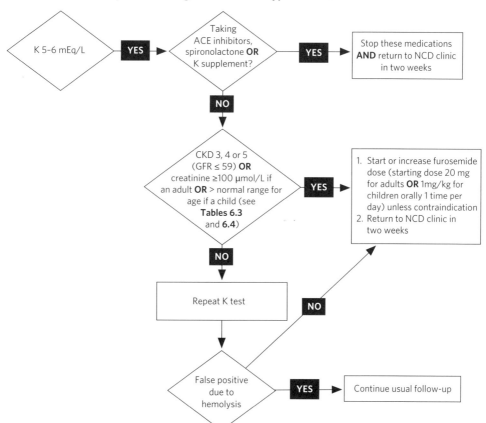

In patients with mild elevations in serum potassium (5–6 mEq/L), several medications can help with the excretion of electrolytes. Furosemide is an effective potassium-wasting diuretic. If the patient does not have heart failure, the dose of this medication should be increased carefully until potassium levels normalize. The patient should be followed every two weeks to monitor for signs of hypovolemia.

Patients with a confirmed K ≥ 6 mEq/dL should be hospitalized to receive treatment that could immediately decrease potassium levels. We do not include ECG testing routinely in this management protocol. Acute therapies include intravenous insulin administered along with glucose, intravenous calcium gluconate, and albuterol. Chronic therapies include furosemide and albuterol. Cation exchange resins such as sodium polystyrene sulfonate are not readily available. We do not discuss hospital management of hyperkalemia in this section. We refer the practitioner to the forthcoming WHO district clinician manual for adult and adolescent medicine.

If the patient has hyperkalemia at baseline in the setting of severe, irreversible renal dysfunction (CKD 4 or 5), the decision about the intensity of therapy should depend on discussion with the patient about the goals of care.

6.6   Palliative Care for Chronic Kidney Disease

Palliative care entails responding to and relieving suffering of any kind, whether physical, psychological, social, or spiritual (see **CHAPTER 2**). PIH's experience in responding successfully to social suffering with social supports—including housing, nutrition, clean water, and daily visits by community health workers—are described in the *PIH Guide to Community-Based Treatment of HIV in Resource-Poor Settings*.[17] This section will focus on the physical and psychological effects specific to advanced chronic kidney disease (CKD).

There is no contradiction between treatment of CKD and palliative care. Every effort should be made to prevent and slow the progression of early-stage chronic kidney disease. At any stage of CKD, pain, dyspnea, and other distressing symptoms should be treated. In the later stages of CKD, many patients will have an increasing need for palliative care, including relief of physical symptoms and psychosocial distress.

The number and severity of physical and psychological symptoms experienced by patients with CKD 5 is similar to those experienced by patients with advanced cancers and other chronic, life-threatening illnesses. Symptoms of patients with CKD 5, their frequency, their known or presumed causes, and recommended treatments are listed in **TABLE 6.6** and **TABLE 6.7**.

TABLE 6.6   Common Physical Symptoms in Advanced Chronic Kidney Disease and Their Treatment[18]

Physical symptom	Cause	Treatment (see CHAPTER 2 for details)
Fatigue and drowsiness 86%	Depression	Assess for depression and treat if found.
	Fluid overload	Diurese for fluid overload, if needed.
	Anemia, poor nutrition, other organ failure, uremia, insomnia	
Itch 84%	Dry skin	Emollients for dry skin.
	Secondary hyperparathyroidism Hyperphosphatemia Anemia Opioids	Antihistamine such as diphenhydramine (can worsen fatigue and delirium). Steroid.

Physical symptom	Cause	Treatment (see CHAPTER 2 for details)
Dyspnea (the most distressing symptom) 80%	Pulmonary edema Pleural effusion Metabolic acidosis Anemia Aspiration Comorbid CHF, COPD, or other lung pathology	If comfort and quality of life are the only goals of care, not preservation of renal function, diurese for symptomatic pulmonary or peripheral edema. Opioid relieves dyspnea of any cause. Renal dosing for morphine (see APPENDIX A).
Delirium (agitated or hypoactive) 76%	Metabolic derangements Hypoxia/hypercapnia Medications	Reduce or eliminate culprit medications, if possible. Haloperidol.
Pain 73%	Bone pain due to 2° hyperparathyroidism Diabetic neuropathy Polycystic kidney disease Calciphylaxis (hemodialysis patients only)	Avoid NSAIDS due to nephrotoxicity and increased risk of bleeding with uremic platelet dysfunction. Paracetamol is safe and requires no dose adjustment for renal failure. Morphine: active metabolite accumulates in CKD 5 and can cause neurotoxicity. Use lower dose and/or longer dosing interval than usual.
Anorexia 71%	Nausea (see below) Diabetic gastroparesis Dry mouth	Anti-emetics (see below). Metoclopramide for gastroparesis. Oral care. Steroid to stimulate appetite.
Swelling in legs/arms 71%	Fluid overload Low oncotic pressure due to proteinuria and malnutrition Comorbid heart failure	Elevate edematous extremities (although this may exacerbate pulmonary edema). Elastic wraps as tolerated. If comfort and quality of life are the only goals of care, not preservation of renal function, diurese for symptomatic peripheral edema or anasarca. This may require higher than normal furosemide doses.
Dry mouth 69%	Intravascular volume depletion (can exist even with total body fluid overload).	Instruct family caregivers to keep mouth moist with sips of liquid or sponge.
Constipation 65%	Medications including opioids and anticholinergics Intravascular volume depletion	Laxative
Nausea with or without vomiting 59%	Uremia Emetogenic medications Diabetic gastroparesis	Reduce or eliminate culprit medications, if possible. Haloperidol for nausea due to endogenous or exogenous emetogenic toxin. Start with low dose. Metoclopramide for gastroparesis.
Cough 47%	Pulmonary edema Aspiration Comorbid COPD or other lung pathology	If comfort and quality of life are the only goals of care, not preservation of renal function, diurese for symptomatic pulmonary edema. Opioid relieves cough of any cause. Renal dosing for morphine.

TABLE 6.7   Common Psychological Symptoms in Advanced Chronic
            Kidney Disease and Their Treatment

Psychological symptom	Treatment
Anxiety 78%	Psychosocial supports Haloperidol Diazepam (can cause delirium and paradoxical agitation)
Feeling sad 65%	Psychosocial supports
Depression Unknown prevalence	Psychosocial supports Antidepressant such as fluoxetine or amitriptyline

Many medications, including those used for palliation, require dose
adjustment for patients with renal failure (see **APPENDIX A**).

6.7   Renal Replacement Therapy (Hemodialysis and Peritoneal Dialysis)

Without renal replacement therapy, patients who have end-stage renal
disease (CKD 5) will die in a matter of days or weeks. Death results from
electrolyte imbalances such as hyperkalemia, which causes fatal cardiac
arrhythmias or suffocation from fluid overload. These deaths can be
witnessed in district hospitals across sub-Saharan Africa. In the days
before death, patients may also suffer intractable nausea and vomiting,
mental status changes, and seizures as a result of the buildup of urea
and other toxins.

Dialysis offers an effective and immediate solution to otherwise im-
minent death from renal failure. Dialysis may be performed by filtering
the blood through a membrane (hemodialysis), or by filtering the blood
across the peritoneum (peritoneal dialysis).

Unfortunately, hemodialysis is technically demanding and the consum-
able costs of both hemodialysis and peritoneal dialysis remain high.
Peritoneal dialysis is a preferable option in resource-limited settings.
Hemodialysis can only be offered at referral centers because of the technical demands of the procedure (including water filtration and equipment maintenance). Peritoneal dialysis can—in theory—be delivered at
local facilities or in the patient's home. The risk of peritoneal infection
in peritoneal dialysis equals the risk of venous catheter infection in
hemodialysis.

Dialysis of either kind is currently performed in Rwanda only at referral
centers. The primary indication is for acute, reversible renal failure. We
do not currently have an estimate of the number of patients in Rwanda
who would require chronic dialysis, if available.

Barriers to more extensive availability of chronic peritoneal dialysis include the costs of the solution. Centers in India have been able to provide even hemodialysis for $2500 per year for twice-weekly sessions. Continuous ambulatory peritoneal dialysis costs $4500 per year for 3 exchanges per day.[19] These examples give hope that this service can be provided at an affordable price, using less expensive consumables.[20,21]

6.8   Renal Transplantation

Renal transplant has been shown to represent a better value than dialysis, in terms of money spent and quality of life gained. Middle-income countries such as India and South Africa provide one avenue for patients in lower-income countries to undergo life-saving renal transplant surgery. This may be possible only if patients have living donors who can travel with them. The high cost of immunosuppressive drugs poses another barrier to successful kidney transplantation. Older immunosuppressives such as cyclosporine are now generic, but annual costs remain around $2000 per year for typical regimens. Other issues still to be resolved are appropriate systems of follow-up for transplanted patients in resource-limited settings.

In our opinion, any transplant program should be conducted nationally to ensure a fair and equitable process of case selection. This is the same strategy used for cardiac surgery patient selection in Rwanda. Given the limited number of transplants needed in a country like Rwanda, the annual cost per capita of such a service may not be prohibitive, if organized efficiently.

6.9   Acute Kidney Failure in Hospitalized Patients

This manual does not address management of acute renal failure in hospitalized patients. We refer to the forthcoming WHO district clinician manual for adolescents and adults.

Chapter 6 References

· ·

1   Arogundade FA, Barsoum RS. CKD prevention in Sub-Saharan Africa: a call for governmental, nongovernmental, and community support. Am J Kidney Dis 2008;51:515-23.

2   Barsoum RS. Chronic Kidney Disease in the Developing World. N Engl J Med 2006;354:997-9.

3   National Kidney and Urologic Diseases Information Clearinghouse. Kidney and Urologic Diseases Statistics for the United States: U.S. Department of Health and Human Services, National Institutes of Health, National Institue of Diabetes and Digestive and Kidney Diseases; 2010 April. Report No.: 10-3895.

4   Atkins R, Perico N, Codreanu I, Peng L, Remuzzi G. Program for Detection and Management of Chronic Kidney Disease, Hypertension, Diabetes and Cardiovascular Disease in Developing Countries: International Society of Nephrology; 2005 February 15.

5   Kirby T. Screening for chronic kidney disease shows promise. Lancet;375:1240-1.

6   Sumaili EK, Krzesinski JM, Cohen EP, Nseka NM. [Epidemiology of chronic kidney disease in the Democratic Republic of Congo: Review of cross-sectional studies from Kinshasa, the capital]. Nephrol Ther 2010;6:232-9.

7   Fabian J, Naicker S. HIV and kidney disease in sub-Saharan Africa. Nat Rev Nephrol 2009;5:591-8.

8   Naicker S, Han TM, Fabian J. HIV/AIDS—dominant player in chronic kidney disease. Ethn Dis 2006;16:S2-56-60.

9   Constantiner M, Sehgal AR, Humbert L, et al. A dipstick protein and specific gravity algorithm accurately predicts pathological proteinuria. Am J Kidney Dis 2005;45:833-41.

10 Cockcroft DW, Gault MH. Prediction of creatinine clearance from serum creatinine. Nephron 1976;16:31-41.

11 Eastwood JB, Kerry SM, Plange-Rhule J, et al. Assessment of GFR by four methods in adults in Ashanti, Ghana: the need for an eGFR equation for lean African populations. Nephrol Dial Transplant 2010;25:2178-87.

12 Levey AS, Stevens LA, Schmid CH, et al. A new equation to estimate glomerular filtration rate. Ann Intern Med 2009;150:604-12.

13 Levey AS, Atkins R, Coresh J, et al. Chronic kidney disease as a global public health problem: approaches and initiatives—a position statement from Kidney Disease Improving Global Outcomes. Kidney Int 2007;72:247-59.

14 Schwartz GJ, Munoz A, Schneider MF, et al. New equations to estimate GFR in children with CKD. J Am Soc Nephrol 2009;20:629-37.

15 Shah S, Price D, Bukhman G, Shah S, Wroe E, eds. The Partners In Health Manual of Ultrasound for Resource-Limited Settings. Boston: Partners In Health; 2011.

16 Moghazi S, Jones E, Schroepple J, et al. Correlation of renal histopathology with sonographic findings. Kidney Int 2005;67:1515-20.

17 Mukherjee JS. The PIH Guide to the Community-Based Treatement of HIV in Resource-Poor Settings. Second Edition. Boston: Partners In Health; 2006 July.

18 Murtagh FE, Addington-Hall J, Edmonds P, et al. Symptoms in the month before death for stage 5 chronic kidney disease patients managed without dialysis. J Pain Symptom Manage 2010;40:342-52.

19   Sakhuja V, Sud K. End-stage renal disease in India and Pakistan: burden of disease and management issues. Kidney Int Suppl 2003:S115-8.

20   White SL, Chadban SJ, Jan S, Chapman JR, Cass A. How can we achieve global equity in provision of renal replacement therapy? Bull World Health Organ 2008;86:229-37.

21   Dirks JH, Levin NW. Dialysis rationing in South Africa: a global message. Kidney Int 2006;70:982-4.

CHAPTER 7
Diabetes
. . . .

Recent discussions about the burden of diabetes in sub-Saharan Africa have focused on the growing epidemic in urban centers, where prevalence has reached as high as 8% in adult populations.[1] The International Diabetes Federation (IDF) has outlined excellent practice guidelines for the African region, and the IDF's Life for a Child program has begun to make medications and supplies freely available to children and young adults around the world.[2-6]

This handbook chapter is based on our experience with a cohort of around 250 patients with diabetes in rural Rwanda. It focuses on integration of diabetes services (including insulin therapy) for predominantly rural populations living on less than a dollar a day. In these populations, diabetes still remains relatively uncommon. The management of these patients is complex, since many of them require insulin. Although successful decentralization of oral therapy for diabetes is increasing in sub-Saharan Africa and other very low-income settings, management of insulin outside of referral centers remains a major challenge.[7-18]

Surveys conducted in rural sub-Saharan Africa over the past 30 years have consistently found a diabetes prevalence of around 1% in those over 15 years old.[1,19-22] Type 1 diabetes accounts for a very small portion of this burden, with an estimated 0.01% prevalence.[23,24] Of course, among subsistence farmers with low body weight, type 2 diabetes as it is known in urbanized populations is uncommon. Type 1 diabetes may also be slightly less common in rural Africa than in Europe and the United States; however, the very high mortality and misdiagnosis of these patients likely also contributes to its low prevalence.

The causes of diabetes in places like rural Rwanda are often different than in industrialized regions. In some cases, malnutrition leads to a unique and poorly understood type of diabetes, characterized by impaired insulin secretion without ketosis.[25,26] In West Africa, another variant has been described as ketosis-prone type 2 diabetes.[27] Patients with this disease do not have circulating islet cell antibodies; however, they can develop transient ketosis requiring admission and insulin therapy. Once stabilized, these patients can later be managed well with oral medications alone. This diabetes variant has recently been linked to human herpesvirus 8 (HHV-8). Another subset of rural African patients develop glucose intolerance as a side effect of antiretroviral (ARV) therapy, particularly stavudine (d4T).[28,29] Pregnancy can also result in a state of insulin resistance. Hyperglycemia during pregnancy can result in a large fetus prone to complications at the time of delivery. Gestational diabetes is uncommon among young women and among those with low BMIs and is therefore likely to be uncommon in rural Rwanda. We discuss issues of gestational and pre-existing diabetes in pregnancy below (see **SECTION 7.7**).

This chapter focuses on the management of diabetes in predominantly rural, subsistence-farming populations. Diabetes care is especially challenging in these settings due to lack of food, systems to monitor glucose, refrigeration for insulin storage, and common knowledge of the disease. An integrated NCD program is well suited to address this complex, yet relatively low-prevalence disease.

In Rwanda, the impact of diabetes on the lives of afflicted individuals is enormous. Although chronic care services for HIV have been decentralized rapidly to the district and health-center level, most diabetes care in Rwanda still occurs at referral centers. The MOH NCD initiative is an effort to remedy this situation. Prior to 2006, Rwandans had already organized a Rwanda Diabetes Association, which receives support from the World Diabetes Foundation, among other philanthropies. The group holds educational workshops for physicians and nurses and sponsors patient associations. The MOH NCD clinic has extended this group's initiatives by integrating tailored protocols for diabetes into the training of NCD providers and other chronic care workers. The number of patients followed by the NCD clinics has grown, and patients with diabetes are now seen on specific days of the week. This has allowed for group education and also made it possible for specialists from referral centers to make supervisory visits on a regular basis.

Management of patients with diabetes who can be controlled with oral hypoglycemics is relatively inexpensive and straightforward. However, approximately 50% of patients in our cohort require insulin. Their management can become costly, largely because of the price of finger-stick glucose testing (see **APPENDIX B.7**). Moreover, optimal insulin regimens, such as glargine (Lantus) and lispro (Humalog), are still patented. Our approach attempts to minimize cost while achieving reasonable glucose control and avoiding hypoglycemia. Efforts to make patented insulins more widely available and to reduce the cost of finger-stick monitoring may allow for more intensive management and better outcomes as these programs develop.

7.1 Opportunistic Identification and Screening for Diabetes in Acute Care Health Center Clinics

As with other chronic diseases, most patients with diabetes initially present to outpatient acute care clinics. A certain percentage of these arrive very ill with severe hyperglycemia or with diabetic ketoacidosis and require immediate hospitalization. Other patients may have more indolent signs of hyperglycemia. Patients with such signs or symptoms require screening for diabetes. We urge all primary and urgent care health workers to consider diabetes in any patient that presents with polyuria, polydipsia, unexplained weight loss, or dehydration. Diabetes should also be considered in those patients with unexplained renal failure, neuropathy, or blindness, as these entities can be manifestations of prolonged hyperglycemia. All health centers should have the ability to check blood glucose (see **PROTOCOL 7.1**).

As with other chronic conditions, such as tuberculosis, programs to combat diabetes should be designed to ensure good outcomes for patients with symptoms (passive case-finding) before searching for asymptomatic patients (active case-finding). Once a program feels comfortable with its diabetes management, initial routine screening might be considered for particular high-risk groups. Traditional risk factors for diabetes include hypertension, age, and overweight.[30] In Rwanda, we have begun by screening all adults with stage 1 hypertension and a BMI ≥ 25 kg/m^2, or stage 2 hypertension, with a random urine glucose. Data from rural Gambia suggest that in those with this cluster of risk factors, diabetes prevalence is between 4%–6% compared with 1% in the general population.[31] Carried out comprehensively, this approach would lead us to screen roughly 1% of the adult population. The sensitivity of this method of screening is between 20%–40% with a specificity of 95%.[32] Patients with any glycosuria then undergo confirmatory testing with either a fasting blood glucose or hemoglobin A1c measurement (see **TABLE 7.1**).[33] In our clinics, adults with hypertension greater than 160/100 mmHg already get regular urine dipsticks to check for proteinuria, and therefore this screening strategy does not add much in terms of cost to the program.

Our protocols use urine glucose as a first-pass screening test for hyperglycemia. Studies have shown that this method will pick up roughly 93% of people with blood glucose levels greater than 200 mg/dL.[34] This form of screening has the advantage of very low cost and universal availability at health center level. It will miss the majority of patients with diabetes who have lower levels of random hyperglycemia (roughly 60%–80% of patients with diabetes), but it should catch those at highest risk of complications.

More aggressive (and more resource-intensive) screening strategies would include random finger-stick blood glucose testing with cut-offs between 110 mg/dL (80% sensitivity) and 150 mg/dL (50% sensitivity) followed by confirmatory fasting blood glucose, HbA1c testing, or an oral glucose tolerance test (see **TABLE 7.1**).[35] Because of the logistical difficulty of glucose tolerance testing, this method is not used frequently in clinical practice. We currently do not perform any of these more intensive screening strategies in our outpatient clinics.

Our protocol for diabetes screening in asymptomatic adults with hypertension can be found in **CHAPTER 8** (**PROTOCOL 8.2** and **PROTOCOL 8.4**). **PROTOCOL 7.1** addresses diabetes diagnosis in patients who present to health centers with symptoms of hyperglycemia. It is important to avoid misdiagnosis of diabetes in acutely ill patients. While diabetes is one cause of hyperglycemia, it should be noted that patients may develop mild to moderate hyperglycemia with severe illness of any kind.

TABLE 7.1   Diabetes Diagnosis: Blood Sugar Measurement and Symptoms

Blood sugar	≥ 126 mg/dL (7 mmol/L) fasting **OR** ≥ 200 mg/dL (11 mmol/L) random with symptoms **OR** ≥ 200 mg/dL (11 mmol/L) with an oral glucose tolerance test
Glycosylated hemoglobin (HbA1c)	≥ 6.5% (using a point-of-care device)
Symptoms of chronic hyperglycemia	Polyuria (excessive urination) Polydipsia (excessive thirst) Weight loss

PROTOCOL 7.1   Diagnosis of Diabetes and Management of Hyperglycemia at Health-Center Level

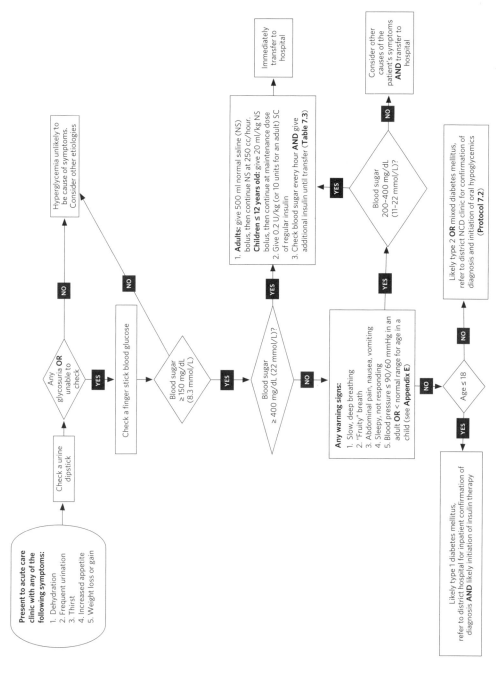

Present to acute care clinic with any of the following symptoms:
1. Dehydration
2. Frequent urination
3. Thirst
4. Increased appetite
5. Weight loss or gain

Check a urine dipstick

Any glycosuria **OR** unable to check

NO → Hyperglycemia unlikely to be cause of symptoms. Consider other etiologies

YES

Check a finger stick blood glucose

Blood sugar ≥ 150 mg/dL (8.3 mmol/L)?

NO → Hyperglycemia unlikely to be cause of symptoms. Consider other etiologies

YES

Blood sugar ≥ 400 mg/dL (22 mmol/L)?

YES →
1. **Adults:** give 500 ml normal saline (NS) bolus, then continue NS at 250 cc/hour. **Children ≤ 12 years old:** give 20 ml/kg NS bolus, then continue at maintenance dose
2. Give 0.2 U/kg (or 10 units for an adult) SC of regular insulin
3. Check blood sugar every hour **AND** give additional insulin until transfer (**Table 7.3**)

→ Immediately transfer to hospital

NO

Any warning signs:
1. Slow, deep breathing
2. "Fruity" breath
3. Abdominal pain, nausea, vomiting
4. Sleepy, not responding
5. Blood pressure ≤ 90/60 mmHg in an adult **OR** < normal range for age in a child (see **Appendix E**)

YES → Blood sugar 200–400 mg/dL (11–22 mmol/L)?

YES → (up to hospital transfer)

NO → Consider other causes of the patient's symptoms **AND** transfer to hospital

NO

Age ≤ 18

NO → Likely type 2 diabetes mellitus, refer to district NCD clinic for confirmation of diagnosis and initiation of oral hypoglycemics (**Protocol 7.2**)

YES → Likely type 1 diabetes mellitus, refer to district hospital for inpatient confirmation of diagnosis **AND** likely initiation of insulin therapy

7.2 Recognition and Treatment of Emergency States (Hyperglycemia and Hypoglycemia)

Providers at all levels in the health system should be aware of danger signs of both hyperglycemia and hypoglycemia. Patients with these signs or symptoms should be treated and referred, if necessary, to the nearest inpatient facility.

7.2.1 Hyperglycemia

The risks associated with hyperglycemia increase in proportion to the degree of glucose elevation. In general, mild to moderate hyperglycemia is not life-threatening (125–199 mg/dL or 6.9–11 mmol/L). However, higher blood glucose levels (≥ 200 mg/dL or 11.1 mmol/L), and the resulting electrolyte shifts, dehydration, and hypovolemia can be very dangerous. Patients with blood sugar greater than 200 mg/dL (11.1 mmol/L) who also have any danger signs of hyperglycemia (see **TABLE 7.2**) should be treated aggressively with fluids and insulin and transferred to the district hospital for admission. Patients with blood sugars greater than 400 mg/dL should always be admitted regardless of symptoms, because at this level of hyperglycemia, dangerous complications are very likely to occur.

TABLE 7.2   Danger Signs in Hyperglycemia

Early findings	Notes
Signs of dehydration	Dry mucus membranes, skin tenting, decreased urine output
Hypotension	From loss of fluids
Slow, deep breathing	From ketosis
Abdominal pain, nausea and vomiting	
Fruity breath	Ketones have a fruity odor
Late findings (neurological)	**Notes**
Focal motor deficits	
Altered mental status	Agitation, sleepiness, eventually coma

Various stressors can increase the amount of insulin needed to transfer glucose out of the bloodstream and into cells. These include infection, trauma, intoxication, and poor medication compliance. As a patient's cells become starved of glucose, they switch to burning fat for fuel (ketosis), leading to an acidosis. This condition is called diabetic ketoacidosis, or DKA. Many patients with type 1 diabetes will present in DKA at the time of diagnosis. Another related condition is called hyperosmolar non-ketotic coma (HONKC), which occurs when blood sugars reach very high levels (usually greater than 800 mg/dL or 44 mmol/L). These lead to hyperosmolality and very dangerous fluid shifts. If left untreated, mortality probably approaches 100%.

Our algorithms do not attempt to differentiate between DKA and HONKC. Our algorithms also do not use blood pH, anion gap or osmolality measurement in the diagnosis or triage of hyperglycemic states. Even at district hospital level, these labs, as a rule, are either unavailable or inaccurate. Therefore, we rely on symptoms, urine dipstick, and finger-stick blood glucose.

TABLE 7.3 Insulin Therapy of Patients with Hyperglycemia (≥ 250 mg/dL) and Danger Signs Awaiting Transfer

Blood sugar	Regular insulin dose (given subcutaneously)	
	For children (≤ 40 kg)	For adults
Initial bolus	0.2 units/kg x 1	10 units
Recheck blood glucose every hour		
≥ 250 mg/dL (13 mmol/L)	0. 1 unit/kg/hour	5 units/hour
150–249 mg/dL (8–13 mmol/L)	0.05 unit/kg/hour	2.5 units/hour
< 150 mg/dL (< 8 mmol/L)	Stop insulin, continue normal saline or lactated ringers	

In our algorithms, any patient with a blood sugar greater than 200 mg/dL (11.1 mmol/L) with danger signs of hyperglycemia, or any patient with a blood sugar greater than 400 mg/dL (18 mmol/L) with or without danger signs, should be hospitalized and given IV fluids and intensive insulin therapy. Treatment with subcutaneous insulin should begin immediately at the health-center level and continue until the patient is transferred. The most important initial step in management of these patients is to establish IV access and begin immediate infusion of normal saline or lactated Ringers. Patients with high levels of hyperglycemia will often be liters of water dehydrated as a result of a hyperglycemic diuresis, and this dehydration is often the most dangerous aspect of the condition.

In addition to giving IV fluids, health center practitioners should give subcutaneous insulin if this medication is available. If transport is to happen immediately, the health center nurse should give a single bolus dose of insulin. If transport is delayed, the clinician should continue to check glucose on an hourly basis and give insulin according to the schedule in **TABLE 7.3**, which outlines insulin therapy in patients with hyperglycemia and danger signs who are awaiting transfer to inpatient district hospital care.

7.2.2   Hypoglycemia

The most dangerous side effect of treatment with either insulin or sulfonylureas (e.g., glibenclamide) is low blood sugar or hypoglycemia. Diabetic patients who don't have enough to eat are at very high risk of developing hypoglycemia and should be identified as particularly vulnerable. Solutions to chronic lack of food are not simple. In the short term, these patients may need direct provision of food. In the medium term, they need social services to help them grow more of their own food, or earn income to buy it reliably.

Kidney or liver problems can also put patients at risk of hypoglycemia. If the cause of the hypoglycemia is ambiguous, these possibilities should be considered and creatinine should be checked. Liver disease usually causes hypoglycemia only in its end stages.

Hypoglycemic symptoms can come in two varieties (see **TABLE 7.4**). One variety is essentially neurological; patients who are not getting enough glucose to their brains can become dizzy, tired, confused, or nauseated. They can also develop seizures or lose consciousness. The other complex of symptoms can result from the body's stress response to low blood sugar. These symptoms include sweating, shaking, palpitations, and anxiety.

Treatments for hypoglycemia are listed in **TABLE 7.4**. Patients with symptoms of hypoglycemia should improve almost immediately with administration of glucose. This should be given orally if the patient is awake and able to swallow. Currently IV glucose (50% solution) is only available in Rwanda at the district and referral level. Note that this is an inappropriate concentration of glucose for IV use in children. The approach to treatment of hypoglycemia following initial resuscitation with glucose depends on the medication at fault. Hypoglycemia can recur until the medication has worn off. The half-life of insulin is relatively short, and patients who have received too much insulin may only require several hours of observation. However, oral hypoglycemics such as sulfonylureas have longer half-lives. Patients who have become hypoglycemic from excessive intake of these medications should be observed for at least 12 hours and receive finger-stick checks every few hours.

TABLE 7.4   Diagnosis and Treatment of Hypoglycemia

Symptoms	Somnolence or agitation
	Confusion
	Lethargy
	Dizziness, nausea
	Seizures
	Stroke-like symptoms
	Sweating
	Tremors
	Palpitations, anxiety
Causes	**Correctable:** Overdose of medication (insulin or orals)
	Increased exercise
	Skipped meals
	Not (easily) correctable: Reduced renal function (diminished clearance of hypoglycemic agents)
	Liver failure (inability to produce glycogen to correct serum hypoglycemia)
Treatment	Juice, soft drink, sugar water (if able to follow commands)
	In adults IV glucose 50% solution (if unable to follow commands)
	In children ≤ 12 give glucose 50% solution by nasogastric tube (if unable to follow commands)
	3–12 hours of frequent finger-stick checks

7.3   Principles and Initial Management of Diabetes

Patients with diabetes in Rwanda will require different levels of care for management. All should be initially referred to the district-level clinic for confirmation of the diagnosis and for initiation of therapy. An intake form should also be filled out (see **APPENDIX D**) and all patients should be screened for renal failure with a creatinine. The majority of patients will be managed with oral medications and can be followed at the health center clinics after the initial diagnosis has been established. These patients will still require occasional visits to the district NCD clinic for yearly creatinine measurement and for opthalmic evaluation every three years. Those patients who require insulin therapy, either because they have failed oral therapy or because they have a history of dangerous hyperglycemia, will be managed initially at the district-hospital level. As health centers gain more experience with integrated chronic care, they can also follow patients on stable regimens of insulin.

For all patients, blood glucose should be checked during each visit. A hemoglobin A1c (HbA1c) test that measures the average level of glycemia over the past 3 months should also be administered every 6 months. While this test is more expensive than a finger-stick, the information gained can help tremendously in management, especially in a setting in which patients are not able to check blood glucose regularly. Point-of-care tests for HbA1c can be inaccurate if the patient has a hemo-globinopathy such as sickle cell anemia or active malaria.[36,37] Rwanda has relatively low prevalence of hemoglobinopathies.[38,39] Furthermore, point–of–care HbA1c machines such as the ones used in Rwanda's NCD clinics are less affected by hemoglobinopathies. However, in other settings with higher prevalence of sickle cell trait, it may be reasonable to examine patients for conjunctival pallor.

TABLE 7.5 outlines glucose control goals. Initially, we aim to keep patients at the higher end of the spectrum so as to avoid problems with hypo-glycemia if they are using insulin or a sulfonylurea. Recent studies call into question the benefits of tighter glucose control relative to potential increase in hypoglycemia and death.[40-43] We feel that initial management should aim for an HbA1c between 7.5% and 8%. This corresponds to an average glucose between 170 and 185 mg/dL (9.4–10.5 mmol/L) and pre-meal glucose levels between 150 and 180 mg/dL (8.3–10 mmol/L). More intensive glucose control reduces the risk of blindness, kidney failure, and neuropathy in both patients with type 1 and type 2 diabetes.[44,45] For this reason, if patients are doing well on initial therapy, it makes sense to pursue a more aggressive target HbA1c of 7.0%–7.5%. HbA1c testing should be carried out twice a year. HbA1c testing is not generally the major driver of cost of care for patients with diabetes in resource-limited settings. However, in patients whose finger-stick blood glucose is routinely above 200 mg/dl (11 mmol/L), HbA1c probably adds little useful information.[46]

TABLE 7.5   Glucose Control Goals

	Reasonable control	More intensive control
Pre-meal and pre-bedtime glucose	150-180 mg/dL (8.3-10 mmol/L)	120-150 mg/dL (6.7-8.3 mmol/L)
Hemoglobin A1c	7.5%-8%: average blood glucose of 170-185 mg/dL (9.4-10.5 mmol/L)	7.0%-7.5%: average blood glucose of 154-170 mg/dL (8.6-9.4 mmol/L)

7.3.1   Oral Hypoglycemic Agents

Even in low-income, low-BMI settings, many patients with diabetes will respond well to oral hypoglycemic medications. These medicines are dramatically cheaper than insulin, easier to use, and less dangerous. Unless the patient is under 18 years old or has had ketoacidosis, oral agents should be tried first. Although their use is likely to be safe, most experts do not recommend use of oral therapy in pregnancy pending further study. **PROTOCOL 7.2** outlines the approach to oral therapy of diabetes.

PROTOCOL 7.2   Treatment of Diabetes with Oral Hypoglycemic Agents (in Adults)

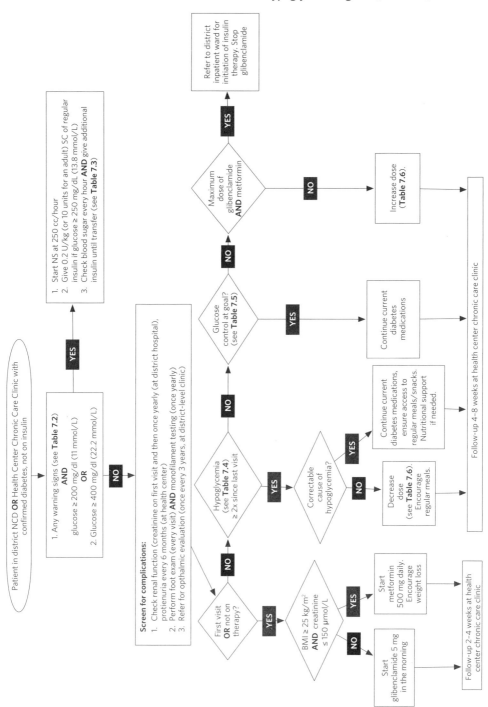

There are two oral hypoglycemic agents available in Rwanda: glibenclamide and metformin. The majority of patients with diabetes in Rwanda have low or normal body weight (BMI ≤ 25 kg/m^2). For these patients, glibenclamide should be the first oral therapy used. This medication, a sulfonylurea, works by increasing pancreatic insulin output. In our experience, most patients with diabetes with normal to low body weight have impaired insulin secretion. However, there is a risk of hypoglycemia with this medication. Dosing for glibenclamide is outlined in **TABLE 7.6**.

For patients who are overweight (BMI ≥ 25 kg/m^2), metformin is a good first choice. This medicine works in part by increasing glucose uptake into cells in response to endogenous insulin. Metformin rarely causes hypoglycemia. However, it can result in stomach upset. When it is administered in low doses and gradually titrated up, stomach side effects can sometimes be avoided. **TABLE 7.6** also shows dosing for metformin. Due to the rare risk of lactic acidosis, most endocrinologists do not recommend the use of metformin in patients with renal failure. In our clinics, patients should have a creatinine checked at the district-level clinic upon confirmation of their diagnosis and then yearly thereafter. We do not use metformin in patients with a creatinine ≥ 150 µmol/L.

It is generally preferable to use the maximum dose of a single agent before adding a second. When a single oral agent is insufficient for maintaing glycemic control (**TABLE 7.5**), adding the second agent, or adding insulin therapy, should be considered. The maximum oral regimen is glibenclamide 10 mg twice per day and metformin 1000 mg twice per day.

TABLE 7.6   Oral Hypoglycemic Therapy

Steps	Metformin		Glibenclamide	
	7 a.m.	7 p.m.	7 a.m.	7 p.m.
1	500 mg	-	5 mg	-
2	500 mg	500 mg	5 mg	5 mg
3	1000 mg	500 mg	10 mg	5 mg
4	1000 mg	1000 mg	10 mg	10 mg
5	Add glibenclamide		Add metformin	

7.3.2   Patient Education

Education is an essential aspect of diabetes care. Group classes can be a useful way to educate patients with diabetes in their own self-care. Diabetes visits are organized in groups that allow similar patients (e.g., children, adults on oral therapy, adults on insulin) to get educated while they are awaiting their clinic visits. Sessions are run by the nurse clinicians.

Patients are given lessons in the storage of insulin, in proper injection technique, and in the recognition of symptoms of hypoglycemia (see **TABLE 7.7** for common causes of hyperglycemia in patients on insulin). Other topics include the importance of foot care, appropriate diet, and physical activity.

TABLE 7.7   Common Causes for Hyperglycemia in Patients on Insulin

Problems with insulin injection and mixing technique
Problems with insulin storage or expiration
Unusual dietary excess
Active infection (e.g., malaria, urinary, skin, or pulmonary)

A frequent misconception among patients is the need to limit how much they eat. Partially as a result of this, patients often present in a malnourished state. Even though most patients consume high-carbohydrate diets, dietary counseling should focus on the need for regular meals rather than on specific restrictions. In the rare case of a patient who is overweight (more common in the urban areas of Rwanda), weight loss and diet modification should be encouraged. Exercise frequently improves blood glucose and should be recommended to all patients, irrespective of weight. However, increases in exercise can result in hypoglycemia if insulin or glibenclamide are being administered. Patients should be made aware of this issue, and practitioners should keep this risk in mind when adjusting drug regimens. Whenever available, community health workers should be used to improve therapeutic adherence and to provide social support.

7.4   Management of Diabetes with Insulin Therapy

Many patients with diabetes—in our cohort, approximately half of patients—need insulin therapy.[47] **TABLE 7.8** lists the indications for insulin. Successful initiation of insulin therapy requires extensive patient counseling (see **SECTION 7.3.2**). We refer all patients in need of insulin to the district hospital for admission. The main goals of hospitalization are patient education and also treatment and prevention of dangerous levels of hyperglycemia. We do not attempt to establish tight control of blood glucose. Insulin requirements in the hospital may differ substantially from those in the community. Food provision in-hospital is variable. Some hospitals in Rwanda provide meals to patients, but most do not. Therefore, patients may be receiving more or less food than they would at home. Often levels of physical activity are also altered in the hospital setting. As a result of these variables, it is safer to discharge patients on the minimum amount of insulin necessary to prevent life-threatening hyperglycemia and titrate their dose afterward. To this end, all patients should be assigned a community health worker (CHW) prior to discharge. The CHW will perform daily home visits to help with insulin

administration and documentation of glucose levels. NCD clinicians then review this information at weekly district NCD clinic visits and make adjustments accordingly. This process continues until a stable insulin regimen is established, usually within several weeks. **PROTOCOL 7.3** outlines the steps taken in initiation and adjustment of insulin therapy.

TABLE 7.8   Indications for Insulin Therapy

Type 1 diabetes
Failed maximum oral therapy
Pregnancy
Creatinine ≥ 150 mmol/L (1.6 mg/dL) (which prevents use of metformin), and unable to control glucose with glibenclamide alone
History of diabetic ketoacidosis
Child ≤ 18 years of age

PROTOCOL 7.3   Initiation and Adjustment of Insulin Regimens

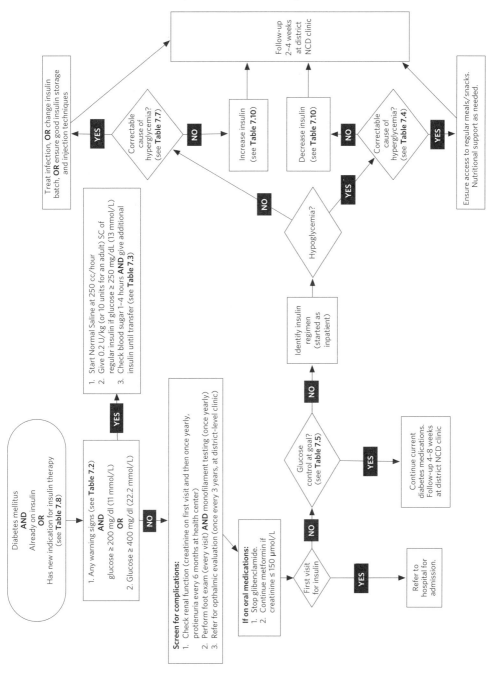

Diabetes mellitus **AND** Already on insulin **OR** Has new indication for insulin therapy (see **Table 7.8**)

1. Any warning signs (see **Table 7.2**) **AND** glucose ≥ 200 mg/dl (11 mmol/L) **OR**
2. Glucose ≥ 400 mg/dl (22.2 mmol/L)

YES →

1. Start Normal Saline at 250 cc/hour
2. Give 0.2 U/kg (or 10 units for an adult) SC of regular insulin if glucose ≥ 250 mg/dL (13 mmol/L)
3. Check blood sugar 1–4 hours **AND** give additional insulin until transfer (see **Table 7.3**)

NO →

Screen for complications:
1. Check renal function (creatinine on first visit and then once yearly, protienuria every 6 months at health center)
2. Perform foot exam (every visit) **AND** monofilament testing (once yearly)
3. Refer for opthalmic evaluation (once every 3 years, at district-level clinic)

If on oral medications:
1. Stop glibenclamide.
2. Continue metformin if creatinine ≤ 150 μmol/L

Glucose control at goal? (see **Table 7.5**)

YES → Continue current diabetes medications. Follow-up 4–8 weeks at district NCD clinic

NO →

First visit for insulin

YES → Refer to hospital for admission.

NO → Identify insulin regimen (started as inpatient)

Hypoglycemia?

NO → Correctable cause of hyperglycemia? (see **Table 7.7**)

YES → Treat infection, **OR** change insulin batch, **OR** ensure good insulin storage and injection techniques

NO → Increase insulin (see **Table 7.10**)

YES → Correctable cause of hyperglycemia? (see **Table 7.4**)

NO → Decrease insulin (see **Table 7.10**)

YES → Ensure access to regular meals/snacks. Nutritional support as needed.

Follow-up 2–4 weeks at district NCD clinic

7.4.1   Initiation of Insulin Therapy

Once the decision to start insulin has been made, patients should be referred to the district hospital for admission. In the hospital, the following steps will be taken:

- **Change in oral medication regimen if already on maximum dose.**

- **Stop glibenclamide.** Since glibenclamide stimulates insulin secretion by the pancreas, its continued use in the setting of insulin therapy can increase the risk of hypoglycemia. For this reason, glibenclamide should be discontinued in all patients on insulin.

- **Continue metformin unless creatinine ≥ 150 µmol/L (1.6 mg/ dL).** Metformin should be continued in patients who are beginning insulin therapy. Metformin causes the body's tissues to better respond to insulin, resulting in decreased hepatic glucose output. Metformin may lower insulin dose requirements.

- **Start insulin.** In the hospital, patients will be started on an insulin regimen that is appropriate for them (see **SECTION 7.4.2**).

- **Provide patient education.** While hospitalized, patients should be given education regarding the appropriate injection of insulin and the importance of regular meals.

- **Ensure good outpatient follow-up plan.** At discharge, a community health worker should be assigned to the patient. This community health worker will visit the patient daily and, during the first 2–3 weeks, check and record daily blood glucose levels. The patient should also be given an appointment for one week after discharge to be examined at the district-level NCD clinic. The importance of follow-up should be emphasized to the patient.

7.4.2   Insulin Regimen Selection

Insulin should be made available at the health-center level, along with appropriate training in its use. For a program that is relatively new in a district, it may be preferable to manage insulin-dependent patients with diabetes at the district level, where nurse clinicians have more extensive training and physicians are available to supervise. However, in most cases, patients live further from the district clinics than from health-center clinics. In such situations, a community health worker is vital to ensuring that patients do not run out of insulin. The community health worker or the patient may refill insulin prescriptions at the health center in the periods between district clinic visits. Eventually, programs may find it possible to decentralize insulin management to the health-center clinic, once a patient has established a stable regimen.

In Rwanda, there are three types of insulin available through public pharmacies (see **TABLE 7.9**): NPH (*insulatard* or *lente*), regular (*insuline* *rapide*), and combination (*mixte* or *mixtard*). NPH is generally considered to be a basal insulin; it provides a long-acting baseline insulin level. On the other hand, regular insulin is shorter-acting, and is thus usually used to treat mealtime glucose surges. Combination insulin is a third option, which consists of a premade mixture of regular and NPH insulin. The most common ratio for pre-mixed insulin is 70/30 (70% NPH, 30% regular).

TABLE 7.9 Properties of Insulin Available in Rwanda

	Regular (*rapide*)	NPH (*insulatard* or *lente*)	Combination (70/30 or *mixte*)
Time to onset	20-30 minutes	1-2 hours	30 minutes
Peak effect	2.5-5 hours	4-12 hours	3-8 hours
Duration	4-12 hours	18-24 hours	18-24 hours
Dosing	20-30 minutes before meals	Once or twice daily, around 7 am and 7 pm (or bedtime)	20-30 minutes before breakfast and/or dinner
Vial appearance (manufacturer-specific)	Clear	Cloudy	Cloudy

The available types of insulin can be used in isolation or in various combinations to achieve the desired effect. Simpler regimens result in looser glucose control than the complex regimens. Of course, more complex regimens are more difficult for patients to follow. For this reason, all patients using insulin should have access to regular assistance from a trained community health worker.

The initial regimen will be determined in the inpatient setting, but it may need to be adjusted after the patient is discharged. The simplest insulin regimen is a single nighttime injection of NPH. This approach targets the fasting blood sugar and can serve as a building block for future adjustments, if needed.

This strategy has been shown to control glucose in roughly half of adult patients with diabetes in a U.S. population.[48] However, in our experience, most patients in rural Rwanda cannot be controlled on a once-a-day regimen. This may be because their insulin secretion is more impaired than in the average patient with type 2 diabetes in an industrialized setting. Most of our patients require twice-daily NPH with regular insulin or twice daily pre-mixed insulin. These regimens avoid severe hyperglycemia due to carbohydrate-rich meals. **TABLE 7.10** outlines the available insulin regimens in order, from simplest to most complex. The most commonly used regimens in Rwanda are highlighted in red. The starting doses of insulin provided here are purposefully on the low side and most patients will require much higher dosing than this over time.

TABLE 7.10 Insulin Regimens

Regimen	Injections	Coverage of basal glycemia	Coverage at meals	Notes	Starting dose type 1	Starting dose type 2
NPH (insulatard or lente) 1x/day	1	Some	None	Most simple, but not good coverage if high-carbohydrate diet	Not appropriate	0.2 units/kg/day or 10 units/day (whichever is less) given at bedtime
NPH (insulatard or lente) 2x/day	2	Good	None	Good for some patients with type 2 diabetes, but again problem with coverage if high-carbohydrate diet	Not appropriate	0.3-0.6 units/kg/day: 60% pre-breakfast, 40% pre-dinner (20-30 minutes before meal)
70/30 (mixte) 2x/day	2	Good	Breakfast and dinner (no lunch coverage)	Post-prandial hyperglycemia. For high-carbohydrate diets, may need closer to a 50/50 mix	Not appropriate	0.3-0.6 units/kg/day: 50% pre-breakfast, 50% pre-dinner (20-30 minutes before meal)
NPH (insulatard or lente) and regular (rapide) Insulin 2x/day	2	Good	Breakfast and dinner. Lunch may be covered by morning NPH	Allows patients to control mix. Patients combine insulin from two vials (NPH and regular) and give the injection 2x/day	0.2-0.3 units/kg; Give 50% of dose as NPH 60% pre-breakfast 40% pre-dinner; Give 50% of dose as regular (split evenly pre-breakfast and pre-dinner, 20-30 minutes before meal)	0.5-0.7 units/kg
Basal/Prandial	3	Good	All meals	Best for large midday meals. Dinner-time NPH and regular combination. Regular alone with breakfast and lunch	0.2-0.3 units/kg; Give 50% of dose as NPH One dose pre-dinner combined with dinner-time regular insulin; Give 50% of dose as regular (split evenly and given 20-30 minutes prior to meals)	0.5-0.7 units/kg

7.5   Insulin Use in the Community

Insulin injection. Typically, insulin injections should be given in the subcutaneous fat of the abdomen. Alternative sites include the subcutaneous fat of the thighs and arms. The abdominal fat is generally thought to be the best site for absorption because it contains a greater fat-to-muscle ratio. However, with repeated injections, many patients develop pain, calluses, or bruising, and sometimes they prefer alternating sites. For this reason, it may be reasonable to recommend that morning injections be given at abdominal sites, and evening injections in the thigh. The emphasis should focus on the consistent use of the site or sites, in order to ensure reliable absorption.

Insulin storage. If insulin is stored improperly, it may not have the desired effect. For patients who have hyperglycemia despite escalating doses of insulin, proper insulin storage should be reviewed with the patient. In an ideal setting, insulin should be refrigerated. However, this is impractical and probably unnecessary in rural Rwanda and in most other limited-resource settings. Alternatively, patients can place the vial in a small container of water, which should be kept in a cool place out of the sun, such as an inside corner of the house on the floor. Clay pots filled with sand and water, allowing for evaporation, are also frequently used. Fortunately, Rwanda has a temperate climate. In other, hotter countries, refrigeration may be available through local soft drink distributors. There is little evidence that problems with insulin storage are currently a major barrier to good outcomes for patients with diabetes in such areas.[49]

TABLE 7.11   Example of Glucose Monitoring Chart

Date	Before breakfast			Before lunch			Before dinner			Before bedtime	
	Blood sugar	Insulin	Symptoms of hyperglycemia/ hypoglycemia	Blood sugar	Insulin	Symptoms of hyperglycemia/ hypoglycemia	Blood sugar	Insulin	Symptoms of hyperglycemia/ hypoglycemia	Blood sugar	Insulin
Day 1	183 mg/dL	2U Regular	None		2U Regular	None	125 mg/dL	7U NPH 2U Regular	None		
Day 2		2U Regular	None	240 mg/dL	2U Regular	None		7U NPH 2U Regular	None	72 mg/dL	
Day 3	170 mg/dL	2U Regular	None		2U Regular	None	150 mg/dL	7U NPH 2U Regular	None		
Day 4		2U Regular	None	204 mg/dL	2U Regular	None		7U NPH 2U Regular	None	57 mg/dL	

Insulin syringe disposal. After use, insulin syringes should always be placed in an appropriate sharps container. These safety containers should be distributed to patients. Patients should be instructed to bring their filled boxes to the local health center for disposal.

Blood glucose monitoring for patients on insulin. After starting insulin therapy, the blood glucose should be monitored closely. In the hospital, a patient's eating and other activities are very different than at home. Hypoglycemia or hyperglycemia can result after discharge. Ideally, patients should be monitored with finger-sticks as often as four times per day (before each meal and before bedtime). However, given the high cost of test strips, we have pursued a strategy to minimize unnecessary use of these consumables.

In our clinics, each community health worker is given a glucometer and test strips to check a patient's blood sugar twice daily for the first 2–3 weeks following discharge. Having data points at different times of the day (see **TABLE 7.11**) can help the practitioner decide which insulin dose needs adjustment. On one day, the patient checks glucose pre-breakfast and pre-dinner; on the next, the patient should check glucose pre-lunch and pre-bedtime. During this period of adjustment, patients should be seen at the district NCD clinic weekly. Once a patient is on a stable regimen, community health workers may teach patients to use twice-daily urine glucose testing to monitor for hyperglycemia. If the patient has two or more positive urine dipsticks per week, home blood glucose monitoring is started again.

7.5.1 Principles of Insulin Adjustment

Insulin can be a life-saving medication. However, if it is administered or dosed incorrectly, serious complications can ensue. Making insulin adjustments can be complicated. Until a stable regimen is achieved, patients should be followed at district level. When there is doubt regarding a change of insulin dose, the decision should be made with the help of a doctor. It is important that specialists from referral centers make regular visits to district hospitals to consult and supervise care. Large changes in regimens (such as switching to a new type of insulin) should happen only in the hospital setting.

Small dose changes. In general, the size of the dose increase should be small (around 1–2 units). Decreases in dosage can be larger (2–4 units). These general guidelines will limit unexpected hypoglycemia in response to an increase in the dose, or severe hyperglycemia in response to a dose reduction. Patients with uncontrolled diabetes have likely been poorly controlled for a long time, so one extra month of hyperglycemia is unlikely to have much of a detrimental impact. If a practitioner is concerned about a particular patient, more frequent follow-up will be needed. However, insulin should continue to be adjusted by small amounts each time.

Start with a simple regimen. For patients beginning insulin, compliance will be more likely if the regimen is simple. As a patient learns how to administer insulin and monitor for side effects, transitioning to a more complex regimen will become easier for the patient. The regimen should be selected and started by the district inpatient physician. The simplest regimen would be a single dose of NPH at bedtime. However, most patients in Rwanda will have high blood sugar spikes at mealtimes because of their carbohydrate-rich diets. For this reason, most patients are started on a more physiologic regimen with a shot of NPH and regular insulin (either as two separate shots or combined) twice daily (see **TABLE 7.10**).

Watch for patterns and tailor the regimen accordingly. After the first week of insulin use in the community, the district-level NCD provider has data on the patient's glucose trends (see **TABLE 7.11**). The thresholds for adjusting the insulin dose are listed in **TABLE 7.5**. Initial control should aim for glucose levels between 150 and 180 mg/dL (8.3–10 mmol/L) prior to meals and at bedtime. The goal HbA1c should be between 7.5% and 8%. There should be roughly 3 or 4 pre-meal and 3 or 4 bedtime measurements available for a given week. The first step is to identify measurements that are outside of the goal range. If there are correctable causes not related to the prescribed medication dose, these should be addressed first (**PROTOCOL 7.3**). If there is no other correctable cause, and at least 2 of the measurements are below the target level (e.g., 150 mg/dL) or there is symptomatic hypoglycemia, the insulin regimen should be adjusted downward. Similarly, if two or more measurements are above the target level (e.g., 180 mg/dL), the insulin regimen should be adjusted upward.

The insulin adjustment strategy depends on the kind of insulin regimen used at baseline. The peak effect of NPH (*lente*) and 70/30 (*mixte*) insulins is experienced 3–12 hours after administration (see **TABLE 7.9**). **TABLE 7.12** shows the recommended adjustment strategy for regimens using only these insulins.

TABLE 7.12   Principles for Adjusting Insulin 70/30 (*Mixte*) or 2x/day NPH Regimens

Timing of hyperglycemia/ hypoglycemia	Hyperglycemia (documented)	Hypoglycemia (documented OR symptoms)
Morning/overnight	Increase dinner-time or evening insulin by 2 units	Decrease dinner-time or evening basal insulin by 4 units or 10%, whichever is greater
Mid-day/evening	Increase morning insulin by 2 units	Decrease morning insulin by 4 units or 10%, whichever is greater

For patients on a regimen involving both NPH and regular insulin, adjusting insulin is slightly more complicated. The pharmacokinetics of regular insulin and NPH must be kept in mind when reviewing the timing of hyperglycemia and hypoglycemia. If hyperglycemia or hypoglycemia occur 3–4 hours after an injection, the effect is likely due to regular insulin. If the symptoms occur 6–12 hours after an injection, the effect is likely due to NPH (see **TABLE 7.13**).

TABLE 7.13   Principles for Adjusting Combined Basal (NPH) and Prandial (Regular Insulin) Regimens

	Hyperglycemia (documented)	Hypoglycemia (documented OR symptoms)
Middle of the night	n/a	Decrease PM Regular 2-4 U
Before breakfast	Increase PM NPH 2 U	Decrease PM NPH 2-4 U
Mid-day	Increase AM Regular 2 U	Decrease AM Regular 2-4 U
Before dinner	Increase AM NPH 2 U	Decrease AM NPH 2-4 U
Before bedtime	Increase Pre-dinner Regular 2 U	Decrease Pre-Dinner Regular 2-4 U

Patients who need to be transitioned to a different regimen altogether should be hospitalized to have this change made. Although physicians in the hospital will make these adjustments, we outline the basic principles below.

All transitions. In transitions from one insulin regimen to another, there are two methods for choosing the starting dose for the new insulin: (1) dosing based on the current dose of insulin, or (2) weight-based dosing. When possible, it is preferable to use an existing insulin dose as a starting point for a new insulin regimen. In general, the dose of insulin should be rounded downward to avoid hypoglycemia.

Dosing based on current dose of insulin. In most patients who are already on insulin, the current total daily dose can be used as a starting point for the new regimen. For instance, if a patient is already taking 20 units of NPH as a single evening dose, this can be transitioned to 20 total units of a combination of NPH and regular insulin given twice daily. Of the 20 units, 50% (or 10 units) can be given as NPH and 50% (10 units) can be given as regular insulin. Of the NPH, 60% (6 units) can be given before breakfast and 40% (4 units) can be given before dinner. The regular insulin can be divided between meals (rounded down to 3 units with each meal for 9 total units of regular insulin per day).

Weight-based dosing. If a patient is not already taking insulin, the initial dosing can be based on weight by using the formulas provided in **TABLE 7.10**. To divide the total daily insulin among multiple administration times, the value can be rounded down to the nearest whole unit so as to avoid hypoglycemia.

Transition to 70/30 insulin. While 70/30 insulin preparations are widely available in many regions, adequate glycemic control is often difficult to achieve in patients with high dietary carbohydrate intake. These preparations can be used if necessary (i.e., when stock-outs leave no other available insulin) and dosing can be based either on a prior insulin regimen or based on weight. If a patient's fasting glucose is controlled with NPH insulin, but the daytime, post-meal glucose measurements are still very high, the patient may benefit from a mealtime dose of regular insulin in addition to NPH. Using insulin 70/30 can help with this. In general, one can use the same dose as insulin NPH 2x/day as the starting dose for insulin 70/30 2x/day. For example, if a patient takes insulin NPH 12 units in the morning and 8 units before dinner, the starting dose of insulin 70/30 can also be 12 units in the morning and 8 units at dinner.

Transition from a 70/30 combination to NPH/regular. Since the ratio of NPH insulin to regular is fixed in insulin 70/30, patients may have persistent midday hyperglycemia (due to an insufficiency of short-acting insulin prior to meals) despite having controlled fasting glucose (due to a correct amount of NPH). Indeed, as the dose of insulin 70/30 is increased, patients may well develop fasting hypoglycemia and midday hyperglycemia. These patients will need to have NPH insulin and regular insulin in a different ratio than that available in fixed-dose preparations. Patients should first be transitioned to NPH and regular insulin at the same dose and in the same ratio as insulin 70/30 (**TABLE 7.14**). Adjustments should then be made as outlined in **TABLE 7.13**. Some patients may also require an extra dose of regular insulin prior to lunch if midday hyperglycemia continues to be a problem (see **TABLE 7.10**).

TABLE 7.14   Example of Transitioning from 70/30 (*Insuline Mixtard*) to NPH/Regular (*Insuline Lente + Rapide*)

Initial dose:	Pre-breakfast	Pre-dinner
70/30 (*Insuline mixtard*)	20 units	10 units
Final dose:	**Pre-breakfast**	**Pre-dinner**
NPH (*Insuline lente*)	14 units (70% of 20 units)	7 units (70% of 10 units)
Regular (*Insulin rapide*)	6 units (30% of 20 units)	3 units (30% of 10 units)

7.6   Adjuvant Therapies and Routine Monitoring for Complications in Patients with Diabetes

Patients with diabetes in rural areas living on less than $1 per day are typically younger (below 40) and have a low prevalence of vascular comorbidities such as obesity, tobacco use, hyperlipidemia, and lack of physical activity. Complications from diabetes in these populations are typically microvascular in origin (retinopathy, diabetic foot, renal failure), rather than macrovascular (strokes and heart attacks).[50,51] The risk of complications is highest in patients who have had their disease untreated for 10 to 20 years. **TABLE 7.15** outlines the most common complications of diabetes and their prevalence in some African cohorts from Ethiopia, Malawi, and Tanzania.

At the time of initial diagnosis, all patients with diabetes should have a blood pressure measurement, a foot exam with a monofilament, a fundoscopic examination by an ophthalmic officer, a creatinine test, and a urine dipstick.

Blood pressure goals for patients with diabetes should be set at less than 130/80 mmHg. For children less than 18 years old, blood pressure goal should be set to less than the 95% percentile for age, sex, and height. We do not check lipid levels routinely, but if patients have diabetes and have BMI greater than 25 kg/m^2, they should also take aspirin daily at a low dose such as 100 mg. Given the low incidence of coronary events in this population, we have not pursued statin therapy.

TABLE 7.15 Common Complications of Diabetes and Their Prevalence in Some African Cohorts

	Prevalence[52-54]	Mode of evaluation	Frequency of evaluation	Action if abnormal
Peripheral neuropathy	35%–70%	Monofilament sensory testing of the feet. If a microfilament is not available, proprioception can be tested. Patients may also complain of neuropathic pain (burning, electrical sensations) in the feet	Once yearly	Intensify treatment regimen if possible. Consider treating neuropathic pain with amitriptyline 25 to 100 mg per day orally (in adults). Shoes if needed. Counsel on foot protection
Foot ulcer	1.7%–10%	Visual inspection, probe evaluation to rule out osteomyelitis	Every visit	Referral to district hospital for possible debridement and broad-spectrum antibiotics
Retinopathy or sight-threatening eye disease	5%–35%	Fundoscopic evaluation or retinal photography	Once every 3 years, performed at a district hospital with an ophthalmic clinical officer. More frequent follow-up if established retinopathy.	Intensify treatment regimen if possible. Referral for evaluation at an ophthalmic center if needed for intervention
Cataracts	8.7%–25%	Fundoscopic evaluation	Once every 3 years performed at a district hospital with an ophthalmic clinical officer	Referral for evaluation at an ophthalmic center for intervention
Albuminuria	18%	Urine dipstick	Every six months	Intensify treatment regimen if possible. Add an ACE inhibitor
Nephropathy	19%–34%	Serum creatinine testing	Yearly	Intensify treatment regimen if possible. Add an ACE inhibitor if no counterindication

Retinopathy and cataracts. Intervention for established diabetic eye disease can reduce the risk of blindness by as much as 50%.[55] Focal photocoagulation is indicated for clinically significant macular edema due to nonproliferative diabetic retinopathy, and panretinal photocoagulation is indicated for severe proliferative diabetic retinopathy.[56] Typically, the yield of patients who will benefit from treatment is around 1% to 4%.[57] Rwanda has trained ophthalmic clinical officers for work at district hospitals and photocoagulation is available at referral–center level.[58] However, the quality of screening for such rare findings may be difficult to control. One solution that has been implemented at many other sites around the world, including South Africa, is use of retinal photography, followed by interpretation at a referral center.[59,60]

Peripheral neuropathy, foot ulcers, and limb sepsis. Peripheral neuropathy is a common complication of diabetes that poses a great risk to patients living in rural areas. Loss of sensation and lack of proper footwear can lead to small cuts and infections, which can result in sepsis or death.[61] One study in Tanzania found that almost 10% of patients with diabetes with foot injuries evaluated at a referral center had evidence of being bitten on the foot by rodents.[62] Prevention of diabetic foot ulcers requires good glucose control and focused education regarding foot care. Care of foot ulcers requires evaluation by providers at district levels with skills in debridement, and also in some cases the use of broad-spectrum antibiotics. Specific training initiatives for diabetic foot care have been established in Africa and India.[63] It is a goal of the Rwandan NCD program to integrate these skills into the competencies of district NCD providers. Patients with diabetes must learn to take seriously even small injuries to the hands or feet, as these may progress quickly to sepsis if not dressed properly.[64]

Proteinuria and nephropathy. Although we do not check routinely for urine microalbumin, urine dipstick is used to screen for more significant proteinuria (see **CHAPTER 8, TABLE 8.2**). A dipstick should be checked twice a year, and a serum creatinine should be checked once per year. The finding of 2+ proteinuria or greater on a dipstick should lead to initiation of therapy with an ACE inhibitor after exclusion of other causes of proteinuria. One contraindication to use of ACE inhibitors is severe renal dysfunction (estimated glomerular filtration rate less than 29 ml/min). A reasonable starting dose of an ACE inhibitor for an adult is 5 mg per day orally. This can be increased at subsequent visits up to a goal dose of 10 mg, and then to 20 mg unless the blood pressure falls too far (less than 100 mmHg systolic) or potassium rises too high (more than 5 mEq/L). For children weighing ≤ 20 kg, a reasonable starting dose of lisinopril is 0.07 mg/kg once per day (maximum dose 5 mg). A reasonable starting dose of captopril in these children is 0.6 mg/kg three times per day (maximum dose 2 mg/kg three times per day).

7.7 Diabetes and Pregnancy

The danger of diabetes in pregnancy is that the fetus may develop birth defects or become unusually large and thus be at increased risk of trauma at birth. Hormonal changes during pregnancy lead to a degree of insulin resistance. So-called gestational diabetes as a result of these changes can arise, but it is rare in women who are younger than 30 who have low to normal body weight. Therefore, we focus on issues specific to pregnant women who had diabetes prior to pregnancy.

Women between the ages of 15 and 45 who have diabetes should be counseled regarding the risks of pregnancy, and should be offered the usual family planning options. Pregnancy may expose women with diabetes to increased risk, particularly those who already have complications due to their diabetes. All contraception options are reasonable, although progestin-only injectables should probably be avoided because of the increased risk of hyperlipidemia.

Women with diabetes who become pregnant should be changed from oral agents to insulin, because the safety of metformin and glibenclamide for the fetus are not well established. Because of the increased risk to fetus of both hypoglycemia and hyperglycemia, treatment should aim for a narrower than usual therapeutic goal. We suggest a goal HbA1c of 7% to 7.5% (see **TABLE 7.5**). Finger-stick glucose monitoring should be performed twice per day with community health worker support during pregnancy. At the time of delivery, glucose levels should be kept below 126 mg/dL (7 mmol/L) to avoid hypoglycemia in the neonate.

7.8   Social Assistance and Community Health Workers

Insulin-dependent patients with diabetes are some of the most vulnerable patients in any health system. Inability to access food or interruption of medication supply can rapidly become life threatening. For this reason, we ensure that our patients on insulin receive a full social work assessment and, if necessary, assistance with food and transport to clinic appointments. In addition, all patients on insulin in our Rwanda clinics are assigned a community health worker.

7.8.1   Community Health Workers and Accompaniment
Taking the right type of insulin in the right dose at the right time can be very difficult for a patient who has no medical training. Community health workers provide assistance. They help ensure that patients are taking their insulin correctly and monitor for symptoms of hyperglycemia and hypoglycemia. They also make sure patients do not miss appointments or run out of medications. Community health workers also serve as the keepers of relatively scarce glucometers; they can intensely monitor a patient's blood glucose while patients are first adjusting to an insulin regimen They can assist patients in checking blood glucose readings, improve compliance and adherence to treatment regimens, and help identify and relay problems patients may be having with their therapies.

7.8.2   Food Assistance
The timing of meals in relationship to the dose of insulin is very important. If a patient takes insulin without eating, hypoglycemia will result. Ensuring that patients on insulin have stable supplies of food is essential.

This may be accomplished by providing food packages to the patient's family or by supporting the family's ability to grow food, either on their own land or on a community plot, through patient associations. A full social work evaluation of the family should be done, as the family of a patient without enough food will often have other malnourished members.

Chapter 7 References

· ·

1   Levitt NS. Diabetes in Africa: epidemiology, management and healthcare challenges. Heart 2008;94:1376-82.

2   Type 2 Diabetes Clinical Practice Guidelines for Sub-Saharan Africa: International Diabetes Federation Africa Region; 2006.

3   Diabetes Education Training Manual for Sub-Saharan Africa: International Diabetes Federation Africa Region; 2007.

4   Bahendeka S. The African Diabetes Care Initiative (ADCI). 2010-2012. South Africa: International Diabetes Federation; 2010.

5   Life for a Child. (Accessed at **http://www.lifeforachild.org**)

6   Mbanya JC, Motala AA, Sobngwi E, Assah FK, Enoru ST. Diabetes in sub-Saharan Africa. Lancet 2010;375:2254-66.

7   Coleman R, Gill G, Wilkinson D. Noncommunicable disease management in resource-poor settings: a primary care model from rural South Africa. Bull World Health Organ 1998;76:633-40.

8   Kengne AP, Sobngwi E, Fezeu L, Awah PK, Dongmo S, Mbanya JC. Setting-up nurse-led pilot clinics for the management of non-communicable diseases at primary health care level in resource-limited settings of Africa. Pan Afr Med J 2009;3:10.

9   Unwin N, Mugusi F, Aspray T, et al. Tackling the emerging pandemic of non-communicable diseases in sub-Saharan Africa: the essential NCD health intervention project. Public Health 1999;113:141-6.

10 Gill GV, Price C, Shandu D, Dedicoat M, Wilkinson D. An effective system of nurse-led diabetes care in rural Africa. Diabet Med 2008;25:606-11.

11 Gill GV, Yudkin JS, Keen H, Beran D. The insulin dilemma in resource-limited countries. A way forward? Diabetologia 2011;54:19-24.

12 Yudkin JS. Insulin for the world's poorest countries. The Lancet 2000;355:919-21.

13 Janssens B, Van Damme W, Raleigh B, et al. Offering integrated care for HIV/AIDS, diabetes and hypertension within chronic disease clinics in Cambodia. Bull World Health Organ 2007;85:880-5.

14 Raguenaud ME, Isaakidis P, Reid T, et al. Treating 4,000 diabetic patients in Cambodia, a high-prevalence but resource-limited setting: a 5-year study. BMC Med 2009;7:33.

15. Amoah AG, Owusu SK, Acheampong JW, et al. A national diabetes care and education programme: the Ghana model. Diabetes Res Clin Pract 2000;49:149-57.

16 Beran D, Silva Matos C, Yudkin JS. The Diabetes UK Mozambique Twinning Programme. Results of improvements in diabetes care in Mozambique: a reassessment 6 years later using the Rapid Assessment Protocol for Insulin Access. Diabet Med 2010;27:855-61.

17 Beran D, Yudkin JS. Looking beyond the issue of access to insulin: what is needed for proper diabetes care in resource poor settings. Diabetes Res Clin Pract 2010;88:217-21.

18 Beran D, Yudkin JS, de Courten M. Access to care for patients with insulin-requiring diabetes in developing countries: case studies of Mozambique and Zambia. Diabetes Care 2005;28:2136-40.

19 McLarty DG, Kitange HM, Mtinangi BL, et al. Prevalence of diabetes and impaired glucose tolerance in rural Tanzania. The Lancet 1989;333:871-5.

20   King H, Aubert RE, Herman WH. Global burden of diabetes, 1995-2025: prevalence, numerical estimates, and projections. Diabetes Care 1998;21:1414-31.

21   Mbanya JC, Cruickshank JK, Forrester T, et al. Standardized comparison of glucose intolerance in west African-origin populations of rural and urban Cameroon, Jamaica, and Caribbean migrants to Britain. Diabetes Care 1999;22:434-40.

22   Levitt NS, Unwin NC, Bradshaw D, et al. Application of the new ADA criteria for the diagnosis of diabetes to population studies in sub-Saharan Africa. American Diabetes Association. Diabet Med 2000;17:381-5.

23   Beran D, Yudkin JS. Diabetes care in sub-Saharan Africa. The Lancet 2006;368:1689-95.

24   Majaliwa ES, Elusiyan BE, Adesiyun OO, et al. Type 1 diabetes mellitus in the African population: epidemiology and management challenges. Acta Biomed 2008;79:255-9.

25   Alemu S, Dessie A, Seid E, et al. Insulin-requiring diabetes in rural Ethiopia: should we reopen the case for malnutrition-related diabetes? Diabetologia 2009;52:1842-5.

26   Abu-Bakare A, Taylor R, Gill GV, Alberti KG. Tropical or malnutrition-related diabetes: a real syndrome? Lancet 1986;1:1135-8.

27   Sobngwi E, Choukem SP, Agbalika F, et al. Ketosis-prone type 2 diabetes mellitus and human herpesvirus 8 infection in sub-Saharan Africans. JAMA 2008;299:2770-6.

28   Tien PC, Schneider MF, Cole SR, et al. Antiretroviral therapy exposure and insulin resistance in the Women's Interagency HIV study. J Acquir Immune Defic Syndr 2008;49:369-76.

29   De Wit S, Sabin CA, Weber R, et al. Incidence and risk factors for new-onset diabetes in HIV-infected patients: the Data Collection on Adverse Events of Anti-HIV Drugs (D:A:D) study. Diabetes Care 2008;31:1224-9.

30   Pramono LA, Setiati S, Soewondo P, et al. Prevalence and predictors of undiagnosed diabetes mellitus in indonesia. Acta Med Indones;42:216-23.

31   van der Sande MA, Milligan PJ, Nyan OA, et al. Blood pressure patterns and cardiovascular risk factors in rural and urban Gambian communities. J Hum Hypertens 2000;14:489-96.

32   Wei OY, Teece S. Best evidence topic report. Urine dipsticks in screening for diabetes mellitus. Emerg Med J 2006;23:138.

33   Standards of medical care in diabetes—2010. Diabetes Care;33 Suppl 1:S11-61.

34   Morris LR, McGee JA, Kitabchi AE. Correlation between plasma and urine glucose in diabetes. Ann Intern Med 1981;94:469-71.

35   Fetita LS, Sobngwi E, Serradas P, Calvo F, Gautier JF. Consequences of fetal exposure to maternal diabetes in offspring. J Clin Endocrinol Metab 2006;91:3718-24.

36   Armor BL, Britton ML. Diabetes mellitus non-glucose monitoring: point-of-care testing. Ann Pharmacother 2004;38:1039-47.

37   Schrot RJ, Patel KT, Foulis P. Evaluation of Inaccuracies in the Measurement of Glycemia in the Laboratory, by Glucose Meters, and Through Measurement of Hemoglobin A1c. Clinical Diabetes 2007;25:43-9.

38   Munyanganizi R, Cotton F, Vertongen F, Gulbis B. Red blood cell disorders in Rwandese neonates: screening for sickle cell disease and glucose-6-phosphate dehydrogenase deficiency. J Med Screen 2006;13:129-31.

39   Mutesa L, Boemer F, Ngendahayo L, et al. Neonatal screening for sickle cell disease in Central Africa: a study of 1825 newborns with a new enzyme-linked immunosorbent assay test. J Med Screen 2007;14:113-6.

40   Currie CJ, Peters JR, Tynan A, et al. Survival as a function of HbA(1c) in people with type 2 diabetes: a retrospective cohort study. Lancet 2010;375:481-9.

41   Nathan DM, Kuenen J, Borg R, Zheng H, Schoenfeld D, Heine RJ. Translating the A1C assay into estimated average glucose values. Diabetes Care 2008;31:1473-8.

42   Yudkin JS, Richter B, Gale EA. Intensified glucose control in type 2 diabetes—whose agenda? Lancet 2010.

43   Ismail-Beigi F, Craven T, Banerji MA, et al. Effect of intensive treatment of hyperglycaemia on microvascular outcomes in type 2 diabetes: an analysis of the ACCORD randomised trial. Lancet 2010;376:419-30.

44   The effect of intensive treatment of diabetes on the development and progression of long-term complications in insulin-dependent diabetes mellitus. The Diabetes Control and Complications Trial Research Group. N Engl J Med 1993;329:977-86.

45   Intensive blood-glucose control with sulphonylureas or insulin compared with conventional treatment and risk of complications in patients with type 2 diabetes (UKPDS 33). UK Prospective Diabetes Study (UKPDS) Group. Lancet 1998;352:837-53.

46   Rotchford AP, Rotchford KM, Machattie T, Gill GV. Assessing diabetic control—reliability of methods available in resource poor settings. Diabet Med 2002;19:195-200.

47   Bliss M. The discovery of insulin. Chicago: University of Chicago Press; 1982.

48   Vaidya A, McMahon G. Initiating Insulin for Type 2 Diabetes: Strategies for Success. Journal of Clinical Outcomes 2009;16:127-36.

49   Gill GV. Viewpoint: stability of insulin in tropical countries. Trop Med Int Health 2000;5:666-7.

50   Kengne AP, Amoah AG, Mbanya JC. Cardiovascular complications of diabetes mellitus in sub-Saharan Africa. Circulation 2005;112:3592-601.

51   Rolfe M. Macrovascular disease in diabetics in Central Africa. Br Med J (Clin Res Ed) 1988;296:1522-5.

52   Ejigu A. Patterns of chronic complications of diabetic patients in Menelik II Hospital, Ethiopia. Ethiop J Health Dev 2000;14:113-16.

53   Cohen DB, Allain TJ, Glover S, et al. A survey of the management, control, and complications of diabetes mellitus in patients attending a diabetes clinic in Blantyre, Malawi, an area of high HIV prevalence. Am J Trop Med Hyg 2010;83:575-81.

54   Neuhann HF, Warter-Neuhann C, Lyaruu I, Msuya L. Diabetes care in Kilimanjaro region: clinical presentation and problems of patients of the diabetes clinic at the regional referral hospital—an inventory before structured intervention. Diabet Med 2002;19:509-13.

55   Frank RN. Diabetic retinopathy. N Engl J Med 2004;350:48-58.

56   Mohamed Q, Gillies MC, Wong TY. Management of diabetic retinopathy: a systematic review. JAMA 2007;298:902-16.

57   Bachmann MO, Nelson SJ. Impact of diabetic retinopathy screening on a British district population: case detection and blindness prevention in an evidence-based model. J Epidemiol Community Health 1998;52:45-52.

58   National Plan for Eliminating Needless Blindness in Rwanda. 2008-2012. Kigali: Ministry of Health, Rwanda; 2008.

59   Benbassat J, Polak BC. Reliability of screening methods for diabetic retinopathy. Diabet Med 2009;26:783-90.

60 Mash B, Powell D, du Plessis F, van Vuuren U, Michalowska M, Levitt N. Screening for diabetic retinopathy in primary care with a mobile fundal camera—evaluation of a South African pilot project. S Afr Med J 2007;97:1284-8.

61 Abbas ZG, Gill GV, Archibald LK. The epidemiology of diabetic limb sepsis: an African perspective. Diabet Med 2002;19:895-9.

62 Abbas ZG, Lutale J, Archibald LK. Rodent bites on the feet of diabetes patients in Tanzania. Diabet Med 2005;22:631-3.

63 Pendsey S, Abbas ZG. The step-by-step program for reducing diabetic foot problems: a model for the developing world. Curr Diab Rep 2007;7:425-8.

64 Gill GV, Famuyiwa OO, Rolfe M, Archibald LK. Tropical diabetic hand syndrome. Lancet 1998;351:113-4.

CHAPTER 8
Hypertension
....

Worldwide, hypertension is a leading cause of preventable end-organ disease. This is true even in rural sub-Saharan Africa, a setting with high levels of physical activity and malnutrition and low levels of obesity and tobacco use.[1] There are no national prevalence studies on hypertension in rural Rwanda, but there are numerous studies of adults in other rural areas of sub-Saharan Africa. These studies show a pattern of low prevalence but severe hypertension, often in isolation from other metabolic risk factors. For example, a study in rural Gambia during the mid-1990s found 6.8% of surveyed participants over the age of 15 had a blood pressure greater than 160/95 mmHg.[2] Roughly half of these cases had systolic blood pressures greater than 180 mmHg. Almost 80% had no other metabolic risk factor. Almost 18% of the population had blood pressures greater than 140/90 mmHg. Other surveys from the past 30 years have produced similar findings.[3,4] As in industrialized countries, most hypertension in sub-Saharan Africa is likely due to essential hypertension.

The Framingham Heart Study began during the 1950s, prior to the widespread use of effective antihypertensives. Back then, 11% of women between the ages of 45 and 75 had blood pressures greater than 180/110 mmHg.[5] By the 1980s, this prevalence had declined to 0.9%. Data from sites like rural Gambia suggest that as much as 2% of the population over age 15 currently has untreated systolic blood pressures greater than 180 mmHg.[2] So far, in Rwanda, we have focused on the chronic care of patients in this category who present to district hospitals. This approach has the advantage of treating first those people most likely to have negative cardiovascular outcomes and establishing good systems on a small scale prior to expanding case-finding.

However, passive case-finding misses most asymptomatic patients, patients whose untreated hypertension leaves them vulnerable to end-organ disease. More active case-finding would involve opportunistic screening for hypertension as part of acute care at the health-center level. This approach raises the controversial question of what level of hypertension necessitates treatment.

Blood pressure is a continuous risk factor and interacts with other variables such as age, tobacco exposure, and lipid and glucose levels. For this reason, many have advocated medication treatment thresholds based not on a single risk factor, but on wider criteria: the patient's absolute risk for a combination of cardiovascular events.[6,7] As we have discussed, most people with high blood pressure in rural sub-Saharan settings have no risk factors for cardiovascular disease beyond their hypertension. Most absolute risk models would calculate the risk of a cardiovascular event for such people at less than 10% over a 5-year period even at very high blood pressures. However, it is unclear how well these models predict the outcomes associated with isolated hypertension at levels above 160/95 mmHg, particularly in sub-Saharan Africa. International hypertension guidelines that embrace the absolute risk approaches have made the caveat that patients with persistent blood pressures above 170/100 mmHg (New Zealand) or 160/95 mmHg (WHO) should receive pharmacologic treatment regardless of their calculated risk.[8,9] Another factor not often included in standard treatment models is the cost to the patient. Facility-based chronic care for hypertension is expensive for patients, especially in rural areas. They must pay for transport to the clinic and also, in most health systems, for the costs of their care. Our protocols offer one attempt to balance the risks associated with untreated hypertension and the significant cost of treatment to patients and society. This approach treats all patients with confirmed blood pressures greater than or equal to 160/95 mmHg. Patients with lower levels of blood pressure are treated only if they also have diabetes, renal failure, or two or more other cardiovascular risk factors, such as advanced age (greater than 65), current tobacco use, or obesity. Given the relatively low risk of developing end-organ damage from mild, lone hypertension and the large health care and direct patient costs of chronic medical therapy, we have adopted a policy of watchful waiting for this group of patients. We believe reducing the facility-based component of care for lower-risk hypertension offers one way of reducing costs and making this intervention more accessible. We have not yet explored an intervention for low-risk hypertension at the community level in rural Rwanda. The reason for this is because community health workers are currently burdened with a host of different tasks, and because the short-term risks for these patients are probably small.

Provision of hypertension treatment at first-level facilities close to patient homes also reduces health system and out-of-pocket costs. Most hypertension is relatively simple to diagnose and treat once a system of chronic care has been established. In Rwanda, most hypertension is managed at the health-center level. At this level, nurses with a basic level of training treat simple NCDs as well as HIV and TB in integrated chronic care clinics. These clinics tend to be closer to patients' homes and cost less to run than those at district level. Patients with severe levels of hypertension are referred to the district hospital or district-level NCD clinic for more specialized treatment.

In some settings, combination tablets (polypills) currently under development may offer another means of reducing treatment costs and increasing compliance, particularly among patients who have previously suffered a myocardial infarction.[10] These combination tablets often mix a hypertension agent with other medications such as aspirin and HMG-CoA reductase inhibitors (statins) to reduce the risk of vascular events among hypertensives. However, non-ischemic events, such as heart failure, renal failure, and hemorrhagic stroke, constitute the primary risks faced by hypertensive patients in settings such as rural Rwanda.[11] For this reason, we do not advocate the routine use of these combination or adjuvant therapies for most hypertensives in our setting. Rather, we reserve the use of aspirin for hypertensive patients with diabetes. Currently, we do not recommend adding statins to the Rwandan formulary for rural facilities because of the low incidence of vascular events.

8.1   Clinic and Community-Based Hypertension Screening

In rural Rwanda, hypertension, HIV, and streptococcal pharyngitis constitute the main drivers of cardiovascular risk. Blood pressure screening in asymptomatic individuals can help identify people with hypertension before they develop end-organ complications. Of course, screening will identify a spectrum of high- and low-risk patients. A strong chronic care system and risk-stratification protocols are needed to avoid overwhelming the fragile health infrastructure with patients who have low levels of hypertension that confer little risk of end-organ disease. Our goal in screening is to identify high-risk individuals who would not otherwise seek treatment before complications arise.

Potential occasions for screening include opportunistic blood pressure measurement at acute care or outpatient department clinics and systematic blood pressure measurement by health workers in the community. In resource-poor settings, lack of equipment, training, and time can pose barriers to implementation of routine blood pressure measurement at any level of the health care system. Given the competing demands on community health workers, we have focused initially on screening at the health-center level. We do this in the context of acute care protocols for the Integrated Management of Adult and Adolescent Illness.[12] At PIH-supported health centers, we encourage practitioners to measure the vital signs, including blood pressure, of everyone over the age of 15 who presents with a routine complaint. We use validated automatic blood pressure machines and we keep manual cuffs available in case the machine malfunctions. Batteries or electricity can power the machines. Accurate measurements require training in appropriate cuff sizes and the procurement of machines compatible with small, regular, and large adult cuffs.

A more or less intensive facility-based screening approach may be appropriate in other settings. A more resource-intensive strategy would be to hire an extra clerk to measure vital signs on all patients and to triage accordingly. A less intensive strategy would be to only measure blood pressure of patients above a certain age (e.g., 40). In some resource-poor settings, community-based screening may be an appropriate adjunct to clinic-based blood pressure measurement. This screening could take place at churches or schools. The utility of community-based screening depends in part on how often adults visit health facilities, or whether they visit them at all. As mentioned above, competing demands for services at the community level may make active detection strategies a lower priority in some contexts. **PROTOCOL 8.1** outlines an approach for this initial screening process.

As mentioned above, hypertension is both very common and relatively simple to treat. Most hypertension patients can be treated at the health-center level. However, the subject becomes more complex when one considers all the diseases encompassed by the diagnosis of hypertension. At low levels of blood pressure elevation, risk to the patient is very low and required treatment is accordingly minimal. At higher levels, hypertension becomes a rapidly deadly disease, requiring very aggressive treatment. In between, there is a range of more and less severe presentations. This heterogeneity results in what may appear to be complex protocols to explain treatment of a simple problem. However, this approach, we believe, represents our best attempt to appropriately tailor treatment according to risk while avoiding unnecessary testing or referrals.

PROTOCOL 8.1 **Initial Screening and Management of Hypertension in Adults in Acute Consultation Clinics**

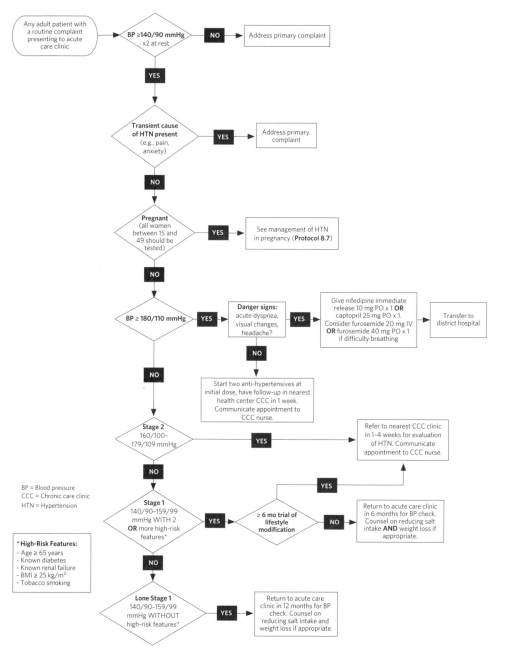

BP = Blood pressure
CCC = Chronic care clinic
HTN = Hypertension

* High-Risk Features:
- Age ≥ 65 years
- Known diabetes
- Known renal failure
- BMI ≥ 25 kg/m²
- Tobacco smoking

In this chapter we give detailed explanations of the reasoning behind each of the protocols for hypertension.

8.1.1 Evaluation of Blood Pressure in Acute Care Clinics

Acute care clinicians should check the blood pressure of any adult
($\geq$ 15 years) patient presenting with a routine complaint. We discuss
evaluation of blood pressure in children in **SECTION 8.6**. If the blood
pressure measures less than 140/90 mmHg, the clinician proceeds with
the visit as usual. If the blood pressure measures $\geq$ 140/90 mmHg, the
clinician rechecks the blood pressure, making sure that the patient is at
rest and that the cuff size is appropriate.

If both measurements are greater than or equal to 140/90 mmHg, the
clinician looks for and addresses any identifiable transient cause of
hypertension (e.g., pain or anxiety).

Female patients between age 15 and 49 are tested for pregnancy. For
management of hypertension in pregnancy, see **PROTOCOL 8.7** and
SECTION 8.9.

The clinician then evaluates the patient's level of hypertension and
treats accordingly.

8.1.2 Identification and Treatment of Emergency Conditions in Acute Consultation

Patients with symptomatic stage 3 hypertension ($\geq$ 180/110 mmHg)
receive fast-acting anti-hypertensive therapy (**TABLE 8.4**) and are
transferred to the district hospital for inpatient management
(see **SECTION 8.4**).

8.1.3 Treatment of Asymptomatic Hypertension by Disease Classification

Asymptomatic stage 3 hypertension patients are started on two antihypertensives and given a follow-up appointment in the nearest health
center integrated chronic care clinic within the next week. **SECTION 8.3**
discusses our rationale for drug choices, and **TABLE 8.2** and **TABLE 8.3**
outline initial antihypertensive treatment for stable patients.

In all cases of referral to the health center integrated chronic care clinic,
the acute care clinician must communicate the referral to the chronic
care clinician, either through a shared written patient log book and/or
through the electronic medical record system.

8.1.3.1 Stage 2 Hypertension (160/100–179/109 mmHg)

Patients with stage 2 hypertension (160/100–180/110 mmHg) are not
started on any medications in the acute setting. They are referred to
the nearest health center integrated chronic care clinic in a non-urgent
fashion. This approach ensures confirmation of the diagnosis prior to
initiation of therapy in patients at low risk for short-term complications.

8.1.3.2   Stage 1 Hypertension (140/90–159/99) with High-Risk Features

Patients with stage 1 hypertension are evaluated for high-risk features that may warrant more aggressive treatment of blood pressure. High-risk features include known diabetes or renal failure, overweight (BMI ≥ 25 kg/m2), tobacco use, or age greater than 65 (**TABLE 8.1**). Clinicians already routinely measure height and weight and use a chart to find the corresponding BMI for all patients as part of adult malnutrition screening in acute care. In addition, patients are asked about tobacco use and previous diagnosis of diabetes. Information on prior diagnoses can often be obtained from the patient-carried medical record.

Each risk factor earns a patient a certain number of points. Risk factors such as diabetes and renal failure confer more risk than the other risk factors and are weighted more heavily. Patients with 2 or more points are considered high risk and are treated more aggressively.

TABLE 8.1   High-Risk Features in Hypertension

High-risk feature	Points
Diagnosis of diabetes	2
Diagnosis of renal failure (creatinine ≥ 100 μmol/L (1.1 mg/dL))	2
Age ≥ 65 years	1
BMI ≥ 25 kg/m2	1
Tobacco smoking	1
A total of 2 or more points is considered high risk and warrants more aggressive treatment.	

Patients with stage 1 hypertension (140/90–159/99 mmHg) who have two or more high-risk features are counseled on reducing salt intake and, if appropriate, on the benefits of weight loss. They are asked to return to acute care in six months. If still hypertensive after a six-month trial of lifestyle modification, the patient is referred to the nearest integrated chronic care clinic within 1 to 4 weeks. The clinician does not initiate anti-hypertensive therapy in the acute care setting.

8.1.3.3   Low-Risk Stage 1 Hypertension

Patients with stage 1 hypertension and fewer than two risk points are at low risk of complications from their hypertension. For this reason, we advocate delaying pharmocologic treatment and/or referral to integrated chronic care clinics for these patients. These patients are counseled to avoid added salt and instructed to return to the acute care clinic in one year for a repeat blood pressure measurement. Patients with a BMI ≥ 25 are also counseled on the benefits of weight loss.

8.2 Initial Management of Newly Referred Adult Hypertension Cases in Health Center Integrated Chronic Care Clinics

PROTOCOL 8.2 outlines the initial management of newly referred hypertension cases in integrated chronic care clinics.

PROTOCOL 8.2 Initial Management of Newly Referred Adult Hypertension Cases in Health Center Integrated Chronic Care Clinics

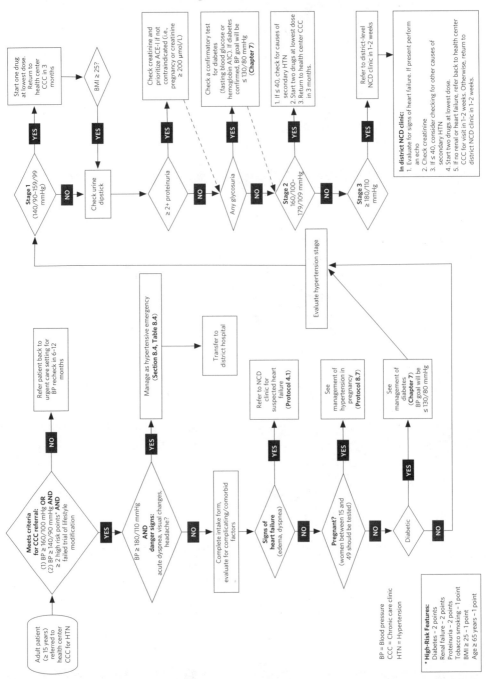

Adult patients referred to the integrated chronic care clinic for elevated blood pressure first undergo confirmation of hypertension. If the patient has a blood pressure < 140/90 mmHg, the patient is reassured and dismissed from the clinic.

If the patient has confirmed hypertension, clinicians further classify patients into levels of risk and initiate therapy accordingly. Only patients who have a blood pressure ≥ 160/100 mmHg confirmed on two separate visits, or who have a blood pressure between 140/90 and 159/99 mmHg with two or more high-risk features (**TABLE 8.1**) despite a 6-month trial of salt reduction and/or weight loss, if indicated, should enroll in an integrated chronic care clinic for pharmacologic treatment. Others should be referred back to the acute care clinic for repeat blood pressure measurement in 6–12 months.

8.2.1 Identification and Treatment of Emergency Conditions in the Health Center Integrated Chronic Care Clinic

Patients with stage 3 hypertension (≥ 180/110 mmHg) should be evaluated for symptoms of hypertensive emergency. Those with signs of end-organ effects from the elevated blood pressure (e.g., acute dyspnea, headache, or visual changes) should receive fast-acting anti-hypertensive therapy (**TABLE 8.4**) and are transferred to the district hospital for inpatient management. See **SECTION 8.4** for management guidelines for hypertensive emergency.

8.2.2 Evaluation for Comorbid Conditions in the Health Center Integrated Chronic Care Clinic

If the patient shows no signs of hypertensive emergency, the chronic care clinician proceeds with the standardized intake form (**APPENDIX D**), which includes information on the presence of complicating or co-morbid factors. This intake process should take approximately five minutes.

Initial patient history and physical exam may reveal signs of heart failure, including increased respiratory rate and peripheral edema. As mentioned earlier, patients with an acute elevation in blood pressure can develop symptoms of heart failure. These patients should be treated according to the guidelines for management of hypertensive emergency (**SECTION 8.4**). However, some patients who have high blood pressure will have chronic heart failure as a result of long-standing hypertension (hypertensive heart disease). Patients with symptoms of chronic heart failure such as chronic dyspnea and edema should be evaluated as suspected heart failure patients (see **CHAPTER 4**).Women between the ages of 15–49 are tested for pregnancy, and pregnant patients are managed according to **PROTOCOL 8.7**.

Patients with known diabetes are at much greater risk of complications from hypertension and will warrant more aggressive treatment. We initiate anti-hypertensive medications in these patients at a blood pressure of ≥ 130/90 mmHg. See **CHAPTER 7** for further detail on management of diabetic patients.

8.2.3   Evaluation of Hypertension Stage in the Health Center Integrated Chronic Care Clinic

After assessing for comorbid/complicating factors and evidence of hypertensive emergency, patients are classified according to hypertension severity. Patients with higher degrees of hypertension and/or comorbid factors receive more aggressive treatment according to the high-risk, point-based system above (**TABLE 8.1**). **TABLE 8.2** outlines the initial treatment strategy based on risk and hypertension category. **SECTION 8.3** and **TABLE 8.3** outline a step-by-step approach to antihypertensive medication selection.

8.2.3.1   Treatment of Higher-Risk Stage 1 Hypertension in the Health Center Integrated Chronic Care Clinic

Patients with higher-risk stage 1 hypertension (BP 140/90–159/99 mmHg and ≥ 2 high risk points; see **TABLE 8.1**) who have failed a six-month trial of lifestyle modification should be started on one antihypertensive at the starting dose (**TABLE 8.3**). Patients with diabetes or renal failure will also fall into this category. These patients should follow up at the health center chronic care clinic for a blood pressure check and medication dose titration in three months.

8.2.3.2   Evaluation of Proteinuria in Stage 2 and Stage 3 Hypertension in the Health Center Integrated Chronic Care Clinic

Patients with stage 2 or greater hypertension (BP ≥ 160/100 mmHg) are at increased risk of developing renal failure. The presence of renal failure in these patients will change treatment strategies. For this reason, we advocate checking a urine dipstick for proteinuria as a rough marker of renal dysfunction. Patients with greater than 2+ proteinuria should be referred to the district hosptial to have their creatinine checked. Patients with a creatinine less than 200 µmol/L and proteinuria should be started on an ACE inhibitor as first-line therapy for its established renal protective effects.

8.2.3.3   Evaluation of Glycosuria in Stage 2 and Stage 3 Hypertension or Overweight Patients in the Health Center Integrated Chronic Care Clinic

Patients with hypertension and overweight are at increased risk for diabetes. Those who are found to have any glucose on their urine dipstick should receive confirmatory testing with either a fasting glucose or a hemoglobin A1C. Patients confirmed to have diabetes should be managed according to the diabetes guidelines in **CHAPTER 7**. They will also have a lower goal blood pressure of ≤ 130/90 mmHg.

8.2.3.4   Treatment of Stage 2 Hypertension in the Health Center
           Integrated Chronic Care Clinic

Patients with stage 2 hypertension (BP 160/100–179/109) should be started on two antihypertensives at starting doses (**TABLE 8.3**). Two drugs are started because this level of hypertension is usually not controlled with one agent alone. These patients should follow up in 3 months at the health center chronic care clinic.

8.2.3.5   Treatment of Asymptomatic Stage 3 Hypertension in the
           Health Center Integrated Chronic Care Clinic

Patients with asymptomatic stage 3 hypertension should likewise be started on two-drug therapy at starting doses (**TABLE 8.3**). Given their degree of hypertension, these patients are at high risk of complications, such as heart and renal failure. They should all be referred to the district level NCD clinic for further evaluation urgently, within 1–2 weeks.

In the district NCD clinic, patients should be re-evaluated for signs of heart failure. Patients with any such signs or symptoms likely have hypertensive heart disease and should have an echocardiograph per-formed (see **CHAPTER 4** and **PROTOCOL 4.1** for diagnosis of heart failure).

All patients should have creatinine levels checked. Patients under 40 who have a normal creatinine should have other causes of secondary hypertension investigated (**PROTOCOL 8.3**).

Patients should be started on two anti-hypertensive medications at the lowest dose. Patients without evidence of heart or renal failure may be referred back to the health center chronic care clinic for ongoing management. There they should continue to be followed closely with follow-up visits every 1–2 weeks until their treatment is stabilized. Pa-tients with evidence of heart or renal failure or those who have second-ary hypertension will require continued follow-up at the district-level NCD clinic.

TABLE 8.2   Initiation of Hypertension Treatment According to Stage and Risk Factors

Stage	Blood pressure range	Treatment	Clinic follow-up
Stage 1 **AND** ≤ 1 high risk point (**TABLE 8.1**)	140/90-159/99 mmHg	Do not start medications. Counsel on salt intake and weight loss if indicated.	12 months in acute care
Stage 1 **AND** ≥ 2 high risk points (**TABLE 8.1**) **AND** No trial of lifestyle modification	140/90-159/99 mmHg	Do not start medications. Counsel on salt intake and weight loss if indicated.	6 months in acute care
Stage 1 **AND** ≥ 2 high risk points (**TABLE 8.1**) **AND** Failed 6-month trial of lifestyle modification	140/90-159/99 mmHg	Start first-line medication at lowest dose	3 months in health center integrated chronic care clinic
Stage 2	160/100-179/109 mmHg	Start first- and second-line medications at lowest dose	3 months in health center integrated chronic care clinic
Stage 3 **WITHOUT** Danger signs*	≥ 180/110+ mmHg	Start first- and second-line medications at lowest dose	1-2 weeks in district level NCD clinic
Stage 3 **WITH** Danger signs*	≥ 180/110+ mmHg	Initiate therapy listed in **TABLE 8.4**. Transfer to district hospital for inpatient management	

* Danger signs include acute dyspnea, visual changes, headaches.

8.3   Recommended Hypertension Medications and Dosing

TABLE 8.3 shows the usual order in which medications should be started for hypertension management in adults. This order was chosen based on safety, side-effect profile, cost, and ease of dosing. Just as some of these factors (such as cost) vary between countries, so may the ordering of preferred anti-hypertensive medications in different settings. **APPENDIX B** lists our cost estimates for each medication.

In the presence of some comorbid conditions, such as proteinuria, renal failure, and pregnancy, different medications may be preferred. These exceptions are noted in the text below and in **TABLE 8.5, TABLE 8.6**, and **TABLE 8.15**.

First-line agents. For most patients, hydrochlorothiazide is the best medication to start initially. It is extraordinarily cheap, taken only once a day, and the incidence of clinically significant side effects such as hypokalemia are low. However, in some circumstances, such as pregnancy, renal failure, or diabetes, a different medication should be used first (see **TABLE 8.5, TABLE 8.6, and TABLE 8.15**).

Second-line agents. When a patient's dose of the first-line medication has been maximized without achieving adequate blood pressure control, another medication must be started. For most patients, this will be an indication for starting a calcium-channel blocker (such as amlodipine or nifedipine). Patients with stage 2 or 3 hypertension will likely need at least 2 medications to achieve blood pressure control. In these situations, patients should be initiated on the starting dose of both the first- and second-line agents at their first visit.

Third-line agents. In many patients, two medications even at their maximum dose may not be enough to achieve blood pressure control. This is particularly true for patients with stage 3 hypertension. ACE inhibitors (lisinopril or captopril) are the preferred third-line agent after the maximum dose of hydrochlorthiazide and amlodipine have been reached. ACE inhibitors are contraindicated in pregnancy and renal failure (creatinine ≥ 200 µmol/L).

Fourth-line agents. Some patients may have hypertension that is particularly resistant to blood pressure medications. Four medications for hypertension may be needed. In general, atenolol is the fourth-line antihypertensive of choice. Although it is inexpensive, the effectiveness of atenolol in reducing central blood pressure and preventing adverse cardiovascular outcomes has been called into question.[13]

Fifth-line agents. These medications should rarely be used for hypertension management in the absence of a specific indication. Although effective, methyldopa and hydralazine require multiple doses per day and cost significantly more than other available medication. Paradoxically, these medications are frequently the most available in resource-poor settings due to their safety in pregnancy (see **SECTION 8.9**).

TABLE 8.3 Recommended Hypertension Medications and Dosing for Most Adult Patients

First-line drug	Starting dose	Increase dose by	Maximum dose	Notes
Hydrochlorothiazide	12.5 mg 1x/day	12.5 mg 1x/day	25 mg 1x/day	Can cause hypokalemia Not effective in the setting of severe renal failure (creatinine ≥ 300 µmol/L)
Second-line drug	**Starting dose**	**Increase dose by**	**Maximum dose**	**Notes**
Amlodipine	5 mg 1x/day	5 mg 1x/day	10 mg 1x/day	Can cause lower-extremity edema
Third-line drug	**Starting Dose**	**Increase dose by**	**Maximum dose**	**Notes**
Lisinopril	5 mg 1x/day	5 mg 1x/day	20 mg 1x/day	Contraindicated in pregnancy and renal failure (creatinine ≥ 200 µmol/L)
Captopril	12.5 mg 3x/day	12.5 mg 3x/day	50 mg 3x/day	Can cause cough
Fourth-line drug	**Starting dose**	**Increase dose by**	**Maximum dose**	**Notes**
Atenolol	25 mg 1x/day	25 mg 1x/day	50 mg 1x/day	Contraindicated if heart rate ≤ 55 bpm Use with caution in renal failure, since atenolol is renally cleared
Fifth-line drug	**Starting dose**	**Increase dose by**	**Maximum dose**	**Notes**
Hydralazine	25 mg 3x/day	25 mg 3x/day	50 mg 3x/day	Safe in pregnancy Headache common side effect of hydralazine
Methyldopa	250 mg 2x/day	250 mg 2x/day	500 mg 2x/day	Safe in pregnancy

8.4 Recognition and Management of Hypertensive Emergency in Adults

Acute rises in blood pressure can result in end-organ damage in a matter of hours. These hypertensive emergencies usually occur at blood pressures above 180 mmHg systolic or 110 mmHg diastolic. Signs of a hypertensive emergency include headache and blurred vision caused by increased intracranial pressure, dyspnea caused by an acute stiffening of the heart and back-up of fluid into the lungs, and hematuria or flank pain caused by injury to the kidneys.

Patients reporting such symptoms with blood pressures of 180/110 mmHg or greater should be treated immediately with medications to lower their blood pressure by approximately 25% in the first hour.

Because the body adjusts to hypertension over time, lowering blood pressure too rapidly can decrease blood flow to the brain and cause clinical deterioration. **TABLE 8.4** lists medications recommended for acute management of hypertensive emergency.

All patients with suspected hypertensive emergency should be transferred to the nearest district hospital for inpatient management.

TABLE 8.4   **Recommended Medications for Management of Hypertensive Emergency (Adult Dosing)**

Medication	Dosing	Notes
Nifedipine (immediate release)	10 mg orally	
Captopril	25 mg orally	Contraindicated in pregnancy and renal failure (Cr ≥ 200 µmol/L)
Hydralazine	25 mg orally	
Furosemide	40 mg orally or 20 mg IV	If evidence of pulmonary congestion

8.5   Renal Dysfunction in Hypertension

Hypertension and renal dysfunction often coexist. When the kidneys no longer work well enough to dispose of excess fluid, blood pressure may increase. Hypertension may also lead to renal failure by putting increased stress on the kidney's filtering system. Controlling blood pressure with antihypertensives can slow the progression of renal disease. However, certain medications are either dangerous or no longer work well in the setting of renal failure, as explained below.

TABLE 8.5   Hypertension Medications and Dosing in Setting of Proteinuria
or Mild Renal Failure (CKD 1-3, Creatinine 100–199 μmol/L)

First-line drug	Starting dose	Increase dose by	Maximum dose	Notes
Lisinopril	5 mg 1x/day	5 mg 1x/day	20 mg 1x/day	Contraindicated in pregnancy and renal failure (creatinine ≥ 200 μmol/L)
Captopril	12.5 mg 3x/day	12.5 mg 3x/day	50 mg 3x/day	Can cause cough
Second-line drug	**Starting dose**	**Increase dose by**	**Maximum dose**	**Notes**
Hydrochlorothiazide	12.5 mg 1x/day	12.5 mg 1x/day	25 mg 1x/day	Can cause hypokalemia Not effective in the setting of severe renal failure (creatinine ≥ 300 μmol/L)
Third-line drug	**Starting dose**	**Increase dose by**	**Maximum dose**	**Notes**
Amlodipine	5 mg 1x/day	5 mg 1x/day	10 mg 1x/day	Can cause lower-extremity edema
Fourth-line drug	**Starting dose**	**Increase dose by**	**Maximum dose**	**Notes**
Atenolol	25 mg 1x/day	25 mg 1x/day	50 mg 1x/day	Contraindicated if heart rate ≤ 55 bpm Use with caution in renal failure as is renally cleared
Fifth-line drug	**Starting dose**	**Increase dose by**	**Maximum dose**	**Notes**
Hydralazine	25 mg 3x/day	25 mg 3x/day	50 mg 3x/day	Safe in pregnancy. Headache common side effect
Methyldopa	250 mg 2x/day	250 mg 2x/day	500 mg 2x/day	Safe in pregnancy

8.5.1   Proteinuria or Mild to Moderate Renal Failure (Creatinine between 100–199 μmol/L)

Proteinuria is an early sign of renal dysfunction. Mild to moderate renal failure (chronic kidney disease stages 1 through 3) is typically present at creatinine levels between 100 and 199 μmol/L in adults. ACE inhibitors help decrease proteinuria and prevent further renal damage in this setting. ACE inhibitors should be started as the first-line agent in all patients with proteinuria or mild to moderate renal failure unless contraindications are present. Contraindications include a creatinine level ≥ 200 μmol/L (≥ 2.3 mg/dL) and pregnancy.

TABLE 8.6   Recommended Hypertension Medications and Dosing in Setting of Severe Renal Failure (Creatinine ≥ 200 μmol/L)

First-line drug		Starting dose	Increase dose by	Maximum dose	Notes
If Cr < 300 μmol/L	Hydrochlorothiazide	12.5 mg 1x/day	12.5 mg 1x/day	25 mg 1x/day	Can cause hypokalemia
If Cr ≥ 300 μmol/L	Furosemide	20 mg 1x/day	20 mg 1x/day	40 mg 1x/day	

Second-line drug	Starting dose	Increase dose by	Maximum dose	Notes
Amlodipine	5 mg 1x/day	5 mg 1x/day	10 mg 1x/day	Can cause lower-extremity edema

Third-line drug	Starting dose	Increase dose by	Maximum dose	Notes
Atenolol	25 mg 1x/day	25 mg 1x/day	100 mg 1x/day	Contraindicated if heart rate ≤ 55 bpm Use with caution in renal failure

Fourth-line drug	Starting dose	Increase dose by	Maximum dose	Notes
Hydralazine	25 mg 3x/day	25 mg 3x/day	50 mg 3x/day	Safe in pregnancy Headache common side effect
Methyldopa	250 mg 2x/day	250 mg 2x/day	500 mg 2x/day	Safe in pregnancy

If a patient is found to have a severely elevated creatinine ≥ 200 μmol/L (≥ 2.3 mg/dL), hydrochlorothiazide should still be the first-line agent. However, in the case of even more severe renal dysfunction (creatinine ≥ 300 μmol/L or 3.4 mg/dL), hydrochlorothiazide loses its efficacy. In this scenario, a loop diuretic (furosemide) should be substituted as the first-line agent. Calcium-channel blockers (amlodipine and nifedipine) are also safe in renal failure, and should be the next choice. Atenolol can also be used, but the dose should not exceed 50 mg/day in these patients. This is because atenolol is excreted by the kidneys. ACE inhibitors and spironolactone should be avoided due to the risk of hyperkalemia. Because these patients are at risk for multiple complications, they should be followed at the level of the district hospital.

8.6 Evaluation and Management of Hypertension in Patients ≥ 15

Most essential hypertension will occur in patients over the age of 40. If a patient presents with moderate to severe hypertension at a younger age, secondary causes of hypertension are more likely to be a cause (see **TABLE 8.7**). **PROTOCOL 8.3** outlines a diagnostic approach to patients between the ages of 15 and 40. **SECTION 8.8** discusses an approach to hypertension in children younger than 15.

PROTOCOL 8.3 Initial Diagnosis and Management of Suspected Secondary Hypertension in Adults (age ≥ 15)

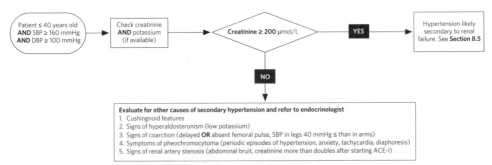

Renal failure, often due to chronic glomerulonephritis, is by far the most common reason for secondary hypertension in settings such as rural Africa. Therefore, adult patients who are under 40 years of age with blood pressure over 160 mmHg systolic or 100 mmHg diastolic should be referred to a health facility where creatinine can be checked. If creatinine is normal, the patient should be evaluated for other signs or symptoms suggestive of a secondary cause of hypertension, and referred accordingly. While investigating the secondary cause of hypertension, treatment may be initiated according to the protocol for hypertension (see **PROTOCOL 8.2**).

TABLE 8.7   Causes of Secondary Hypertension

Cause	Findings	Management
Renal failure	Elevated creatinine (≥ 200 µmol/L or 2x normal creatinine for age in children)	See **SECTION 8.5** for adults and **SECTION 8.8.4** for children
Cushing's syndrome (hypercortisolism)	Truncal obesity, round face, extremity wasting, hypokalemia	Refer to tertiary referral center for endocrinology consultation
Hyperaldosteronism	Hypokalemia	Refer to tertiary referral center for endocrinology consultation
Pheochromocytoma	Periodic episodes of hypertension, anxiety, tachycardia, diaphoresis	Refer to tertiary referral center for endocrinology consultation
Coarctation	Delayed or absent femoral pulse; SBP in legs 40 mmHg ≤ than SBP in arms	Refer to tertiary referral center for echocardiography and cardiology consultation
Renal artery stenosis	Abdominal bruit; creatinine more than doubles after starting ACE inhibitor	Refer to tertiary referral center for renal ultrasound and nephrology consultation

8.7   Follow-Up Treatment for Hypertension in Adults

PROTOCOL 8.4 outlines an approach to ongoing management of adult patients who are followed in the chronic care clinics for hypertension.

PROTOCOL 8.4   Follow-Up Visit for Chronic Hypertension in Adults at Health Center Integrated Chronic Care Clinic

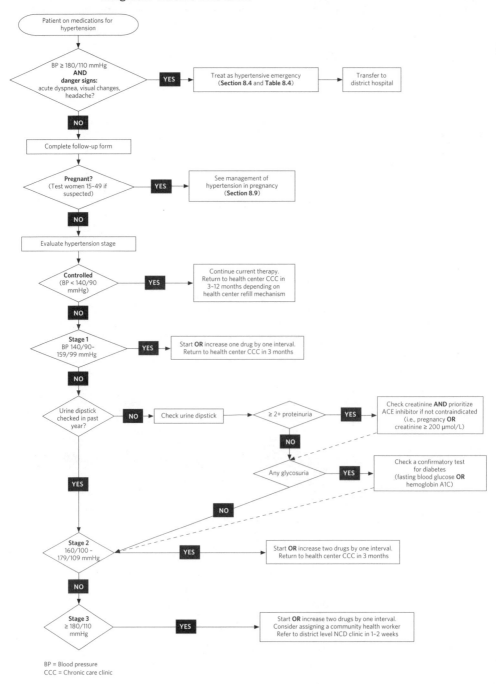

BP = Blood pressure
CCC = Chronic care clinic

On return visits, the clinician should re-evaluate the patient, first for signs of hypertensive emergency, and then for any change in complicating or comorbid factors. The clinician should then review the effectiveness and appropriateness of the current medication regimen.

8.7.1   Management of Well-Controlled Hypertension on Follow-Up

Patients with well-controlled hypertension should have their current regimen continued. These patients do not need to be seen in the clinic very often. However, it may be difficult for the pharmacy to give patients multi-month supplies of medication without causing stock-outs. Therefore, the time between clinic visits will depend mostly on the dispensing capacity of the pharmacy and the refill policy of the health center.

8.7.2   Follow-Up of Stage 1 Hypertension

For patients with stage 1 hypertension (between 140/90 and 159/99 mmHg), the blood pressure medication should be increased by one interval (see **TABLE 8.3**).

8.7.3   Follow-Up of Stage 2 Hypertension

Patients with stage 2 hypertension (between 160/100 and 179/109 mmHg) should have two medications started or increased by one interval (see **TABLE 8.3**). Patients in this category should have a urine dipstick checked once a year. Patients with proteinuria and a creatinine level < 200 µmol/L should have an ACE inhibitor started as part of their regimen. Patients with any glycosuria should undergo a confirmatory test for diabetes, such as a hemoglobin A1C or a fasting glucose finger-stick.

8.7.4   Follow-Up of Stage 3 Hypertension

Patients with stage 3 hypertension (≥ 180/110 mmHg) should also have two medications started or increased by one interval (see **TABLE 8.3**). Patients in this category should also have a urine dipstick checked once a year, and patients with proteinuria should have an ACE inhibitor started as part of their regimen. Patients with any glycosuria should undergo a confirmatory test for diabetes, such as a hemoglobin A1C or a fasting glucose finger-stick. In addition, patients in this category need closer follow-up and should be given an appointment within 1–2 weeks. Some of these patients may benefit from a community health worker to provide support and ensure good medication adherence.

8.8   Diagnosis and Management of Hypertension in Children (Age < 15)

Hypertension in children (defined here as ≥ 95th percentile systolic or diastolic blood pressure for age) is rare, but when present often signals serious disease. Most hypertension in children is due to secondary causes (see **TABLE 8.7**). The most common secondary cause is renal failure.

8.8.1 Initial Diagnosis of Hypertension in Children

PROTOCOL 8.5 outlines an approach to the initial management of pediatric patients found to have hypertension. Blood pressure is not routinely measured on all children presenting to health-center acute care clinics. Children only need to have blood pressure checked if there are signs or symptoms that are concerning for either elevated or low blood pressure. These should include any child presenting to the health center with edema or complaints about changes in urine color. Children who have new onset seizures or are ill-appearing should also have their blood pressure checked. Health centers must be stocked with functioning pediatric cuffs. In cases in which a pediatric cuff is not available, clinicians should use the small adult cuff (the standard cuff for a low BMI population) as a thigh cuff. Appropriate cuff size is when 100% of the bladder of the cuff wraps around the circumference of the arm. When in doubt, choose the larger cuff size, as too small a cuff will give falsely high BP readings. Table 8.8 lists blood pressure percentiles for age for children (< 15 years). This information is also listed in **APPENDIX E.** We define hypertension in a child as a systolic or diastolic blood pressure ≥ 95th percentile for age.

PROTOCOL 8.5 Initial Diagnosis and Management of Hypertension in Children in the Acute Care Clinic

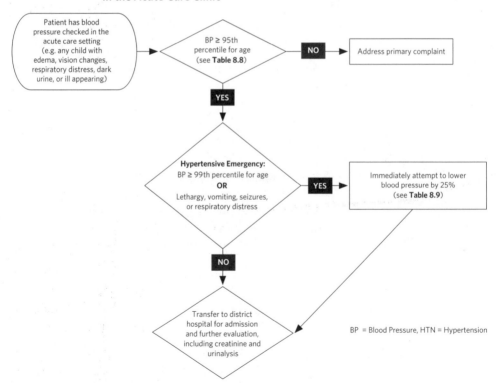

TABLE 8.8   Blood pressure ranges for children

Age (year)		Blood pressure percentile (mmHg) (for 25th percentile of height)			
		50th percentile	90th percentile	95th percentile	99th percentile
1	Systolic	83	97	101	108
	Diastolic	36	51	55	63
2	Systolic	87	100	104	111
	Diastolic	41	56	60	68
3	Systolic	89	103	107	114
	Diastolic	45	60	64	72
4	Systolic	91	105	109	116
	Diastolic	49	64	68	76
5	Systolic	93	106	110	118
	Diastolic	52	67	71	79
6	Systolic	94	108	112	119
	Diastolic	54	69	73	81
7	Systolic	95	109	113	120
	Diastolic	56	71	75	83
8	Systolic	97	110	114	122
	Diastolic	58	72	77	85
9	Systolic	98	112	116	123
	Diastolic	59	74	78	86
10	Systolic	100	114	117	125
	Diastolic	60	74	79	86
11	Systolic	102	115	119	127
	Diastolic	60	75	79	87
12	Systolic	104	118	122	129
	Diastolic	61	75	80	88
13	Systolic	106	120	124	131
	Diastolic	61	76	80	88
14	Systolic	109	123	127	134
	Diastolic	62	77	81	89
15	Systolic	112	125	129	136
	Diastolic	63	78	82	90

8.8.2 Recognition and Management of Hypertensive Emergency in Children

Patients with a very high blood pressure (≥ 99th percentile for age) and/or signs of severe end-organ damage, such as lethargy, severe headaches or vision changes, seizures or respiratory distress, should have their blood pressure lowered by 25% if possible while transport is being arranged. **TABLE 8.9** lists medications and dosing to acutely reduce blood pressure in pediatric patients. As in adults, dropping blood pressure too quickly can be very dangerous. If correct dosing is not available for smaller children, the clinician should focus on fast transfer and avoid over-medication.

TABLE 8.9 Recommended Medications and Dosing for Pediatric Patients For Hypertensive Emergency (BP ≥ 99th percentile or ≥ 95th percentile with symptoms)

	< 10 kg	10 kg	15 kg	20 kg	30 kg	≥ 40 kg
Hydralazine 50 mg tablet	See mg/kg dosing*	See mg/kg dosing*	See mg/kg dosing*	12.5 mg ¼ tab x 1	12.5 mg ¼ tab x 1	25 mg ½ tab x 1
Initial dose: 0.5 mg/kg/dose. **Maximum dose:** 25 mg/dose.						
Nifedipine 10 mg tablet	See mg/kg dosing*	2.5 mg ¼ tab x 1	5 mg ½ tab x 1	10 mg 1 tab x 1	10 mg 1 tab x 1	10 mg 1 tab x 1
Initial dose: 0.25-0.5 mg/kg/dose. **Maximum dose:** 10 mg/dose.						
Captopril 25 mg tablet	See mg/kg dosing*	6.25 mg ¼ tab x 1	6.25 mg ¼ tab x 1	12.5 mg ½ tab x 1	12.5 mg ½ tab x 1	25 mg 1 tab x 1
Initial dose: 0.3-0.5 mg/kg/dose. **Maximum dose:** 3 mg/kg/dose.						

* Note that dosing medications for small children may require crushing pills and diluting. This should only be done under the supervision of an experienced clinician.

8.8.3 Initial Management of Children with Hypertension

Children with newly diagnosed hypertension (≥ the 95th percentile for age) who are not in a hypertensive crisis do not need their blood pressure acutely decreased before being admitted to the hospital. However, these children should still be hospitalized for an evaluation of the cause of the hypertension and initiation of treatment.

In the inpatient setting, renal function should be evaluated with a creatinine and urinalysis. Most children will be found to have signs of renal dysfunction due to post-streptococcal glomerulonephritis, nephrotic syndrome, or untreated severe urinary tract infection. If renal function is normal, other causes of secondary hypertension should be investigated. These secondary causes are similar to those seen in young adults with hypertension (see **TABLE 8.7**).

8.8.4   Follow-Up of Children with Hypertension

After discharge, children should follow up in the district NCD clinic within 1–2 weeks for blood pressure evaluation and medication adjustment (see **PROTOCOL 8.6**).

On a follow-up visit, the child should be evaluated for level of blood pressure as well as signs and symptoms of organ dysfunction. If there has been a change in clinical status, creatinine should be checked, if available. Children and their family members should be asked about medication adherence. Some children may benefit from a community health worker if adherence is a problem.

Children who have well-controlled blood pressure (< 90th percentile for age) should be kept on their current regimen. Care for these children may be transferred to the health-center level for at least some of their visits if this is more convenient for the patient and family. As a general rule, these children should be seen every 1–3 months at the health center and 2 times per year in the district NCD clinic. Children with difficult-to-control blood pressure or renal failure should continue to be followed primarily at the district hospital, where electrolytes can be monitored.

If the patient has a persistently elevated blood pressure and signs or symptoms of a hypertensive emergency, the child should be managed as described above (**SECTION 8.8.2**, **TABLE 8.9**) and re-hospitalized.

Children with mildly to moderately elevated blood pressure (≥ 90th percentile for age) despite good adherence to their medication regimen should have their antihypertensive medication dosing increased (see **TABLE 8.10**). As with adults, one medication should be increased until either the maximum dose is reached or side effects are encountered. At this point, a second agent should be added. Children should have follow-up visits every 2–4 weeks in the district NCD clinic until blood pressure is controlled.

PROTOCOL 8.6 Outpatient Follow-Up of Children with Hypertension

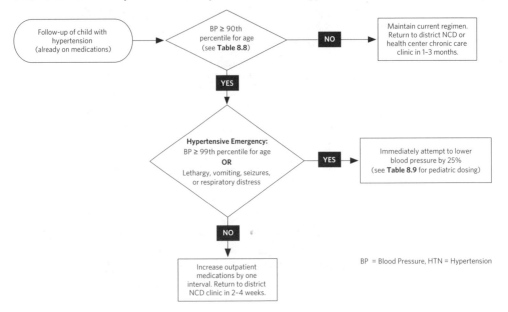

TABLE 8.10 Recommended Medications and Dosing for Pediatric Patients with Chronic Hypertension (BP ≥ 95th percentile)

First-line drug						
Starting doses	≤ 10 kg	10 kg	15 kg	20 kg	30 kg	≥ 40 kg
Hydrochlorothiazide 25 mg tablet	See mg/kg dosing*	12.5 mg ½ tab daily	12.5 mg ½ tab daily	25 mg 1 tab daily	25 mg 1 tab daily	25 mg 1 tab daily

Initial dose: 1 mg/kg/day as one daily dose.

Maximum dose: 3 mg/kg/day as one daily dose, up to 25 mg/day.

Notes: May cause hypokalemia. Doses higher than 25 mg increase risk of hypokalemia without much additional blood pressure control. Use with caution in newborns, as they are more sensitive to electrolyte shifts. Should be stopped if progressive renal failure occurs.

Second-line drug						
Starting doses	≤ 10 kg	10 kg	15 kg	20 kg	30 kg	≥ 40 kg
Amlodipine 10 mg tablet	See mg/kg dosing*	2.5 mg ¼ tab daily	2.5 mg ¼ tab daily	2.5–5 mg ¼–½ tab daily	2.5–5 mg ¼–½ tab daily	5–10 mg ½–1 tab daily

Initial dose: 0.1 mg/kg/day.

Maximum dose: 10 mg once daily.

Notes: Not well studied in children less than 6 years of age.

Third-line drug						
Starting doses	**≤ 10 kg**	**10 kg**	**15 kg**	**20 kg**	**30 kg**	**≥ 40 kg**
Lisinopril 10 mg tablet	See mg/kg dosing*	See mg/kg dosing*	See mg/kg dosing*	2.5–5 mg ¼–½ tab daily	2.5–5 mg ¼–½ tab daily	5–10 mg ½–1 tab daily

Initial dose: 0.07 mg/kg/day as one daily dose.

Maximum dose: 0.6 mg/kg/day or 20 mg as one daily dose.

Notes: Contraindicated in pregnancy and renal failure (creatinine ≥ 2x normal for age). Can cause cough.

Captopril 25 mg tablet	See mg/kg dosing*	6.25 mg ¼ tab 2x/day	6.25 mg ¼ tab 2x/day	6.25–12.5 mg ¼–½ tab 2x/day	6.25–12.5 mg ¼–½ tab 2x/day	12.5–25 mg ½–1 tab 2x/day

Initial dose: 0.3–0.5 mg/kg/dose given 2 times/day.

Maximum dose: 6 mg/kg/day divided into 2 doses/day.

Notes: Contraindicated in pregnancy and renal failure (creatinine ≥ 2x normal for age). Can cause cough.

Fourth-line drug						
Starting doses	**≤ 10 kg**	**10 kg**	**15 kg**	**20 kg**	**30 kg**	**≥ 40 kg**
Atenolol 50 mg tablet	See mg/kg dosing*	12.5 mg ¼ tab daily	12.5 mg ¼ tab daily	12.5–25 mg ¼–½ tab daily	25 mg ½ tab daily	25–50 mg ½–1 tab daily

Initial dose: 0.5–1 mg/kg/day as one daily dose.

Maximum dose: 2 mg/kg/day as one daily dose, up to 100 mg/day.

Notes: Contraindicated if heart rate ≤ normal HR range for age. In renal failure, use half of normal recommended dose.

Add if edema or Stage 4 chronic kidney disease (CKD 4)						
	≤ 10 kg	**10 kg**	**15 kg**	**20 kg**	**30 kg**	**≥ 40 kg**
Furosemide 40 mg tablet	See mg/kg dosing*	10 mg ¼ tab daily	10–20 mg ¼ tab daily	20 mg ½ tab daily	20–40 mg ½–1 tab daily	20–80 mg ½–2 tabs daily

Oral

Initial dose: 1–2 mg/kg/day as 1–2 doses. Do not start at more than 20 mg/dose.

Maximum dose: 4 mg/kg/dose given 2–4 times/day.

Increase by: 1 mg/kg/dose.

Note: Need to give higher dose range in renal failure.

* Dosing medications for small children may require crushing pills and diluting. This should only be done under the supervision of an experienced clinician.

8.8.5 Management of Hypertension in Children with Renal Failure

The management strategy for children with both hypertension and renal failure is very similar to that in adults. As with adults, treatment of blood pressure with appropriate medication in children can slow the progression of renal disease. **CHAPTER 6** discusses the diagnosis and management of renal failure in greater detail.

TABLE 8.11 lists medications in the order of preference in renal failure.

TABLE 8.11   Recommended Hypertension Medications for Pediatric
Patients with Renal Failure

For CKD 1-3 (GFR ≥ 30, creatinine < 2x normal value for age)*	
First-line drug	Lisinopril or Captopril
Second-line drug	Hydrochlorothiazide
Third-line drug	Amlodipine
Fourth-line drug	Atenolol**
For CKD 4 or 5 (GFR < 30, creatinine ≥ 2x normal value for age)*	
First-line drug	Furosemide
Second-line drug	Amlodipine
Third-line drug	Atenolol**

* See TABLE 8.10 for dosing.
** In renal failure, use half of normal recommended dose.

For mild to moderate renal dysfunction (proteinuria, creatinine < 2x normal value for age, CKD 1-3), an ACE inhibitor is recommended as a first-line agent in children. Medications should be increased incrementally to reach desired blood pressure (< 90th percentile for age) as described above. See **TABLE 8.10** for medication dosing. Note that atenolol dosing is reduced in renal failure, as the medication is excreted through the kidneys. Dosing should be half of that used for children without renal failure.

ACE inhibitors are not safe for use in children with severe renal failure, defined here as a creatinine ≥ 2x normal value for age, roughly corresponding with a GFR < 30 (CKD 4-5). At this level of renal failure, the risks of hyperkalemia become too high to justify its use in our setting. **TABLE 8.11** lists medications in order of preference in severe renal failure. Most of these children will need to be followed at the district-level health center for electrolyte and creatinine monitoring.

8.9   Hypertension in Pregnancy

Hypertensive disorders account for approximately 9% of total maternal mortality in Africa.[14] The management of these conditions is complicated by the fact that many common antihypertensives cause birth defects. Few clinical trials have investigated treatment of hypertension in pregnancy. As a result, there is significant disagreement on the subject, and most current guidelines rely on expert opinion rather than well-designed studies.

Hypertension in pregnancy can be pre-existing (chronic) or caused by the pregnancy itself.[15] In normal pregnancy, blood pressure tends to fall. In this context, blood pressures above 140 mmHg systolic or 90 diastolic are considered elevated; blood pressures greater than 160 mmHg systolic or 110 mmHg diastolic are considered severely elevated.[16]

TABLE 8.12 outlines the categories of hypertensive disorders in pregnancy. Treatment of hypertension does not alter the course of hypertensive disorders of pregnancy, given that anti-hypertensive medications do not affect the underlying pathophysiology of the disease. The one proven benefit of treating blood pressure in pregnancy is stroke prevention.[16] Providing magnesium to patients with severe preeclampsia has been shown to decrease the risk of seizures.

Proteinuria is a defining feature of preeclampsia. The gold standard for signficant proteinuria is the presence of 300 mg of protein in urine collected over a 24-hour period. Random protein-to-creatinine measurements with a ratio ≥ 0.19 correlate well with 24-hour urine protein measurements ≥ 300 mg. However, these tests may be impractical for wide-scale use in settings without well-developed lab infrastructure. Urine dipsticks are quick and inexpensive, but they are less sensitive and specific in detecting significant protein excretion in patients with suspected preeclampsia. Specificity improves with more strongly positive dipstick results. WHO's Integrated Management of Pregnancy and Childbirth (IMPAC) guidelines recommend using 3+ proteinuria as a marker of severe proteinura, and 2+ proteinuria as the threshold for diagnosing significant proteinuria. In our protocols, we have adopted the same proteinuria thresholds.[17,18]

Definitions of hypertensive disorders in pregnancy also incorporate the gestational age of pregnancy. However, accurate pregnacy dating can be difficult in resource-poor settings. Ultrasound offers the best estimation of gestational age, and several studies have shown these measurements can be easily taught.[19] In settings in which an ultrasound is not available and last menstrual period is not accurately known, fundal height may be used as a proxy for gestational age.[20,21] Since most complications of hypertension in pregnancy occur at greater than 34 weeks of gestational age, using a convervative threshold of 20 cm fundal height (typically equivalent to 20 weeks gestational age) should guarantee acceptable sensitivity.

The choice of antihypertensives is limited in pregnancy by the known potential for birth defects with ACE inhibitors, and lack of safety data for most other agents except for methyldopa, hydralazine, and nifedipine. Recommended agents include those that have been shown to be safe and effective. These are listed in order of preference in **TABLE 8.15**. ACE inhibitors are contraindicated in pregnancy.

Traditionally, diastolic blood pressure has been used to guide treatment initiation in pregnancy, as it seems to better correlate with risk of developing seizures.[17] However, recent studies show that systolic blood pressure correlates better with risk of maternal stroke.[16] In our protocols, we have included both diastolic and systolic blood pressure as criteria for treatment initiation.

TABLE 8.12 Hypertensive Disorders of Pregnancy

Classification	Definition	Risks	Role of antihypertensives
Chronic hypertension	BP ≥ 140/90 mmHg **AND** Diagnosis of hypertension prior to pregnancy or before 20 weeks of gestation	≥ 20% will develop preeclampsia[22] Placental abruption Intrauterine growth retardation	Does not reduce the risk of developing preeclampsia May reduce risk of maternal cerebral hemorrhage
Gestational hypertension	BP ≥ 140/90 mmHg **AND** Diagnoses or progression of hypertension after 20 weeks of gestation **WITHOUT** Significant proteinuria Defined as ≥ 2+ on a urine dipstick	50% will develop preeclampsia[23] 10% will develop severe preeclampsia	Does not reduce the risk of developing preeclampsia May reduce risk of maternal cerebral hemorrhage
Preeclampsia	BP ≥ 140/90 mmHg **AND** Diagnosis or progression of hypertension after 20 weeks of gestation **AND** Significant proteinuria Defined as ≥ 2+ on a urine dipstick	25% will develop severe preeclampsia Eclampsia (seizures) Maternal stroke	Does not reduce the risk of developing severe preeclampsia May reduce risk of maternal cerebral hemorrhage
Severe preeclampsia	Preeclampsia **AND** BP ≥ 160/110 mmHg **OR** ≥ 3+ proteinuria **OR** Any symptom of end-organ damage (oliguria, right-upper-quadrant pain, severe persistent headache, cerebral hemorrhage, nausea, pulmonary edema, low platelets [≤ 100,000], severe intrauterine growth restriction, or transaminitis [≥ twice normal])	Eclampsia (seizures) Maternal stroke	Does not reduce the risk of developing severe preeclampsia May reduce risk of maternal hemorrhage

PROTOCOL 8.7 outlines an algorithm for management of hypertension in pregnancy, defined as a confirmed blood pressure greater or equal to 140/90 mmHg on two separate occasions. At PIH-supported Rwanda MOH sites, prenatal providers manage hypertension in pregnancy; however, this may be a function appropriate for an integrated chronic care clinic in other settings.

PROTOCOL 8.7   Management of Hypertension in Pregnancy

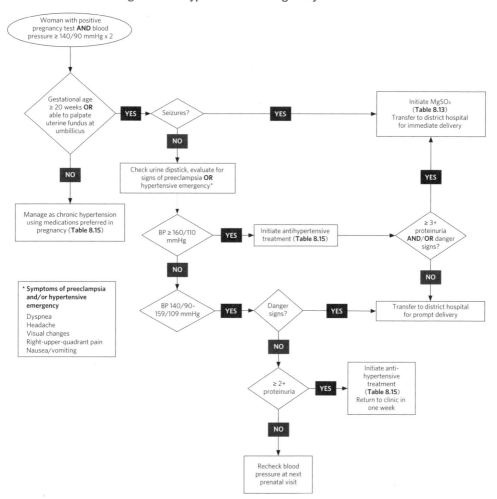

All women between the ages of 15 and 49 who present to either the acute care or the integrated chronic care clinic with hypertension are tested for pregnancy. Pregnant patients are referred to the prenatal clinic. Likewise, all pregnant women presenting for prenatal care should have their blood pressure measured at every visit.

8.9.1   Hypertension in Early Pregnancy (Chronic Hypertension)

Pregnancy-induced hypertension usually occurs in the third trimester. Therefore, patients with hypertension in the earlier stages of pregnancy likely have pre-exisiting hypertension. Here, we use a cut-off of less than 20 weeks gestational age and/or a fundal height less than 20 cm as the definition of early pregnancy. The management of these patients is similar to that of non-pregnant hypertensives, with the exception that different medications are preferred (see **TABLE 8.15**). These patients are at increased risk of developing preeclampsia and should be seen more frequently in the later stages of pregnancy.

8.9.2   Hypertension in Later Pregancy (Gestational Hypertension and Preeclampsia)

Patients who develop hypertension, or whose hypertension progresses at greater than 20 weeks gestational age, are at higher risk of pre-eclampsia and eclampsia. **PROTOCOL 8.7** outlines an adaptation of the IMPAC algorithim for evaluation and treatment of these patients.[18]

8.9.3   Recognition and Management of Emergent Conditions

Patients who are actively seizing or have had seizures during late pregnancy should be immediately started on magnesium and transferred to the nearest district hospital for immediate delivery. See **TABLE 8.13** for loading and maintenance dosing.

TABLE 8.13 Loading and Maintenance Dosing of Magnesium Sulfate in Eclampsia and Severe Preeclampsia (Adapted from IMPAC)[17,18]

Start with loading dose: Inject 4 grams (20 ml of 20% concentration) by IV over 20 minutes. **AND** Inject 5 grams (10 ml of 50% concentration) mixed with 1 ml of 1%–2% lidocaine IM in each buttock (for a total of 10 grams). If unable to establish IV, give only IM dose as loading dose.
If seizures recur after 15 minutes, give reloading dose: Inject 2 grams of 20% concentration IV over 5 minutes.
Follow with maintenance dose: Inject 5 grams of 50% concentration IM mixed with 1 ml of 1%–2% lidocaine in alternate buttocks every four hours.
Maximum total dose: 40 g every 24 hours
Side-effect monitoring: Monitor for respiratory depression (respiratory rate ≤ 16), loss of reflexes and decreased urinary output (≤ 100 ml/4 hrs). Injecting the magnesium too quickly increases the risk of respiratory or cardiac depression. Stop the therapy if the respiratory rate falls below 16 per minute, patellar reflexes are absent, or urinary output is less than 100 mL over 4 hours. For respiratory depression, give calcium gluconate 1 g IV (10 ml of 10% solution) over 10 minutes
Other safety considerations Do not leave the patient by herself. Place her on her left side. Transfer immediately to district hospital unless delivery is imminent

8.9.4 Screening for Preeclampsia

Patients with no history of seizure activity should be screened for pre-eclampsia with a urine dipstick and evaluation of symptoms of end-organ damage. These symptoms include right-upper-quadrant pain, headaches, visual changes (e.g., seeing spots), or lower-extremity edema.

8.9.5 Treatment of Preeclampsia According to Disease Classification

Severe preeclampsia. Severe preeclampsia is preeclampsia with a blood pressure ≥ 160/110 mmHg, or symptoms of end-organ damage, or greater than or equal to 3+ proteinuria. These patients should be started on antihypertensives and receive a loading dose of magnesium for seizure prophylaxsis, while being prepared for immediate transfer to the nearest district hospital for prompt delivery. Nifedipine is the fastest-acting antihypertensive that is safe in pregnancy. The second-line agent, methyldopa, has a longer onset of action (**TABLE 8.14**).

Severe gestational hypertension. Patients with severe hypertension (≥ 160/110 mmHg) without proteinuria or other signs of preeclampsia should be started on antihypertensives and transferred to the nearest district hospital for admission (**TABLE 8.14**). Likewise, pregnant women with mild blood pressure elevation with any sign that could indicate preeclampsia (dyspnea, headache, vision changes, right-upper-quadrant pain, nausea, or vomiting) should be hospitalized for observation.

TABLE 8.14 Recommended Medications for Management of Hypertension in Severe Preeclampsia

Medication	Dosing	Notes
Nifedipine (immediate release)	10 mg orally	Fast acting
Methyldopa	250 mg orally	Slower acting

8.9.5.1   Mild to Moderate Preeclampsia

Mild to moderate preeclampsia is defined by a blood pressure ≥ 140/90 but < 160/110 mmHg, and ≥ 2+ proteinuria and no signs or symptoms of severe preeclampsia. These patients should be started on antihypertensives and followed closely in the prenatal clinic (**TABLE 8.15**). If a woman is already on antihypertensives, she should have her medication dosage increased, with a goal blood pressure of 140–150/90–100 mmHg. Ideally, she will be admitted for observation for at least a 24-hour period and she should be given strict precautionary instructions to return to care immediately if she develops any of the symptoms of severe preeclampsia or has decreased fetal movement.

8.9.5.2   Mild to Moderate Gestational Hypertension

Women with mild hypertension should not be started on medications. Patients already on medications should continue antihypertensive treatment with drugs appropriate for pregnancy.

TABLE 8.15 Recommended Hypertension Medications and Dosing in Pregnancy

First-line drug	Starting dose	Increase dose by	Maximum dose	Notes
Methyldopa	250 mg 2x/day	250 mg 2x/day	500 mg 2x/day	Best-proven safety in pregnancy, cheap, widely available
Second-line drug	**Starting dose**	**Increase dose by**	**Maximum dose**	**Notes**
Nifedipine (immediate release)	10 mg 3x/day	20 mg 3x/day	60 mg 3x/day	Can cause lower-extremity edema
Amlodipine	5 mg 1x/day	5 mg 1x/day	10 mg 1x/day	
Third-line drug	**Starting dose**	**Increase dose by**	**Maximum dose**	**Notes**
Atenolol	25 mg 1x/day	25 mg 1x/day	100 mg 1x/day	Contraindicated if heart rate ≤ 55 bpm
Fourth-line drug	**Starting dose**	**Increase dose by**	**Maximum dose**	**Notes**
Hydralazine	25 mg 3x/day	25 mg 3x/day	50 mg 3x/day	Headache common side effect. Expensive, requires thrice-daily dosing

Chapter 8 References

· ·

1   Ezzati M, Vander Hoorn S, Lawes CM, et al. Rethinking the "diseases of affluence" paradigm: global patterns of nutritional risks in relation to economic development. PLoS Med 2005;2:e133.

2   van der Sande MA, Milligan PJ, Nyan OA, et al. Blood pressure patterns and cardiovascular risk factors in rural and urban Gambian communities. J Hum Hypertens 2000;14:489-96.

3   Opie LH, Seedat YK. Hypertension in sub-Saharan African populations. Circulation 2005;112:3562-8.

4   Addo J, Smeeth L, Leon DA. Hypertension in sub-Saharan Africa: a systematic review. Hypertension 2007;50:1012-8.

5   Mosterd A, D'Agostino RB, Silbershatz H, et al. Trends in the prevalence of hypertension, antihypertensive therapy, and left ventricular hypertrophy from 1950 to 1989. N Engl J Med 1999;340:1221-7.

6   Jackson R, Lawes CM, Bennett DA, Milne RJ, Rodgers A. Treatment with drugs to lower blood pressure and blood cholesterol based on an individual's absolute cardiovascular risk. Lancet 2005;365:434-41.

7   Gaziano TA, Young CR, Fitzmaurice G, Atwood S, Gaziano JM. Laboratory-based versus non-laboratory-based method for assessment of cardiovascular disease risk: the NHANES I Follow-up Study cohort. Lancet 2008;371:923-31.

8   Mann J, et al. The assessment and management of cardiovascular risk: New Zealand Guidelines Group; 2003.

9   World Health Organization. Prevention of Cardiovascular Disease. Guidelines for Assessment and Management of Cardiovascular Risk. Geneva: World Health Organization; 2007.

10 Law MR, Wald NJ, Morris JK, Jordan RE. Value of low dose combination treatment with blood pressure lowering drugs: analysis of 354 randomised trials. BMJ 2003;326:1427.

11 Sliwa K, Wilkinson D, Hansen C, et al. Spectrum of heart disease and risk factors in a black urban population in South Africa (the Heart of Soweto Study): a cohort study. Lancet 2008;371:915-22.

12 IMAI Palliative Care Guideline Module. Geneva, Switzerland: World Health Organization; 2009.

13 Wiysonge CS, Bradley H, Mayosi BM, et al. Beta-blockers for hypertension. Cochrane Database Syst Rev 2007:CD002003.

14 Khan KS, Wojdyla D, Say L, Gulmezoglu AM, Van Look PF. WHO analysis of causes of maternal death: a systematic review. Lancet 2006;367:1066-74.

15 Sibai BM. Treatment of hypertension in pregnant women. N Engl J Med 1996;335:257-65.

16 Martin JN, Jr., Thigpen BD, Moore RC, Rose CH, Cushman J, May W. Stroke and severe preeclampsia and eclampsia: a paradigm shift focusing on systolic blood pressure. Obstet Gynecol 2005;105:246-54.

17 Raise Initiative. Emergency Obstetric Care: Protocols. Clinical Training for Reproductive Health in Emergencies. London, Nairobi and New York: Reproductive Health Access Information and Services in Emergencies Initiative; 2008.

18 World Health Organization. Integrated management of pregnancy and childbirth. Pregnancy, childbirth, postpartum and newborn care: A guide for essential practice. Geneva; 2006.

19   Shah S, Teismann N, Zaia B, et al. Accuracy of emergency physicians using ultrasound to determine gestational age in pregnant women. Am J Emerg Med;28:834-8.

20   Traisathit P, Le Coeur S, Mary JY, Kanjanasing A, Lamlertkittikul S, Lallemant M. Gestational age determination and prevention of HIV perinatal transmission. Int J Gynaecol Obstet 2006;92:176-80.

21   Jehan I, Zaidi S, Rizvi S, et al. Dating gestational age by last menstrual period, symphysis-fundal height, and ultrasound in urban Pakistan. Int J Gynaecol Obstet;110:231-4.

22   Lindheimer MD, Taler SJ, Cunningham FG. ASH position paper: hypertension in pregnancy. J Clin Hypertens (Greenwich) 2009;11:214-25.

23   Barton JR, O'Brien J M, Bergauer NK, Jacques DL, Sibai BM. Mild gestational hypertension remote from term: progression and outcome. Am J Obstet Gynecol 2001;184:979-83.

CHAPTER 9
Rheumatic Heart Disease Prevention
· ·

In most reviews of hospitalizations in sub-Saharan Africa, and in our own experience, rheumatic heart disease (RHD) accounts for around one-third of admissions due to heart failure. In its terminal form, it is a wasting disease that kills young adults and women disproportionately.

RHD is frequently preventable, and is now almost eradicated in the United States. However, it affects more than 60–70 million people worldwide and accounts for at least 1.4 million deaths per year, by one conservative estimate.[1,41] Ninety-five percent of these deaths take place in the developing countries.

In **CHAPTER 4** and **CHAPTER 5** of this handbook, we address both the medical management of patients with RHD, including those with mitral stenosis, as well as post-surgical care for those who have required valve replacement or repair. We have shown how integration of these services is possible as part of chronic care for other advanced non-communicable diseases. We also believe that cardiac surgery is an essential service in the poorest countries. This kind of care, known as tertiary prophylaxis (or prevention of death and suffering), will always be needed because of the imperfections of all known prevention strategies, discussed below.

In this chapter, we focus on the role that district NCD leaders can play in the prevention of advanced RHD. We insist on integration of RHD prevention into the job descriptions of health workers tasked with a cluster of related issues.

9.1 Prevention of Acute Rheumatic Fever: Management of Sore Throat

Rheumatic heart disease (RHD) is the deadly complication of rheumatic fever (RF). RF is largely a disease of school-aged children (ages 5 to 15) in which the body's immune system attacks its own organs, including the heart, the joints, the brain, and the skin. The annual incidence of first attacks of RF in school-aged children is not well characterized in sub-Saharan Africa. Iran has documented the world's highest incidence rate (25 per 100,000 schoolchildren).[2]

RF is thought to result from a reaction to Group A Streptococcal (GAS) throat infections. In susceptible individuals, these bacteria evoke an immune response against the body itself. RHD chiefly involves the cardiac valves, resulting in variable degrees of regurgitation or stenosis. The best kind of prevention for RHD is prevention of RF.

The need for prevention of RF in low-income countries, also known as primary prophylaxis, may seem obvious, but it has been a surprisingly controversial subject in the expert community. One issue has been the challenge of evaluating and diagnosing GAS pharyngitis. Others have called into question the belief that GAS pharyngitis is the major cause of RF, pointing to recent data on the role of skin infections (pyoderma) in RF among Australian Aborigines.[3] Moreover, early cost models for pharyngitis suggested that primary prophylaxis was not a good value for the money.[4] Despite these disputes, most authorities now recommend integration of pharyngitis and pyoderma management into primary health care protocols such as the Integrated Management of Childhood Illness (IMCI).[5]

In this section, we assume that GAS pharyngitis is the underlying driver of RF in most settings. This is an issue of daily importance for acute care clinicians working at health centers and in the community. District NCD clinicians should also acquire a solid understanding of the issues involved in pharyngitis care.

Controlled trials have repeatedly shown 70% risk reductions in RF incidence through individual treatment of pharyngitis with penicillin and other antibiotics.[6] Countries such as Costa Rica have seen rapid reductions in RF incidence following expansion of primary care services that included sore throat management.[7] Good sore throat management can also reduce symptom time and prevent both pharyngeal abscesses and the dangers of traditional healing. There is also speculation that treating pharyngitis can prevent transmission of GAS infections among school-aged children.

Worldwide, the reported number of sore throat episodes per year per school-aged child varies from as few as 0.02 to as many as 7.[8] **FIGURE 9.1** shows the typical fraction of pharyngitis due to GAS in a high–RHD prevalence setting, along with the typical fraction of GAS cases that provoke an attack of acute RF. Even in a setting with such high RF incidence, 250 sore throats would have to be evaluated in order to prevent 1 case of RF.

FIGURE 9.1   Progression from Pharyngitis to Rheumatic Fever

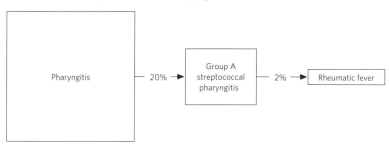

In many resource-poor settings, at least two barriers exist to effective evaluation and treatment of sore throats. The first is clinical: the difficulty of distinguishing GAS from other, more common causes of pharyngitis such as viral infections. Secondly, parents may not take children to a health care provider for a sore throat. Predictable reasons include the distance to the nearest health facility, user fees, and the sometimes-subtle presentation of pharyngitis. Often parents may find it more convenient to seek care from traditional healers.

One approach to address the limitations of facility-based sore throat management is for community health workers to treat or refer pharyngitis cases using clinical criteria. This approach could be integrated into community-based IMCI. We believe that the need for such an aggressive strategy to manage sore throats depends in part on the underlying prevalence of RHD in the population. Because this prevalence may vary even within a country, national surveys would be helpful. Because Rwanda has not yet undertaken such a survey, sore throat management remains a facility-level issue for now.

It is possible, however, to describe a practical, community-based approach to pharyngitis management for high–RHD prevalence settings. The threshold for determining high prevalence (for example, 0.5% of at least moderate echocardiographic regurgitation in school-aged children) will vary among countries.[9] There are no standards in this regard. We discuss the issues involved in determining RHD prevalence in the section on echocardiographic screening below (see **SECTION 9.3.1**).

There is a need for an improved set of clinical decision rules to distinguish GAS from other causes of pharyngitis. More than 80% of sore throats in most settings are not due to GAS. Giving antibiotics to these patients costs money, and risks toxicity and allergic reactions without any benefit. Giving penicillin to such patients may breed resistance to other organisms, such as those that commonly cause pneumonia (*Streptococcus pneumoniae*). The problem of diagnosis can't be solved by rapid streptococcal antigen tests, which are currently too insensitive to be relied upon, and culture methods are too cumbersome for routine use in under resourced settings. Clinical criteria (decision rules) for treatment of sore throats with antibiotics have been derived in Egypt, Brazil, the United States, and other countries.[10-12] These rules vary in their sensitivity and specificity, however. Additionally, there is probably some variation among countries in the clinical presentation of GAS, and yet not every country can afford to develop its own decision rules.[13]

We have recommended that settings with high RF incidence favor clinical criteria that will result in treatment of most individuals with GAS, even at the risk of some overtreatment. We have also tried to simplify the decision process as much as possible. **TABLE 9.1** shows the properties of three decision rules in a pharyngitis population with 24% GAS.

TABLE 9.1   Clinical Decision Rules for Treatment of Pharyngitis

	% with GAS not treated	% without GAS overtreated
Rule 1: WHO[14] Pharyngeal exudate + tender and enlarged cervical lymph nodes	88%	6%
Rule 2: Steinhoff[12] Pharyngeal exudate OR enlarged cervical lymph nodes	10%	60%

Rule 1 is supported by WHO in its IMCI adaptation guidelines for children under 5 years old.[11] This rule avoids overtreatment of those without GAS, but undertreats in 88% of cases.

Rule 2, developed by Steinhoff and colleagues in Egypt, only misses 10% of GAS cases, but results in treatment of 60% of patients without GAS.

We have developed a rule based on data from the Egyptian experience in school-aged children, and also a Canadian clinical decision rule tested in populations between the ages of 3 and 76 (**PROTOCOL 9.1**).

PROTOCOL 9.1   Evaluation and Management of Pharyngitis

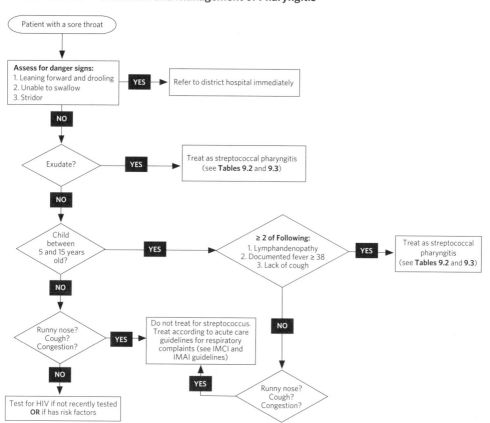

This approach begins with treatment of all patients with pharyngeal or tonsillar exudate. This step alone will identify 80% of those with GAS. We believe that the remaining 20% of patients with GAS on culture may well be streptococcal carriers without active infection, and therefore at less risk of developing acute RF. Rather than calling for treatment of all remaining patients who have enlarged cervical lymph nodes, we have recommended a focus on those between the ages of 5–15. If these school-aged children have a combination of two of the following three findings, we would recommend treatment: enlarged or tender cervical lymph nodes, fever ≥ 38°C, or absence of cough and rhinorrhea.

Clinical decision rules should probably be re-evaluated in each particular country. Given the logistical difficulties of obtaining throat cultures, some sites have used rapid streptococcal antigen tests as a gold standard.[15]

The choice of which antibiotic regimen to use depends on the clinical setting. At the facility level, intramuscular Benzathine Penicillin G is the best option, as it requires only a single injection. This drug carries a small risk of anaphylaxis, and epinephrine should be available. In the community setting, oral therapy is a better choice, although frequently children will stop taking their medication once symptoms improve. If adherence with oral therapy is felt to be poor, community health workers should continue follow-up of these cases until the antibiotic regimen is completed. **TABLE 9.2** and **TABLE 9.3** show typical regimens for pharyngitis treatment and their associated costs and risks.

TABLE 9.2 Antibiotic Regimens for Streptococcal Pharyngitis (Adults and Adolescents Dosing, Weight ≥ 27 kg)

	Regimen	Doses	Cost	Allergic Reactions[16,17]	
Oral penicillin VK	500 mg, two times per day for 10 days	20	$0.66	Cutaneous	1%–2%
Intramuscular benzathine penicillin G	1.2 million units, single dose	1	$0.14	Cutaneous	1%–2%
				Anaphylaxis	0.02%
				Death	0.003%
Oral erythromycin (75 kg adult)	250 mg, four times per day	12	$6.38		

TABLE 9.3 Antibiotic Regimens for Streptococcal Pharyngitis (Pediatric Dosing, Weight ≤ 27 kg)

	Regimen	Doses	Cost
Oral penicillin VK	250 mg, two times per day for 10 days	20	$0.33
Intramuscular benzathine penicillin G	600,000 units, single dose	1	$0.09
Oral erythromycin	12.5 mg/kg, three times per day for 3 days	9	$0.27

9.2 Preventing Rheumatic Heart Disease: Management of Acute Rheumatic Fever and Secondary Prophylaxis for Rheumatic Fever

Rheumatic fever is a disease that primarily affects school-aged children (ages 5 to 15). There are no treatments shown to improve the outcome. However, diagnosis and follow-up is important because chronic antibiotic therapy can prevent RF recurrence. This intervention probably reduces the risk of RF recurrence by more than 50%.[18]

Secondary prophylaxis for RHD should be integrated into chronic care services at the health center level. District NCD clinicians play a critical role in secondary prophylaxis of RHD. These providers have the basic echocardiography skills to rule-out cardiomyopathies, dramatic endocarditis, or alternative causes of significant murmurs. These providers can also organize patients for evaluation by specialists.

Cardiologists or echocardiographers working at referral centers are essential to confirm the diagnosis of RHD echocardiographically and evaluate patients for possible cardiac surgery. Registration of RHD cases should be done as part of an integrated electronic medical record system at both district and referral center levels.

9.2.1 Acute Rheumatic Fever: Diagnosis and Follow-Up

For the most part, acute care clinicians staffing general consultation clinics identify RF cases. Patients are then referred to the nearest district hospital for admission. At discharge, patients are sent to their nearest chronic care clinic for follow-up.

There is no blood test or imaging study to diagnose acute rheumatic fever. Clinical criteria are based on experience in the United States. These criteria, named after T. Duckett Jones, have gone through at least 5 revisions. Over time, the criteria became increasingly stringent to avoid overdiagnosis of RF, since the incidence of the disease was declining.[19-22] The most recent recommendations require confirmation of at least two major criteria, or a combination of one major and at least two minor criteria (**TABLE 9.4**). The guidelines also require objective evidence of a preceding group A streptococcal infection (including elevated or rising ASO titers, or positive microbiologic tests).

The 2007 Australian guidelines for RF and RHD have modified the Jones criteria for use among high-risk groups such as the Aborigines.[23] The Australian guidelines add two additional major criteria: monoarthritis and evidence of subclinical carditis by echocardiography. The guidelines assume access to complete echocardiography and microbiologic testing.

TABLE 9.4   Modified Jones Criteria for High-Risk Groups[21,23,24]

Major criteria (five)	Minor criteria (four)
1. Carditis or subclinical (echocardiographic) carditis	**Clinical**
2. Polyarthritis or monoarthritis	1. Fever $\geq 38\,^{\circ}C$
3. Chorea	2. Arthralgia
4. Erythema marginatum	**Laboratory**
5. Subcutaneous nodules	3. Elevated acute phase reactants (erythrocyte sedimentation rate ≥ 30 mm/h)
	4. PR-interval prolongation

There are several problems with even these modified Jones criteria in low-resource environments with a high incidence of acute RF. First, it may be difficult to fulfill the requirement that there be objective evidence of a preceding streptococcal infection. Neither rapid streptococcal antigen tests nor antistreptolysin O titers alone are particularly sensitive, and neither is available at the district hospital level. Throat culture is also unavailable and has a long turn-around time. The Jones criteria did not require evidence of a streptococcal infection until the 1965 revision.

Second, there is a need for simplified guidance based on the most common presentation of the disease.

In our experience, a great deal of weight should be put on the finding of overt carditis with loud murmurs in the age group at risk (5 to 25 years old). A review of initial RF cases in India found that one-third had carditis at the time of presentation.[25] In our experience, the majority of RF cases in sub-Saharan Africa present with carditis. Erythema marginatum and subcutaneous nodules are rare manifestations. Patients with the finding of clinical carditis or of chorea who otherwise meet the Jones criteria should not require confirmation of a streptococcal infection.

Endocarditis is an important alternative diagnosis to consider. All patients should have basic echocardiography performed at the district level as well as referral for complete echocardiography.

Patients with polyarthritis or monoarthritis as their sole major criteria are more challenging to diagnose with acute RF. The differential diagnosis includes viral as well as gonococcal arthritis. Diagnosis of RF in these cases should probably require evidence of streptoccocal infection—even in resource-limited settings.

There are no therapies shown to improve the outcome of acute rheumatic fever.[26] However, the studies on this subject date back to the 1950s and 1960s. Due to the lack of high-quality evidence, decision-making in this area relies on expert opinion. Our practice is to hospitalize all patients with suspected acute RF for several weeks. We administer IM benzathine penicillin G (see **TABLE 9.3**). For patients with carditis, we administer prednisone at a dose of 1 mg per kg, divided over 2 doses.

Once patients are discharged, they are referred to the NCD clinic, and penicillin is continued chronically. Patients are given the option of either oral penicillin V or benzathine penicillin G, given on a monthly basis (see **TABLE 9.5**). Treatment should be continued for 10 years, or until age 21, whichever is longer. For those with severe disease, or those who have undergone cardiac surgery, treatment should continue indefinitely.

One practice is to follow the erythrocyte sedimentation rate (ESR) on a weekly basis and begin to taper the steroid dose once the ESR has normalized (≤ 20 mm/hr).

TABLE 9.5 Antibiotic Regimens for Secondary Prophylaxis of Rheumatic Fever

	Adults (≥ 27 kg)	Children (≤ 27 kg)
Oral penicillin VK	500 mg, two times per day	250 mg, two times per day
Intramuscular benzathine penicillin G	1.2 million units, once every 4 weeks	600,000 units, once every 4 weeks
Oral erythromycin (penicillin allergy)	250 mg, two times per day	10 mg/kg, twice per day

For decades, benzathine penicillin G administered monthly has been the standard of care for secondary prophylaxis of RHD. There have been concerns about compliance with oral regimens and studies dating back to the 1950s have shown the superiority of intramuscular injections. In practice, however, compliance with intramuscular regimens has been poor.[27,28]

We believe that, given the seriousness of RHD, care of this disease merits the support of community health workers. As others have noted, the studies comparing oral and IM penicillin were conducted prior to the introduction of oral penicillin V.[18] Additionally, studies have shown that penicillin levels decline in blood two weeks after benzathine injection.[29,30] Given the difficulty of twice-monthly injections, we believe there is a strong case for directly observed therapy with oral penicillin V.

9.3 Rheumatic Heart Disease Screening

We have already discussed some of the challenges in RHD prevention. For example, a community survey in rural Pakistan found that only 19 percent of those with findings of RHD on echocardiography were aware of their disease.[31] Almost half of those identified with RHD could not recall symptoms consistent with acute rheumatic fever. Fewer than half of those individuals aware of their disease were receiving antibiotic prophylaxis.

The presentation of GAS pharyngitis may be subtle, and acute RF may be difficult recognize. By the time that patients with RHD present for care, the disease may be so advanced that secondary prophylaxis is of limited value. Patients with milder forms of the disease stand to benefit most from chronic penicillin, but these patients are least likely to be identified. Given these considerations, there have been efforts to screen high-risk groups—school-aged children, primarily—for RHD for more than half a century.[32]

However, screening is not yet an established approach to RHD prevention for several reasons. Because there are no blood tests to diagnose RHD, screening relies on either listening for murmurs, or looking for disease with cardiac ultrasound. Dramatic disease (at least moderate in severity) is not very prevalent. Milder disease is difficult to differentiate from normal variation using these tests, and the natural history of this disease is unknown. Trials of penicillin prophylaxis were performed in individuals who had recently experienced an episode of acute RF, not in asymptomatic populations identified through screening. In fact, screening in the United States became less popular as the prevalence of the disease declined, and concerns about misdiagnosis grew.[33,34]

In developing countries, screening has been promoted, but has never contributed substantially to case finding. The 1986 to 1990 WHO program for the prevention of RHD incorporated school-based screening—mainly listening for murmurs—as part of its case-finding activities.[27] These surveys identified 3135 suspected RHD cases out of more than 1.4 million children screened (0.2%). Screening, however, only accounted for 9% of the total RHD cases registered during this period (mainly through review of existing records).

9.3.1 Echocardiographic Screening for Rheumatic Heart Disease
Since the introduction of echocardiography in the 1980s, it has become increasingly apparent that listening for heart murmurs is not a reliable way to identify mild valvular disease. This technique consistently identifies problems in children who do not have any actual disease. For example, a study in Pakistan has shown that more than a third of RHD cases initially identified through auscultation did not have any signs of heart disease by echocardiography.[35] Another study found that a quarter of school-aged children have some kind of heart murmur. Only 2% of those thought to have murmurs actually had suspected RHD by echocardiography.[36,37]

At the same time, screening with echocardiography has its own problems. Investigators in Kenya published the first pilot study of primary echocardiographic screening for RHD in 1996.[38] Unclear as to the significance of the trivial lesions identified by ultrasound in around 6% of schoolchildren, the group initially randomized these patients to penicillin prophylaxis, but the project stopped prematurely due to logistical difficulties.

Since that time, groups in Mozambique, Cambodia, Fiji, Tonga, and other sites have been honing echocardiographic screening techniques.[36,39-41]

Recent echocardiographic prevalence studies have found a variable rate of definite RHD in school-aged children (see **TABLE 9.6**). These patients generally had mild disease with an uncertain prognosis. Assuming a prevalence of 0.5%, it would take at least a working week for an echocardiographer to identify one definite case of RHD (assuming 10 minutes per study, 5 hours a day, 5 days a week). This kind of effort could be justified given the seriousness of the disease (around $600 per case found), but training in even basic echocardiography is rare in sub-Saharan Africa.

TABLE 9.6   **Echocardiographic Prevalence of Definite and Possible RHD in School-Aged Children**

	Country	N	Setting	Population	Definite or probable RHD	Possible RHD
Paar et al. 2010 [41]	Nicaragua	3150	Rural and urban	Community	0.6%	2.4%
Steer et al. 2009 [37]	Fiji	3462	Rural and urban	School-based	0.8%	n/a
Carapetis et al. 2008 [39]	Tonga	5053	Rural and urban	School-based	3.3%	0.5%
Marijon et al. 2007 [36]	Cambodia	3677	Urban	School-based	3.0%	n/a
Marijon et al. 2007 [36]	Mozambique	2170	Urban	School-based	2.1%	n/a
Anabwani and Bonhoeffer 1996 [42]	Kenya	1115	Rural and urban	School-based	0.3%	7.3%

The clinical viability of echocardiographic screening depends on efforts to increase diagnostic yield. One strategy may be to focus on screening of older schoolchildren who appear to have a higher prevalence of disease. Another important observation has been that an additional 2% to 4% of schoolchildren have borderline echocardiographic abnormalities consistent with possible RHD. At present, the benefit of penicillin in these cases is unclear, and the harm is evident. Groups are currently at work to define standard diagnostic criteria for possible RHD, and to design trials of penicillin prophylaxis for these individuals. Arguably, criteria for definite RHD should be more conservative than those used in many studies.

If echocardiographic screening develops into an attractive prevention strategy, we believe that district NCD clinicians could be a valuable resource. These clinicians have basic echocardiographic skills and could spend a small portion of their time doing school outreach.

9.3.2   Studies of RHD Prevalence

Despite the limitations of echocardiographic diagnosis for mild RHD, some sense of the prevalence of RHD in the community is critical for the design of prevention strategies. For example, in some settings it might make sense to allow community health workers to assess and treat sore throats directly. Countries should engage in echocardiographic screening to obtain prevalence data as part of efforts like the ASAP (Awareness, Surveillance, Advocacy, and Prevention) initiative in Africa.[43]

Countries should consider integration of these studies into larger school health surveys if there are gaps in this area more generally.

There have been a variety of proposed criteria for diagnosis of asymptomatic RHD (see **TABLE 9.7**).[24,44,45] Criteria vary in whether they put more weight on valvular regurgitation or thickening. Some criteria have also insisted on the presence of an audible murmur in addition to echocardiographic findings. None of these criteria have been evaluated prospectively. The vast majority of suspected RHD identified by these criteria is trivial or mild. For example, only 11% of RHD thought definite in one echocardiographic survey was of moderate or greater severity.[39]

TABLE 9.7 Echocardiographic Features of Left-Sided Heart Valves Thought Consistent with Rheumatic Heart Disease in High-Prevalence Settings by Three Sets of Criteria

	World Health Organization 2001 [24]	Marijon et al. 2009 [44]	Preliminary World Health Organization/United States National Institutes of Health 2005 [37]	
Properties of regurgitant jet	Holosystolic (mitral) or holodiastolic (aortic) regurgitation visible in at least two color planes with ≥ 1 cm extension and a velocity ≥ 2.5 m/s	Any degree in two planes	Definite	Probable
			≥ 2 cm, otherwise meeting World Health Organization 2001 criteria*	≥ 2 cm, otherwise meeting World Health Organization 2001 criteria*
Morphologic abnormalities	Not required	Required**	Required***	Not Required***†
Pathologic murmurs	Not required	Not Required	Required	Required

* ≥ 1 cm of jet length is sufficient for aortic regurgitation.
** Any two of the three that include leaflet tethering, leaflet thickening, or sub-valvular thickening.
*** For mitral regurgitation, these include thickening of the valve or a hockey-stick/elbow deformity of the anterior leaflet; in addition, for mitral stenosis, these also include tethering of the posterior leaflet, commissural thickening and calcification with a mean gradient ≥ 4 mmHg; for aortic regurgitation without obvious non-rheumatic causes, these include morphologic abnormalities of the mitral valve.
† Either significant left-sided valvular regurgitation, morphologic abnormalities, or mitral stenosis in the presence of pathologic murmurs.

Because of uncertainty about the importance of mild lesions on echocardiography, we propose that prevalence surveys place more weight on definite disease. At the same time, auscultation alone is not helpful and emphasis should be put on echocardiographic diagnosis (see **TABLE 9.8**).

TABLE 9.8   Proposed Criteria for Definite and Possible RHD

	Definite	Possible
Properties of regurgitant jet	At least mild-to-moderate regurgitation. Regurgitation visible in at least two color planes	Any degree in two planes
Morphologic abnormalities	Required*	Required*
Pathologic murmurs	Not required	Not Required

PROTOCOL 9.2   Screening for Rheumatic Heart Disease (and Other Conditions of School-Aged Children)

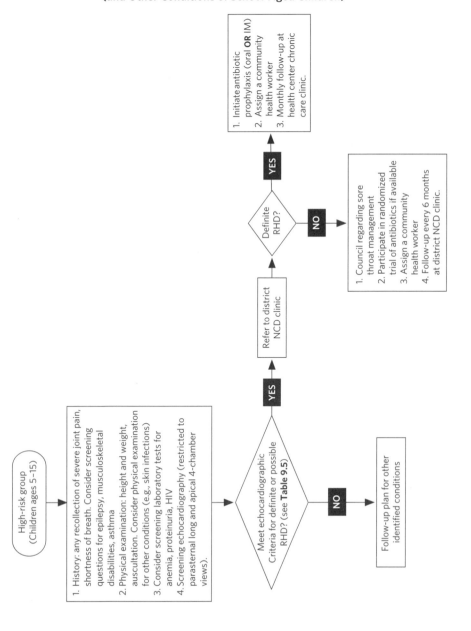

High-risk group (Children ages 5–15)

1. History: any recollection of severe joint pain, shortness of breath. Consider screening questions for epilepsy, musculoskeletal disabilities, asthma
2. Physical examination: height and weight, auscultation. Consider physical examination for other conditions (e.g., skin infections)
3. Consider screening laboratory tests for anemia, proteinuria, HIV
4. Screening echocardiography (restricted to parasternal long and apical 4-chamber views).

Meet echocardiographic Criteria for definite or possible RHD? (see **Table 9.5**)

NO → Follow-up plan for other identified conditions

YES → Refer to district NCD clinic

Definite RHD?

YES →
1. Initiate antibiotic prophylaxis (oral **OR** IM)
2. Assign a community health worker
3. Monthly follow-up at health center chronic care clinic.

NO →
1. Council regarding sore throat management
2. Participate in randomized trial of antibiotics if available
3. Assign a community health worker
4. Follow-up every 6 months at district NCD clinic.

Finally, there should be a plan in place to follow up for individuals identified with borderline lesions. One approach may be more vigilant treatment of pharyngitis episodes rather than continuous RF prophylaxis. Another approach may be to enroll these patients in randomized trials of prophylaxis strategies. **PROTOCOL 9.2** shows a proposed approach for RHD prevalence studies.

Chapter 9 References

1 Carapetis JR, Steer AC, Muholland EK, Weber M. The global burden of group A streptococcal diseases. Lancet Infect Dis 2005;5:685-94.

2 Tibazarwa KB, Volmink JA, Mayosi BM. Incidence of acute rheumatic fever in the world: a systematic review of population-based studies. Heart 2008;94:1534-40.

3 McDonald M, Currie BJ, Carapetis JR. Acute rheumatic fever: a chink in the chain that links the heart to the throat? Lancet Infect Dis 2004;4:240-5.

4 Strasser T. Cost-effective control of rheumatic fever in the community. Health Policy 1985;5:159-64.

5 World Health Organization. Integrated Management of Adolescent and Adult Illness. Guidelines for First-Level Facility Health Workers at Health Centre and District Outpatient Clinic. 2009.

6 Robertson KA, Volmink JA, Mayosi BM. Antibiotics for the primary prevention of acute rheumatic fever: a meta-analysis. BMC Cardiovasc Disord 2005;5:11.

7 Arguedas A, Mohs E. Prevention of rheumatic fever in Costa Rica. J Pediatr 1992;121:569-72.

8 Nandi S, Kumar R, Ray P, Vohra H, Ganguly NK. Group A streptococcal sore throat in a periurban population of northern India: a one-year prospective study. Bull World Health Organ 2001;79:528-33.

9 Steer AC, Carapetis JR, Nolan TM, Shann F. Systematic review of rheumatic heart disease prevalence in children in developing countries: the role of environmental factors. J Paediatr Child Health 2002;38:229-34.

10 Centor RM, Witherspoon JM, Dalton HP, Brody CE, Link K. The diagnosis of strep throat in adults in the emergency room. Med Decis Making 1981;1:239-46.

11 Rimoin AW, Hamza HS, Vince A, et al. Evaluation of the WHO clinical decision rule for streptococcal pharyngitis. Arch Dis Child 2005;90:1066-70.

12 Steinhoff MC, Abd el Khalek MK, Khallaf N, et al. Effectiveness of clinical guidelines for the presumptive treatment of streptococcal pharyngitis in Egyptian children. Lancet 1997;350:918-21.

13 Rimoin AW, Fischer Walker CL, Chitale RA, et al. Variation in clinical presentation of childhood Group A streptococcal pharyngitis in four countries. J Trop Pediatr 2008;54:308-12.

14 Organization WH. Integrated Management of Childhood Illness. IMCI Adaptation Guide. Geneva: Department of Child and Adolescent Health and Development; 2002 June.

15 Joachim L, Campos D, Jr., Smeesters PR. Pragmatic scoring system for pharyngitis in low-resource settings. Pediatrics 2010;126:e608-14.

16 Allergic reactions to long-term benzathine penicillin prophylaxis for rheumatic fever. International Rheumatic Fever Study Group. Lancet 1991;337:1308-10.

17 Idsoe O, Guthe T, Willcox RR, de Weck AL. Nature and extent of penicillin side-reactions, with particular reference to fatalities from anaphylactic shock. Bull World Health Organ 1968;38:159-88.

18 Manyemba J, Mayosi BM. Penicillin for secondary prevention of rheumatic fever. Cochrane Database Syst Rev 2002:CD002227.

19 Bhattacharya S, Tandon R. The diagnosis of rheumatic fever—evolution of the Jones criteria. Int J Cardiol 1986;12:285-94.

20   Jones TD. The diagnosis of rheumatic fever. JAMA 1944;126:481-87.

21   Guidelines for the diagnosis of rheumatic fever. Jones Criteria, 1992 update. Special Writing Group of the Committee on Rheumatic Fever, Endocarditis, and Kawasaki Disease of the Council on Cardiovascular Disease in the Young of the American Heart Association. JAMA 1992;268:2069-73.

22   Ferrieri P. Proceedings of the Jones Criteria workshop. Circulation 2002;106:2521-3.

23   Carapetis JR, Brown A, Wilson NJ, Edwards KN. An Australian guideline for rheumatic fever and rheumatic heart disease: an abridged outline. Med J Aust 2007;186:581-6.

24   WHO Expert Consultation on Rheumatic Fever and Rheumatic Heart Disease. Rheumatic fever and rheumatic heart disease. World Health Organ Tech Rep Ser 2004;923:1-122, back cover.

25   Sanyal SK, Thapar MK, Ahmed SH, Hooja V, Tewari P. The initial attack of acute rheumatic fever during childhood in North India; a prospective study of the clinical profile. Circulation 1974;49:7-12.

26   Cilliers AM, Manyemba J, Saloojee H. Anti-inflammatory treatment for carditis in acute rheumatic fever. Cochrane Database Syst Rev 2003:CD003176.

27   WHO Cardiovascular Diseases Unit and principal investigators. WHO programme for the prevention of rheumatic fever/rheumatic heart disease in 16 developing countries: report from Phase I (1986-90). Bull World Health Organ 1992;70:213-8.

28   Gunther G, Asmera J, Parry E. Death from rheumatic heart disease in rural Ethiopia. Lancet 2006;367:391.

29   Kassem AS, Zaher SR, Abou Shleib H, el-Kholy AG, Madkour AA, Kaplan EL. Rheumatic fever prophylaxis using benzathine penicillin G (BPG): two-week versus four-week regimens: comparison of two brands of BPG. Pediatrics 1996;97:992-5.

30   Kaplan EL, Berrios X, Speth J, Siefferman T, Guzman B, Quesny F. Pharmacokinetics of benzathine penicillin G: serum levels during the 28 days after intramuscular injection of 1,200,000 units. J Pediatr 1989;115:146-50.

31   Rizvi S, Khan M, Kundi A, Marsh D, Samad A, Pasha O. Status of rheumatic heart disease in rural Pakistan. Heart 2004;90:394-9.

32   Weiss MM. The incidence of rheumatic and congenital heart disease among school children of Louisville, KY. Am Heart J 1941;22:112-15.

33   Bergman AB, Stamm SJ. The morbidity of cardiac nondisease in schoolchildren. N Engl J Med 1967;276:1008-13.

34   Bergman AB. The menace of mass screening. Am J Public Health 1977;67:601-2.

35   Sadiq M, Islam K, Abid R, et al. Prevalence of rheumatic heart disease in school children of urban Lahore. Heart 2009;95:353-7.

36   Marijon E, Ou P, Celermajer DS, et al. Prevalence of rheumatic heart disease detected by echocardiographic screening. N Engl J Med 2007;357:470-6.

37   Steer AC, Kado J, Wilson N, et al. High prevalence of rheumatic heart disease by clinical and echocardiographic screening among children in Fiji. J Heart Valve Dis 2009;18:327-35; discussion 36.

38   Anabwani GM, Bonhoeffer P. Prevalence of heart disease in school children in rural Kenya using colour-flow echocardiography. East Afr Med J 1996;73:215-7.

39   Carapetis JR, Hardy M, Fakakovikaetau T, et al. Evaluation of a screening protocol using auscultation and portable echocardiography to detect asymptomatic rheumatic heart disease in Tongan schoolchildren. Nat Clin Pract Cardiovasc Med 2008;5:411-7.

40   Singh PI, Carapetis JR, Buadromo EM, Samberkar PN, Steer AC. The high burden of rheumatic heart disease found on autopsy in Fiji. Cardiol Young 2008;18:62-9.

41   Paar JA, Berrios NM, Rose JD, et al. Prevalence of Rheumatic Heart Disease in Children and Young Adults in Nicaragua. Am J Cardiol 2010;105:1809-14.

42   Anabwani GM, Book W, Bonhoeffer P. Echocardiographic findings in Eldoret: retrospective study. East Afr Med J 1996;73:714-6.

43   Mayosi B, Robertson K, Volmink J, et al. The Drakensberg declaration on the control of rheumatic fever and rheumatic heart disease in Africa. S Afr Med J 2006;96:246.

44   Marijon E, Celermajer DS, Tafflet M, et al. Rheumatic heart disease screening by echocardiography. The inadeququacy of World Health Oganization criteria for optimizing the diagnosis of subclinical disease. Circulation 2009;120:663-668.

45   Marijon E, Tafflet M, Jouven X. Time to use ultrasound and not stethoscopes for rheumatic heart disease screening. Nat Clin Pract Cardiovasc Med 2008;5:E1-3.

CHAPTER 10
Chronic Respiratory Disease

10.1   The Burden of Chronic Respiratory Disease in Rural Rwanda

The main forms of chronic respiratory disease (CRD) in Rwanda are asthma, chronic obstructive pulmonary disease (COPD), and bronchiectasis. Chronic care clinics in three Rwandan districts support more than 500 patients with CRD, most of whom are followed at the health center level, mostly for asthma. Prior to treatment, these patients complained of being limited in their ability to carry out farming or other chores that are vital to a successful rural existence. Acute exacerbations of asthma are also a significant cause of hospitalization and can be fatal. There is no data available regarding population prevalence of CRD in rural Rwanda.

More generally, there is relatively little data on the prevalence of CRD in sub-Saharan Africa, and almost all of this data is regarding asthma in urban centers.[1-4] Studies have found that rural areas on the continent probably have a lower prevalence of asthma (around 4% in school-aged children) than cities do (around 10% in the same population).[5] Despite wide discussion of the so-called hygiene hypothesis, the reason for this difference is unknown.[6] There is some evidence that asthma in rural areas is actually associated with malnutrition.[7]

10.1.1   The Impact of Biomass Fuels and Tuberculosis on Chronic Respiratory Disease

Although in much of the world, tobacco is the main risk factor for CRD, tobacco use in rural Rwanda is low both in prevalence and intensity. The 2005 Demographic Health Survey found that only about 7% of the adult population smoked cigarettes.[8] In order to prevent an epidemic of tobacco use, Rwanda has become a party to the Framework Convention on Tobacco Control, and is in the process of passing a ban on smoking in public places.[8]

Pulmonary tuberculosis (even after treatment), and exposure to particulates from biomass fuels such as wood-burning stoves are probably much more significant risk factors for CRD in Rwanda than tobacco.[9,10] In rural Rwanda, as in other areas of sub-Saharan Africa, nearly 90% of cooking is done with biomass fuels, and women and children may spend up to 7 hours a day exposed to the smoke. Rwanda has moved to disseminate improved cooking stoves in the entire country.

10.2 Integration of Chronic Respiratory Disease Management at Health-Center Level

Many resources exist for sub-Saharan African countries seeking to improve services for chronic respiratory disease at the health-center level.[11-16] These resources include practice guidelines from the Global Initiative for Asthma and the Global Initiative for Chronic Obstructive Lung Disease.[17,18] The International Union Against Tuberculosis and Lung Disease (IUATLD) has prepared guidelines and training materials for asthma management in resource-poor settings.[19] The IUATLD has also established an asthma drug facility that provides inhaled corticosteroids at lower cost than what is often available on the market in many countries.[20,21] The Stop TB department in the World Health Organization (WHO) has incorporated a program called the Practical Approach to Lung Health (PAL) as part of its strategy to improve case-finding for pulmonary tuberculosis.[22]

This chapter adapts existing approaches to CRD care integration to the Rwandan setting. There are a couple of aspects of this strategy that are unique. First, the evaluation of severe CRD takes place within a chronic care system capable of basic echocardiography. This probably avoids some misdiagnosis. Second, a network of chronic care community health workers is available to support adherence in advanced cases.

10.2.1 Initial Evaluation for Chronic Respiratory Disease at Health-Center Level

Resource-poor settings face several challenges in the diagnosis and management of CRD. Dyspnea and chronic cough are at once very common and very non-specific complaints. Tuberculosis and other infectious diseases, as well as heart failure, anemia, and parasitic infections, may all cause symptoms that mimic the presentation of asthma (shortness of breath, cough, or wheezing). Even after other causes have been excluded, confirming chronic respiratory pathology can be difficult. Asthma is an intermittent disease, and patients may not have symptoms at the time of presentation to the clinic. Even in developed countries, asthma is a clinical diagnosis, though spirometry is helpful when available. Somatization and anxiety are common in settings such as post-genocide Rwanda, and often feature shortness of breath.[23] Furthermore, diagnostic tools such as spirometry are often unavailable, and simpler methods such as peak flow measurement are prone to high rates of error.

In our model, most chronic respiratory disease management will take place at the level of the health center integrated chronic care clinic. These clinics also see patients with a variety of chronic illnesses with relatively simple treatment algorithms, such as most cases of hypertension, epilepsy, non-insulin dependent diabetes, tuberculosis, and HIV.

PROTOCOL 10.1 outlines the approach adopted at PIH-supported sites for the initial diagnosis and management of chronic respiratory complaints that present to acute care clinics at health centers.

PROTOCOL 10.1   Initial Management of Chronic Cough or Shortness of Breath at Health Center Acute Care Clinics

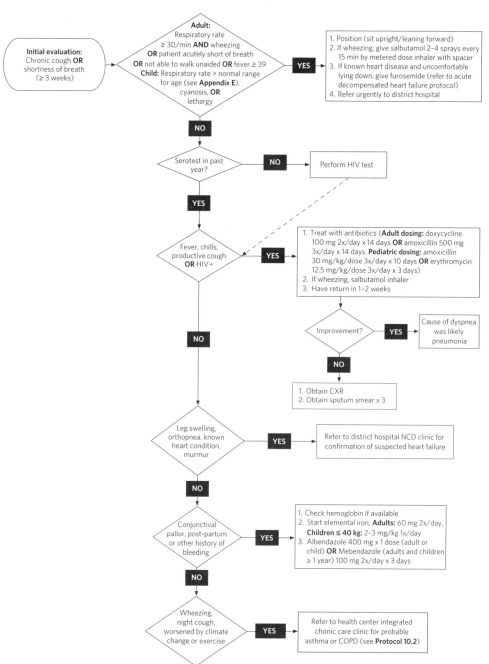

10.2.2 Identification and Treatment of Emergency Conditions

Clinicians must first determine whether the patient is in acute respiratory distress (see **TABLE 10.1**). Clinicians should try to stabilize these patients with available tools: patient positioning, a beta-agonist and steroids if there are signs of bronchospasm, and furosemide if heart failure is suspected. We also recommend that all patients receive a dose of antibiotics until infection has been ruled out. It is preferable to use an agent that does not have anti-tuberculous activity, such as doxycycline, ampicillin, erythromycin, or trimethoprim-sulfamethoxazole (TMP-SMX), in case sputum smears are necessary to rule out tuberculosis. Once stabilized, all patients in respiratory distress should be referred urgently to the district-hospital level for inpatient admission.

TABLE 10.1 Evaluation of Asthma Attack Severity (Adapted from IUATLD Guidelines)[19]

Symptoms	Mild asthma attack	Moderate asthma attack	Severe asthma attack	Imminent respiratory failure
Dyspnea	With physical exertion	With speaking	All the time	All the time
Can speak in	Full sentences	Phrases	Words	Unable to speak
Mental status	Normal	Normal or agitated	Agitated	Somnolent or confused
Respiratory rate	Normal to fast	Fast	Very fast ($\geq$30 breaths/min)	Very fast ($\geq$30 breaths/min)
Pulse (ranges apply to adults)	$\leq$ 100	100–120	$\geq$120	Bradycardic
Peak expiratory flow (PEF) after salbutamol (% of patient's best PEF or predicted PEF , see **APPENDIX E**)	$\geq$ 70%	50%–70%	$\leq$ 50% or $\leq$ 100 liters/min	Cannot measure

10.2.3 Exclusion of Causes Other Than Asthma and COPD

In the rural health center clinic, lack of diagnostic tools and high prevalence of infectious respiratory disease necessitate exclusion of other diseases before making the diagnosis of COPD or asthma. For the most part, this can be done by taking a careful history of symptoms. Certain symptoms should prompt further testing. **TABLE 10.2** outlines the common causes of chronic respiratory symptoms (lasting more than 3 weeks) seen at our clinics.

TABLE 10.2 Causes of Chronic Dyspnea or Chronic Cough (≥ 3 Weeks)

System	Disease	Evaluate for
Respiratory	Asthma	Episodic wheezing
	COPD	Progressively worsening dyspnea
	Bronchiectasis	Large volume of purulent sputum
	Acute bronchitis/pneumonia	Fever, acute dyspnea, productive cough
	Pulmonary tuberculosis	Cough, hemoptysis, fevers, night sweats, weight loss
Cardiovascular	Congestive heart failure	Edema, orthopnea, rales
	Pulmonary hypertension and right heart failure	Edema, ascites
Gastrointestinal	Gastroesophageal reflux disease	Symptoms of reflux, heartburn
Hematologic	Anemia	Conjunctival pallor, measure hemoglobin
Ear, nose, throat	Allergic or non-allergic rhinitis	Nasal congestion, itchy/watery eyes
	Sinusitis (subacute/chronic)	Postnasal drip, headache, rhinorrhea
Psychological	Anxiety	Dyspnea and chest tightness in social situations, palpitations, sweating, tingling in arms or fingers
Medication	ACE inhibitors	Usually non-productive cough shortly after starting the medication, though can occur at any time

For obvious public health reasons, tuberculosis should be the first diagnosis to consider in all patients presenting with chronic respiratory symptoms. Other infections such as pneumonia are also common causes. HIV is the major risk factor for tuberculosis in Rwanda, and all patients presenting with respiratory symptoms should have a test for HIV unless one has been administered within the past year. Patients who have recently been tested should be retested if they have a chronic cough (greater than 3 weeks) plus fever, significant weight loss, hemoptysis or night sweats. These patients as well as those with HIV and respiratory symptoms should be treated empirically for a bacterial pneumonia with an antibiotic that does not have anti-tuberculous activity, such as doxycycline, erythromycin, TMP-SMX, or amoxicillin.

Patients may also have concomitant asthma and/or bronchospasm as a result of infection. These patients should also be given a short-acting beta agonist inhaler. Patients should return within 2–3 days to ensure that they are improving. If they have not improved, sputum smears should be performed to rule out active tuberculosis. The patient should be referred at this point to a district hospital for a chest x-ray. Patients with active tuberculosis in Rwanda are referred to the integrated chronic care clinic at health center for treatment.[24]

Patients without signs of an infectious process should be evaluated for signs of other etiologies of chronic respiratory symptoms, such as heart failure and anemia.

Patients with typical signs and symptoms of asthma or COPD should be referred to the health center integrated chronic care clinic for diagnostic confirmation and initiation of treatment.

10.3 Diagnosis and Initial Management of Chronic Respiratory Disease in Health Center Integrated Chronic Care Clinics

All patients referred to the health center chronic care clinic for chronic respiratory symptoms should first be evaluated for signs of respiratory decompensation and treated appropriately (see **SECTION 10.2.2**).

Patients who are not in acute respiratory distress should next have a complete history taken and be given a physical examination. The exam should aim to confirm the diagnosis and to classify patients by disease severity (see **PROTOCOL 10.2**). The clinician should suspect an alternative diagnosis, including anxiety/hyperventilation, among patients without classic symptoms (see **TABLE 10.3**). Patients in whom the diagnosis is uncertain may be given a bronchodilator and instructed to return in several weeks or a month to determine whether the intervention is helpful or not. Practitioners must instruct patients in the correct use of inhalers and directly observe patients' inhaler technique at each visit to ensure that the medication is being properly delivered to the lungs. Some patients who are not responding may in fact be using the inhaler incorrectly. If available, spacers (usually made from plastic water bottles) should be given to each patient who is using any kind of inhaler.

PROTOCOL 10.2 Initial Management of Asthma or COPD at Integrated Chronic Care Clinics

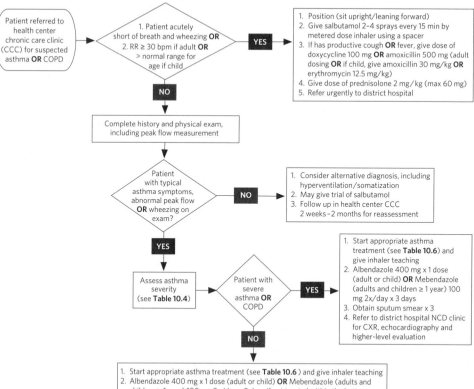

TABLE 10.3 Common Signs and Symptoms of Asthma

Symptoms are intermittent	
Symptoms triggered by changes in weather, exposure to dust, exhaust, exercise or cooking smoke	
Dyspnea	
Wheezing	
Cough	Nonproductive
	Nighttime
Chest tightness	
Reduced PEF in setting of symptoms, 20% improvement with bronchodilators	

Patients for whom the diagnosis of asthma is likely should be classified according to disease severity (see **TABLE 10.4**). Since asthma is characterized mainly by functional limitation, assessing the severity of a patient's asthma via symptoms can be very useful, especially in determining an initial medication regimen. At subsequent visits, an assessment should be made of how well the patient's symptoms are controlled on the current regimen. Our clinic uses questions based on the asthma control test (see **TABLE 10.5**).[25] The assessment should help determine whether the patient needs therapy increased, decreased, or maintained at the same level. All patients should have a chest x-ray performed within the first 3–4 months of diagnosis to rule out any structural cause of dyspnea (such as scarring, bronchiectasis, foreign body aspiration, or anatomic abnormalities).

TABLE 10.4 Classification of Asthma Severity at Initial Visit[26]

Components of severity		Intermittent	Persistent		
			Mild	*Moderate*	*Severe*
Impairment	*Symptoms*	≤ 2 days/week	≥ 2 days/week but not daily	Daily	Throughout the day
	Nighttime awakenings	None	1-2x/month	3-4x/month	≥ 1x/week
	Salbutamol use for symptom control	≤ 2 days/week	≥ 2 days/week but not daily	Daily	Several times per day
	Interference with normal activity	None	Minor limitation	Some limitation	Extremely limited
Risk	Exacerbations requiring oral systemic corticosteroids (prednisolone)	0-1/year	≥ 2 exacerbations in 6 months requiring oral systemic corticosteroids, **OR** ≥ 4 wheezing episodes/year lasting ≥ 1 day **AND** risk factors for persistent asthma		
			Consider severity and interval since last exacerbation. Frequency and severity may fluctuate over time. Exacerbations of any severity may occur in patients in any severity category.		

TABLE 10.5 Asthma Control Test[25]

Maximum score is 25 (points are 1–5 in order as below) ≤ 19 means asthma may not be well controlled		
In the past 4 weeks, how much of the time did your asthma keep you from getting as much done at work, school, or home?	1	All of the time
	2	Most of the time
	3	Some of the time
	4	A little of the time
	5	None of the time
During the past 4 weeks, how often have you had shortness of breath?	1	More than once a day
	2	Once a day
	3	3–6 times a week
	4	Once or twice a week
	5	Not at all
During the past 4 weeks, how often did your asthma symptoms (wheezing, coughing, shortness of breath, chest tightness or pain) wake you up at night or earlier than usual in the morning?	1	4 or more nights a week
	2	2 or 3 nights a week
	3	Once a week
	4	Once or twice
	5	Not at all
During the past 4 weeks, how often have you used your rescue inhaler (salbutamol)?	1	3 or more times per day
	2	1 or 2 times per day
	3	2 or 3 times per week
	4	Once a week or less
	5	Not at all
How would you rate your asthma control during the past 4 weeks?	1	Not controlled at all
	2	Poorly controlled
	3	Somewhat controlled
	4	Well controlled
	5	Completely controlled

Our approach does not ask clinicians to differentiate between COPD and asthma. To do so would likely be impractical in the rural Rwandan chronic care clinic. Risk factors for COPD in our setting are not well understood. Tobacco smoking, the main cause of COPD in industrialized regions, is relatively rare in Rwanda and, when present, is rarely of an intensity or duration likely to cause COPD. Possible causes of COPD, such as repeated exposure to cooking smoke, are hard to quantify. While spirometry may be available at some district hospital clinics, results are both effort-dependent and potentially misleading. Furthermore, we assert that the same simplified strategy can successfully manage both conditions in our setting. With the exception of long-acting beta agonists and anticholinergics, both of which are not readily available in settings such as rural Rwanda, the treatment of these two conditions is similar. As with asthma, patients with suspected COPD should be referred to social work for assessment of indoor air pollution and possible cooking stove improvement.

10.3.1   Step Therapy for Asthma or COPD at Health Centers

Once disease severity has been established, patients should be started on the appropriate therapy (see **TABLE 10.6** and **TABLE 10.7**). We have adapted the step therapy model promoted by the Global Initiative for Asthma (GINA) to the Rwandan setting using the following principles:

- **Patient education:** All patients should receive education about avoidance of triggers, as well as education on the use of the inhaler pumps. Ability to correctly use inhalers should be confirmed by whomever is instructing the patient, and confirmed again at each appointment, particularly if symptoms are not controlled. Where possible, patients should be given spacers (made from plastic water bottles) to be used with their inhalers.

- **Rescue medications:**
  Short-acting beta-agonist—For all patients with asthma, salbutamol should be used as a rescue therapy to control crisis symptoms. Patients should be educated that this medication helps to stop an attack. While oral or injectable salbutamol is widely available, we do not recommend its use. Systemic use of beta-agonists can cause dangerous rises in heart rate and blood pressure due to their non-selective effects. The effect of inhaled salbutamol is relatively limited to the airways without much systemic absorption.

  Oral steroids—For patients in the midst of an acute, severe attack, or for patients with persistent uncontrolled symptoms, a prednisolone burst can be given. We recommend a short burst (0.5 mg/kg twice a day for adults or 2 mg/kg once a day for children < 30 kg for 5 days) as a trial. If this fails to control symptoms or if symptoms rebound, a longer steroid taper (7–14 days) may be given.

- **Controller medications:**
  For all patients with persistent symptoms (mild, moderate, or severe), treatment should include medications to reduce the frequency of attacks. Patients should be educated that these medications need to be taken on a daily basis for effective prevention. Patients using steroid inhalers should be instructed to rinse their mouths out with water after each use, since the medication can land in their mouths and sometimes lead to thrush.

Inhaled steroids—An inhaled steroid such as beclomethasone should be the first controller medication added. The dose of beclomethasone depends on the severity of the patient's symptoms (see **TABLE 10.7**).

Aminophylline—Aminophylline is widely available and can be used as a second-line medication in adults if symptoms are not controlled with inhaled corticosteroids.[27,28] However, if taken at high doses, aminophylline can have toxic effects (particularly nausea, headache, low blood pressure, and seizures). Doses less than 10 mg/kg/day in adults are generally well tolerated.[29] Aminophylline also interacts with many common medications (particularly cimetidine, fluconazole, erythromycin, and ritonavir), and the dose should be reduced if there is potential for drug-drug interaction. Oral aminophylline should not be used for acute exacerbations. Aminophylline should not be used in pregnancy.[30] We also do not use aminophylline in children. In the future, other, safer agents may help to replace aminophylline as the second-line agent of choice for asthma and COPD.

Long-acting beta-agonists—Long-acting preparations of beta-agonist drugs can help prevent and control asthma symptoms when taken on a daily basis. Currently, these medications are not available in Rwanda, but they may be an option in the future.

- **Medication adjustment:** As a patient's symptoms stabilize, monitoring on the current regimen should continue for about 3–6 months. If symptoms remain stable, the therapy can be reduced. The protocol will depend in part on how severe symptoms were initially. Sometimes patients will need controller therapy for a few years or even for the rest of their lives. Others may have symptoms only in the setting of a respiratory infection. Some cases will not fit neatly into the protocol. In such cases, providers should use their best judgments, provided these are based on the underlying principles for managing asthma. If uncertainty persists, the patient should be seen in consultation with a doctor.

- **Level of care and frequency of visits:** Patients with severe disease should be evaluated at the district hospital NCD clinic and receive an extensive work-up for alternative diagnoses, such as tuberculosis or heart failure. Patients with mild or moderate symptoms will be managed at the health center NCD clinic. Follow-up interval should also depend on symptom severity.

- **Adjunctive medications:**
  Anti-helminthics—Although likely not a common cause of asthma symptoms, parasitemia (especially *Strongyloides stercoralis*) can cause wheezing and other respiratory symptoms. Treatment is both inexpensive and effective. Therefore, we recommend treating

all newly diagnosed patients with albendazole 400 mg x 1 dose or Mebendazole 100 mg 2x/day for 3 days, if they have not already been treated for parasites within the last year.

Acid-controllers—Gastroesophogeal reflux disease (GERD) can occasionally cause or exacerbate asthma symptoms. If patients report symptoms of GERD, the clinician may consider a trial of an H2-blocker (cimetidine, ranitidine) or a proton pump inhibitor (omeprazole). If after 2–4 weeks symptoms have improved, the clinician should consider continuing the medication long term. Patients should also be instructed on ways to reduce GERD, such as making sure to stay upright 30–60 minutes after meals, not eating before going to bed, and sleeping with the head and torso propped up.

Antihistamines—Patients suspected of having asthma should also be asked about symptoms of allergic rhinitis, such as itchy or watery eyes, itchy or runny nose, itchy ears, post-nasal drip, and frequent sneezing or cough without concomitant infection. Although the prevalence of allergic rhinitis in the Rwandan population is not known, it is common worldwide and has been reported to be common in other African countries, including Nigeria, Zimbabwe, and South Africa.[1,31-33] Allergic rhinitis often exacerbates asthma. Treating patients with allergic rhinitis who also have asthma can decrease exacerbation and hospitalization rates by 80%.[34] Treatment can be initiated with antihistamines (chlorpheniramine).

TABLE 10.6 Asthma Step Therapy

STEP-UP when poor control / STEP-DOWN when doing well	Asthma severity	Salbutamol	Beclomethasone	Aminophylline (for use only in non-pregnant adults)	Prednisone
	Step 5: Severe uncontrolled	Yes	High dose	Yes	Yes
	Step 4: Severe persistent	Yes	High dose	Yes	No
	Step 3: Moderate persistent	Yes	Medium dose	No	No
	Step 2: Mild persistent	Yes	Low dose	No	No
	Step 1: Intermittent	Yes	No	No	No

TABLE 10.7 Asthma Medication Dosing

	Salbutamol 100 mcg (inhaler)	Beclomethasone 50 and 250 mcg (inhaler) Always use a spacer	Aminophylline 100 mg tab	Prednisone 5 mg tab
Adults and children ≥ 30 kg	1-2 puffs, 3x/day as needed	**High:** 1500 mcg (3 puffs 2x/d) **Medium:** 1000 mcg (2 puffs 2x/d) **Low:** 500 mcg (1 puff 2x/d)	100 mg 3x/day	1-2 mg/kg/day (max 60 mg) x 5 days. If no response, can do a taper over 7-14 days. **Note:** If new CRD diagnosis, first, rule out TB (smear x 3, CXR)
Children 10-30 kg (always use spacers)	1-2 puffs, 3x/day as needed	**High:** 1000 mcg/d (2 puffs 2x/d) **Medium:** 500 mcg/d (1 puff 2x/d) **Low:** 250 mcg/d (1 puff 1x/d)	n/a	2 mg/kg once per day x 5 days (max 60 mg). If no response, can do a taper over 7-14 days.
Children ≤ 10 kg	**REFER TO PHYSICIAN** Very small children should use a metered-dose inhaler with a spacer, or a nebulizer if available.			

10.4 Follow-Up Management of Asthma

PROTOCOL 10.3 outlines subsequent management of patients with an established diagnosis of asthma.

As with other visits, the follow-up visit should first focus on identifying signs of acute respiratory distress and treating accordingly.

Next, the clinician should ask the patients about frequency of symptoms. Questions from the Asthma Control Test (see **TABLE 10.5**) can be used. Vital signs, a lung exam, and peak flow measurement should be performed. Using this data, the clinician should consider how well controlled the patient's symptoms are and decide whether therapy should be continued, increased, or decreased.

PROTOCOL 10.3 Follow-Up Management of Asthma or COPD at Health-Center Level

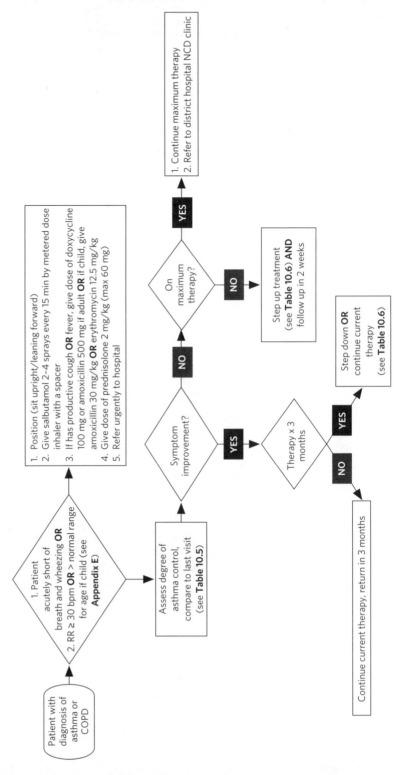

Patient with diagnosis of asthma or COPD

1. Patient acutely short of breath and wheezing **OR**
2. RR ≥ 30 bpm **OR** > normal range for age if child (see **Appendix E**)

1. Position (sit upright/leaning forward)
2. Give salbutamol 2–4 sprays every 15 min by metered dose inhaler with a spacer
3. If has productive cough **OR** fever, give dose of doxycycline 100 mg or amoxicillin 500 mg if adult **OR** if child, give amoxicillin 30 mg/kg **OR** erythromycin 12.5 mg/kg
4. Give dose of prednisolone 2 mg/kg (max 60 mg)
5. Refer urgently to hospital

Assess degree of asthma control, compare to last visit (see **Table 10.5**)

Symptom improvement?

NO → On maximum therapy?

On maximum therapy? **YES** → 1. Continue maximum therapy
2. Refer to district hospital NCD clinic

On maximum therapy? **NO** → Step up treatment (see **Table 10.6**) **AND** follow up in 2 weeks

Symptom improvement? **YES** → Therapy x 3 months

Therapy x 3 months **YES** → Step down **OR** continue current therapy (see **Table 10.6**)

Therapy x 3 months **NO** → Continue current therapy, return in 3 months

Most patients should improve within 3–6 months of receiving consistent, adequate treatment.

Patients whose symptoms are not well controlled may need more intensive therapy. Before intensifying treatment, the clinician should make sure that the patient is adherent to the medications and can demonstrate good inhaler technique. If the clinician believes a worsening of symptoms is due to a temporary exacerbating factor (viral infection or exposure to a known allergen), then intensification of controller medications may not be necessary, or can be employed for a short period only. Patients who are still uncontrolled after a trial of maximum therapy should be referred to the district hospital NCD clinic for evaluation by a physician.

Patients who have achieved symptom control after at least 3–6 months of therapy may be eligible for a reduction in therapy intensity. This should be undertaken with care, in stages. Further reductions should be pursued only after a 3–6 month trial at the new level of treatment. If patients worsen on the less intensive treatment, the higher intensity treatment should be resumed and maintained for one to two years before reduction is again attempted.

Patients well controlled on a stable regimen will require less frequent clinic visits. Some patients may only require visits every 6 (or even 12) months.

10.5 Bronchiectasis

Bronchiectasis is abnormal and irreversible dilatation of the airways, usually due to scarring from previous infection, especially tuberculosis, pneumonia, and pertussis, as well as from other infections. HIV can predispose people to bronchiectasis, most likely from recurrent infections.[35,36] People with bronchiectasis usually have chronic productive cough, shortness of breath, and recurrent infections. Often they also have chest pain (usually pleuritic) and hemoptysis. Occasionally they have wheezing. Diagnosis can be made by CXR, which can reveal thickened airways or evidence of scarring. CT scans, if available, reveal dilated and thickened airways. Symptoms of exacerbations include increased sputum production, fever, shortness of breath, and cough. Exacerbations should be treated with antibiotics (such as doxycyline) for at least 7–10 days, sometimes for as long as 14 days. Anti-pseudomonals, such as ciprofloxacin, may be needed if the patient does not improve. It may be beneficial to give inhaled steroids on a continuing basis. In some studies, this approach led to decreased airway inflammation and clinical improvement.[37,38] It is not unreasonable to try inhaled beta-agonists and continue them if there is symptomatic improvement. Ongoing sputum clearance techniques, such as chest percussion, breathing techniques, and postural drainage, are effective and can be an important means for staving off exacerbations.[39] Such interventions can be performed by a patient's family members or by a community health worker, if the patient has one.

Chapter 10 References

· ·

1   Ait-Khaled N, Pearce N, Anderson HR, Ellwood P, Montefort S, Shah J. Global map of the prevalence of symptoms of rhinoconjunctivitis in children: The International Study of Asthma and Allergies in Childhood (ISAAC) Phase Three. Allergy 2009;64:123-48.

2   Ait-Khaled N, Odhiambo J, Pearce N, et al. Prevalence of symptoms of asthma, rhinitis and eczema in 13- to 14-year-old children in Africa: the International Study of Asthma and Allergies in Childhood Phase III. Allergy 2007;62:247-58.

3   Buist AS, McBurnie MA, Vollmer WM, et al. International variation in the prevalence of COPD (the BOLD Study): a population-based prevalence study. Lancet 2007;370:741-50.

4   Mehrotra A, Oluwole AM, Gordon SB. The burden of COPD in Africa: a literature review and prospective survey of the availability of spirometry for COPD diagnosis in Africa. Trop Med Int Health 2009;14:840-8.

5   Odhiambo JA, Ng'ang'a LW, Mungai MW, et al. Urban-rural differences in questionnaire-derived markers of asthma in Kenyan school children. Eur Respir J 1998;12:1105-12.

6   Wjst M, Boakye D. Asthma in Africa. PLoS Med 2007;4:e72.

7   Berntsen S, Lodrup Carlsen KC, Hageberg R, et al. Asthma symptoms in rural living Tanzanian children; prevalence and the relation to aerobic fitness and body fat. Allergy 2009;64:1166-71.

8   Pampel F. Tobacco use in sub-Sahara Africa: estimates from the demographic health surveys. Soc Sci Med 2008;66:1772-83.

9   Salvi SS, Barnes PJ. Chronic obstructive pulmonary disease in non-smokers. Lancet 2009;374:733-43.

10 Kurmi OP, Semple S, Simkhada P, Smith WC, Ayres JG. COPD and chronic bronchitis risk of indoor air pollution from solid fuel: a systematic review and meta-analysis. Thorax;65:221-8.

11 World Health Organization. Prevention and Control of Chronic Respiratory Diseases in low- and middle-income African countries: a preliminary report based on the Meetings in Montpellier, France, 27-28 July 2002 and Paris, France, 10 June 2003. Gevena: World Health Organization; 2003.

12 Kengne AP, Sobngwi E, Fezeu LL, Awah PK, Dongmo S, Mbanya JC. Nurse-led care for asthma at primary level in rural sub-Saharan Africa: the experience of Bafut in Cameroon. J Asthma 2008;45:437-43.

13 Coleman R, Gill G, Wilkinson D. Noncommunicable disease management in resource-poor settings: a primary care model from rural South Africa. Bull World Health Organ 1998;76:633-40.

14 Bheekie A, Buskens I, Allen S, et al. The Practical Approach to Lung Health in South Africa (PALSA) intervention: respiratory guideline implementation for nurse trainers. Int Nurs Rev 2006;53:261-8.

15 English RG, Bateman ED, Zwarenstein MF, et al. Development of a South African integrated syndromic respiratory disease guideline for primary care. Prim Care Respir J 2008;17:156-63.

16 World Health Organization. Global Alliance Against Chronic Respiratory Diseases. Action Plan 2008-2013. Geneva: World Health Organization; 2008.

17 Bateman ED, Hurd SS, Barnes PJ, et al. Global strategy for asthma management and prevention: GINA executive summary. Eur Respir J 2008;31:143-78.

18 Rabe KF, Hurd S, Anzueto A, et al. Global strategy for the diagnosis, management, and prevention of chronic obstructive pulmonary disease: GOLD executive summary. Am J Respir Crit Care Med 2007;176:532-55.

19 Ait-Khaled N, Enarson DA, Chen-Yuan C, Marks G, Bissell K. Management of Asthma. A Guide to the Essentials of Good Clinical Practice. Third Edition. Paris: International Union Against Tuberculosis and Lung Disease; 2008.

20 Billo NE. Good news: asthma medicines for all. Int J Tuberc Lung Dis 2010;14:524.

21 Billo NE. Do we need an asthma drug facility? Int J Tuberc Lung Dis 2004;8:391.

22 Murray JF, Pio A, Ottmani S. PAL: a new and practical approach to lung health. Int J Tuberc Lung Dis 2006;10:1188-91.

23 Hagengimana A, Hinton DE. Culture and panic disorder. In: Hinton DE, Good B, eds. Stanford, Calif.: Stanford University Press; 2009:xxi, 272 p.

24 Gasana M, Vandebriel G, Kabanda G, et al. Integrating tuberculosis and HIV care in rural Rwanda. Int J Tuberc Lung Dis 2008;12:39-43.

25 Nathan RA, Sorkness CA, Kosinski M, et al. Development of the asthma control test: a survey for assessing asthma control. J Allergy Clin Immunol 2004;113:59-65.

26 National Heart Lung and Blood Institute, National Asthma Education and Prevention Program. Expert Panel Report 3: Guidelines for the Diagnosis and Management of Asthma. Bethesda, MD: U.S. Department of Health and Human Services; 2007.

27 Seddon P, Bara A, Ducharme FM, Lasserson TJ. Oral xanthines as maintenance treatment for asthma in children. Cochrane Database Syst Rev 2006:CD002885.

28 Watson JP, Lewis RA. Is asthma treatment affordable in developing countries? Thorax 1997;52:605-7.

29 Makino S, Adachi M, Ohta K, et al. A prospective survey on safety of sustained-release theophylline in treatment of asthma and COPD. Allergol Int 2006;55:395-402.

30 Nuhoglu Y, Nuhoglu C. Aminophylline for treating asthma and chronic obstructive pulmonary disease. Expert Rev Respir Med 2008;2:305-13.

31 Falade AG, Olawuyi JF, Osinusi K, Onadeko BO. Prevalence and severity of symptoms of asthma, allergic rhinoconjunctivitis, and atopic eczema in 6- to 7-year-old Nigerian primary school children: the international study of asthma and allergies in childhood. Med Princ Pract 2004;13:20-5.

32 Sibanda EN. Inhalant allergies in Zimbabwe: a common problem. Int Arch Allergy Immunol 2003;130:2-9.

33 Zar HJ, Ehrlich RI, Workman L, Weinberg EG. The changing prevalence of asthma, allergic rhinitis and atopic eczema in African adolescents from 1995 to 2002. Pediatr Allergy Immunol 2007;18:560-5.

34 Corren J, Manning BE, Thompson SF, Hennessy S, Strom BL. Rhinitis therapy and the prevention of hospital care for asthma: a case-control study. J Allergy Clin Immunol 2004;113:415-9.

35 Holmes AH, Trotman-Dickenson B, Edwards A, Peto T, Luzzi GA. Bronchiectasis in HIV disease. Q J Med 1992;85:875-82.

36 Bard M, Couderc LJ, Saimot AG, et al. Accelerated obstructive pulmonary disease in HIV-infected patients with bronchiectasis. Eur Respir J 1998;11:771-5.

37 Tsang KW, Ho PL, Lam WK, et al. Inhaled fluticasone reduces sputum inflammatory indices in severe bronchiectasis. Am J Respir Crit Care Med 1998;158:723-7.

38 Tsang KW, Tan KC, Ho PL, et al. Inhaled fluticasone in bronchiectasis: a 12 month study. Thorax 2005;60:239-43.

39 Eaton T, Young P, Zeng I, Kolbe J. A randomized evaluation of the acute efficacy, acceptability and tolerability of flutter and active cycle of breathing with and without postural drainage in non-cystic fibrosis bronchiectasis. Chron Respir Dis 2007;4:23-30.

EPILOGUE

We believe that the right to insulin, and to every other effective tool of public health and medicine, is a fundamental human right. Tragically, it is a right rarely enjoyed by the poor. Our clinical practice, as well as the integrated research, teaching, advocacy, and health systems–strengthening efforts to which it is inextricably linked, has focused on addressing this grotesque inequity.

This manual reminds us, first of all, that the poor deserve our highest discernment and attention. It reminds us that heart disease, to name just one affliction, is a problem not only in wealthy societies but also in the poorest, and that it can be caused not just by tobacco but also by microbes festering unchecked among those who can't afford to buy sufficient food.

Infections often have long, painful, and debilitating aftermaths, as do a host of endemic, non-communicable diseases. The long tails of disease, of rheumatic fever as well as of cancer, are terrible afflictions among the poor—and have been too long neglected. This manual distills four years of work in partnership with the Rwandan national health system, strengthening its ability to address chronic afflictions. It is a collaboration between international medical specialists and Rwandan health professionals, including the country's own growing cadre of community health workers, nurses, and university-based specialists. Their combined efforts have saved the lives and relieved the pain of many Rwandans.

The text describes protocols focused on the essential interventions often deemed too complex to be delivered to the rural poor as well as comprehensive technical strategies shown to be both efficient and effective for managing chronic disease. It encompasses the essentials of cardiology, diabetology, epileptology, pulmonology, nephrology, and palliative care. This manual systematically addresses the needs of the sickest patients first; focuses on developing indigenous leadership in district hospitals; and offers a sound basis for the training, mentoring, and supervision of health professionals.

The PIH Guide to Chronic Care Integration for Endemic NCDs – Rwanda Edition is focused mainly on ambulatory care performed by advanced nurses, clinical officers, and generalist physicians. We expect that over the next decade, many of us will be engaged in further defining the roles of community health workers, family and community medicine physicians, gynecologic nurses, pathologists, and medical and surgical specialists. But this volume will, we hope, offer a starting point for the creation of a system of care for non-communicable diseases: one blueprint for fulfilling, in Rwanda, an essential part of a fundamental human right.

Paul E. Farmer, MD, PhD

Kolokotrones University Professor, Harvard University

Chair, Department of Global Health and Social Medicine, Harvard Medical School

Chief, Division of Global Health Equity, Brigham and Women's Hospital Co-founder, Partners In Health

February 2011

APPENDIX A

Essential Equipment and Medicines[1,2]

A.1 Essential Equipment

Essential equipment	Health center	District hospital	Referral center
Automatic sphygmomanometer (blood pressure machine) with pediatric, small adult, and adult cuffs, and AC adapter	x	x	x
Glucometer with test strips and lancets	x	x	x
Electrocardiography equipment		x	x
Lab: Chemistry testing (point-of-care) including electrolytes and creatinine		x	x
Lab: HbA1c testing (point-of-care)		x	x
Lab: Hemoglobin testing	x	x	x
Lab: HIV testing	x	x	x
Lab: PT/INR testing (point-of-care)		x	x
Lab: Urine dipstick	x	x	x
Lab: Urinalysis		x	x
Monofilament	x	x	x
Multifunction ultrasound machine (with abdominal, cardiac, and obstetric probes) with ultrasound gel		x	x
Nebulizer		x	x
Peak flow meter	x	x	x
Scale	x	x	x
Tape measure/ruler	x	x	x
Water bottle spacers (for inhaler)	x	x	x

A.2   Essential Medicines

x = Currently recommended by Rwanda MOH
* = Recommended for chronic care integration

Pregnancy categories	
Category A	Controlled studies show no risk, OK to use
Category B	No evidence of risk in humans, OK to use
Category C	Risk cannot be ruled out, use only if there is no alternative. Potential benefit may outweigh potential risk
Category D	Positive evidence of risk, avoid use
Category X	Contraindicated in pregnancy, do not use

Palliative care	Pregnancy category	Health center	District hospital	Referral center
Analgesia				
Acetaminophen/paracetamol 250 mg suppository 500 mg tablet 125 mg/5 mL syrup	B	x	x	x
Amitriptyline 25 mg tablet	C		x	x
Diazepam 5 mg tablet 5 mg/mL injectable	D	x	x	x
Diclofenac 50 mg tablet 50 mg suppository	C	x	x	x
Ibuprofen 200 mg tablet 100 mg/5 mL syrup	B	x	x	x
Morphine, powder	C		*	*
Morphine, liquid prepared at district level from powder 50 mg/5 mL 5 mg/5 mL	C	*	*	*
Morphine, injectable 10 mg/mL	C		x	x
Phenytoin (Dilantin) 100 mg capsule	D		x	x
Prednisolone 5 mg tablet	C	x	x	x
Dexamethasone, injectable 4 mg/mL	C	x	x	x

Palliative care	Pregnancy category	Health center	District hospital	Referral center
Anti-emetics				
Chlorpheniramine 4 mg tablet	B	x	x	x
Dexamethasone, injectable 4 mg/mL	C	x	x	x
Haloperidol 2 mg, 5 mg tablets 5 mg/mL injectable	C		x	x
Metoclopramide 10 mg tablet 5 mg/mL	B	x	x	x
Promethazine 10 mg tablet 5 mg/5 mL syrup 25 mg/2 mL injectable	C	x	x	x
Constipation				
Bisacodyl	C	x	x	x
Glycerine suppository 2, 4 mg	C	x	x	x
Lactulose syrup 3.33 grams/5 mL	B	x	x	x
Naloxone 400 mcg/mL	B	*	x	x
Diarrhea				
Hyoscine butylbromide 10 mg tablet 20 mg/1 mL	C	x	x	x
Pruritus				
Betamethasone cream 0.1% cream 0.1% lotion 0.1% ointment	C	x	x	x
Permethrin 5% cream 1% lotion	B	*	x	x
Other				
Fluoxetine 20 mg tablet	C	*	x	x

Heart failure, cardiac surgery, hypertension, anticoagulation, and chronic kidney disease	Pregnancy category	Health center	District hospital	Referral center
Amlodipine 10 mg tablet	C	*	x	x
Aspirin 100 mg, 500 mg tablet	C–D	x	x	x
Atenolol 50 mg tablet	D	*	x	x
Captopril 25 mg tablet	D	*	x	x
Carvedilol 6.25 mg, 25 mg tablet	C	*	*	*
Erythromycin 250 mg tablet 125 mg/5 mL syrup	B	x	x	x
Furosemide (Lasix) 40 mg tablet	C	*	x	x
Furosemide (Lasix) 10 mg/mL	C		x	x
Hydralazine 50 mg tablet	C	*	x	x
Hydralazine, injectable 20 mg/mL	C		x	x
Isosorbide dinitrate 10 mg tablet	C	*	*	x
Lisinopril 10 mg tablet	D	*	*	*
Magnesium sulfate, injectable 500 mg/mL	A	*	*	x
Methyldopa 250 mg tablet	A	*	x	x
Nifedipine 10 mg tablet	C	*	x	x
Penicillin G benzathine, injectable 2 million and 5 million UI vials	B	x	x	x
Penicillin V 250 mg tablet	B	x	x	x
Propranolol 20, 40 mg tablet	C	*	x	x

Heart failure, cardiac surgery, hypertension, anticoagulation, and chronic kidney disease	Pregnancy category	Health center	District hospital	Referral center
Spironolactone (Aldactone) 25 mg tablet	D	*	x	x
Warfarin 1, 5 mg tablet	X		*	*
Diabetes	Pregnancy category	Health center	District hospital	Referral center
Amitriptyline 25 mg tablet	C	*	x	x
Glibenclamide (Daonil) 5 mg tablet	C	x	x	x
Insulin *Lente* (NPH) 100 UI/mL	B	x	x	x
Insulin *Rapide* (Regular) 100 UI/mL	B	x	x	x
Insulin *Mixte* (70/30) 100 UI/mL	B	x	x	x
Metformin 500 mg tablet	B	x	x	x
Chronic respiratory disease	Pregnancy category	Health center	District hospital	Referral center
Aminophylline 100 mg tablet	C	x	x	x
Beclomethasone inhaler 50 mcg/dose, 250 mcg/dose inhalers	C	*	*	x
Chlorpheniramine 4 mg tablet	B	x	x	x
Doxycycline 100 mg tablet	D	x	x	x
Prednisolone 5 mg tablet	C	x	x	x
Salbutamol inhaler 100 mcg/dose inhaler	C	x	x	x
Salbutamol nebulized 5 mg/mL solution	C		x	x

Appendix A References

1   National Essential Medicines List. 5th Edition. Kigali: Ministry of Health, Rwanda; 2009.

2   Lacy CF, Armstrong LL, Golman MP, Lance LR, eds. Lexi-Comp's Drug Information Handbook 2010-2011: A Comprehensive Resource for All Clinicians and Healthcare Professionals. 19th Edition. 2010-2011. Hudson, Ohio: Lexi-Comp; 2010.

APPENDIX B
Cost Models
· ·

The prices for medications listed here are the lowest obtained by
Partners In Health in Rwanda for generics through several different
suppliers. These are actual prices paid. Lower prices may be achievable
through larger-scale purchases and through direct negotiation with
manufacturers.

B.1   Summary of Operational Cost Models

The following cost model projects the estimated marginal costs of national chronic care integration for selected endemic non-communicable
diseases in Rwanda. The model assumes a level of case-finding achievable through decentralization of chronic care services for NCDs down
to the district-hospital level in all districts. The model also shows the
marginal operational costs of a national cardiac surgical program per-
forming 300 surgeries per year.

The estimated time to move from a system with 10% NCD chronic care
coverage at district level to a system with 100% coverage at this level is
approximately 2 years based on current training approaches.

As chronic care services are decentralized to the health-center level,
case-finding rates will increase, as will service utilization and per capita
costs. At the same time, the country's internal sources of revenue will
continue to increase as well.

Condition	Case-finding rate	Population prevalence*	Cases found	Average annual cost		
				Total	Per patient	Per capita
Cardiomyopathy	30%	0.2%	6,000	$2,009,506	$334	$0.20
Cardiac surgical follow-up	3%	0.1%	300	$3,709	$412	$0.012
Screening and follow-up for HIV nephropathy	100%	0.1%	9,000	$46,873	$5	$0.005
Diabetes	50%	0.44%	22,000	$3,806,655	$173	$0.38
Hypertension (160/90 threshold)	100%	4%	400,000	$7,632,542	$9	$0.76
Chronic respiratory disease	15%	2%	24,900	$1,453,695	$57	$0.14
Chronic care integration subtotal				**$3,655,917**		**$1.50**
Cardiac surgery (initial surgery)**	3%	0.1%	300	$1,164,000	$3,880	$0.12
TOTAL				**$819,917**		**$1.62**

* Prevalence given for the entire population.
** 300 cases per year.

B.2 Cardiomyopathy

B.2.1 Cost Inputs

Individual medication costs	Price per tablet	Goal regimen	Annual cost
Furosemide 40 mg tablets	$0.0029	40 mg 2x/d	$2.08
Lisinopril 10 mg tablets	$0.01	20 mg 1x/d	$7.37
Carvedilol 25 mg tablets	$0.035	25 mg 2x/d	$25.6
Isosorbide dinitrate (IDN) 10 mg tablets	$0.025	10 mg 3x/d	$27.2
Hydralazine 50 mg tablets	$0.023	25 mg 3x/d	$23.9
Spironolactone 25 mg tablets	$0.020	25 mg 1x/d	$7.3

B.2.2 Annual Regimen Costs Per Patient

Regimen	Annual cost
FLC: Furosemide 40 mg 2x/d, lisinopril 20 mg 1x/d, carvedilol 25 mg 2x/d	$40.25
FHIC: Furosemide 40 mg 2x/d, hydralazine 50 mg 3x/d, IDN 20 mg 3x/d, carvedilol 25 mg 2x/d	$90.46

Other program costs (per patient)	Annual cost
Laboratory testing (point-of-care chemistries @ $9.8 during 5 visits)	$59
Transport (12 visits per year @ $3 per visit)	$48
Community health workers (@ $30 per month divided over 5 patients)	$72
NCD nurse (@ $10,000 base; 12 visits)	$33
Marginal cost of hospitalization (5 days per year at $15 per day)	$75
Subtotal	$287

B.2.3 Population Age Distribution and Case-Finding (Catchment Area: 350,000)

Estimated cardiomyopathy prevalence	0.2%
Case-finding	30%
Total cardiomyopathy population	700
Total cardiomyopathy patients enrolled in program	210

B.2.4 Total Marginal Costs Per Capita

	Annual cost
Medication costs per patient (85% on FLC and 15% on FHIC)	$47.8
Other program costs per patient	$287
Total costs per patient	$334
Marginal annual program cost	$70,333
Marginal annual cost per capita	$0.20

B.3 Cardiac Surgery
B.3.1 Cost Inputs
B.3.1.1 Follow-Up Cost Inputs

Medication	Price per unit/tablet	Goal regimen	Annual cost
Warfarin 5 mg tablets	$0.13	5 mg 1x/d	$46
Warfarin 1 mg tablets	$0.06	1 mg 1x/d	$21
INR cartridge	$3	16 test/yr	$48

B.3.1.2   Surgical Cost Inputs (At 300 Cases Per Year)

Item	Unit cost	Number	Total annual cost
Operating supplies	$800	300	$240,000
ICU costs	$500	300	$150,000
Hospitalization costs	$600	300	$180,000
Mechanical valves (2 out of 3 cases)	$1000	200	$200,000
Facility cost	fixed	fixed	$50,000
Equipment depreciation annual	fixed	fixed	$20,000
Surgeon salary	$72,000	2	$144,000
Perfusionist salary	$12,000	2	$24,000
Scrub nurse salary	$9,000	2	$18,000
Circulating nurse salary	$9,000	2	$18,000
Anesthesiologist salary	$40,000	2	$80,000
ICU nurse salary	$10,000	4	$40,000
Total surgical cost			$1,164,000
Total surgical per patient cost			$3,880

B.3.1.3   Average Cardiac Surgical Costs as a Function of the Number
of Annual Operations

The figure below shows how the average cost of cardiac surgery decreases
as the number of operations per year increases.

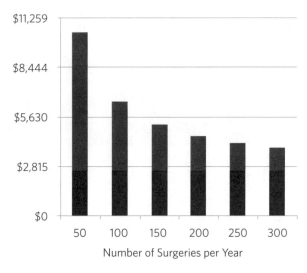

Number of Surgeries per Year

■ average fixed cost/patient   ■ average variable cost/patient

B.3.1.4   Regimen and Follow-Up Costs

	Visits per year	Cost per visit	Annual cost per patient
INR cartridge	16	3	$48
Transport	16	3	$48
Echocardiography	2	72	$144
Community health worker	N/A	N/A	$72
Warfarin 5 mg 1x/d	N/A	N/A	$67
NCD nurse (@ $10,000 base), 12 visits	12	$2.78	$33.3
Subtotal			**$412**

B.3.2   Population Age Distribution and Case-Finding

Population of Rwanda	10,000,000
Estimated population prevalence of advanced RHD	0.1%
Total advanced RHD population in need of surgery	10,000

B.3.3   Total Marginal Costs Per Capita (At 300 Cases Per Year)

Total surgical cost per patient cost	$3,880
Total follow-up cost per patient per year	$412.1
Marginal annual follow-up cost	$160,439
Annual per capita cost	$0.13

B.4   Screening for HIV Nephropathy

B.4.1   Cost Inputs

Medication or lab	Price per unit	Goal regimen	Annual cost
Lisinopril 10 mg tablets	$0.01	5 mg 1x/d	$1.84
Urine dipstick	$0.02	N/A	N/A
Creatinine	$3	N/A	N/A

B.4.2   Marginal Follow-Up Costs

Other program costs (per patient enrolled)	Annual cost
Laboratory testing (point-of-care chemistries @ $9.8 x 6 visits)	$58.8

B.4.3   Population Age Distribution and Case-Finding

Total population size	350,000
HIV population prevalence (all ages)	2%
HIV proteinuria prevalence	6%
Total HIV+ population	5,250
Total with HIV and proteinuria	315

B.4.4   Total Marginal Costs Per Capita

Cost to screen population	Cost
Urine dipstick for screening population	$112.88
Creatinine for patients with proteinuria	$945
Total	$1,057.9

Total costs	
Screening laboratory cost	$1,057.88
Medication cost	$580.62
Follow-up costs	$58.8
Total annual program cost	$1,697.30
Marginal per capita program cost	$0.005

B.5   Diabetes

B.5.1   Cost Inputs

Medication	Price per unit/tablet	Goal regimen	Units/tablets per day	Annual cost
Insulin 70/30 (mixte) 100 IU/mL, 10 mL	$0.009	15 U 2x/d	30	$99
Insulin regular (rapide) 100 IU/mL, 10 mL	$0.010	10 U 2x/d	20	$72
Insulin NPH (lente) 100 IU/mL, 10 mL	$0.010	15 U 2x/d	30	$109
Syringes (1 mL, 26 g needle)	$0.088	2x/d	2	$65
Metformin 500 mg tablets	$0.010	1000 mg 2x/d	4	$15
Glibenclamide 5 mg tablets	$0.003	5 mg 2x/d	2	$2
Lisinopril 10 mg tablets	$0.01	5 mg 1x/d	0.5	$2

Testing supply	Units per package	Package price	Price per test
Finger-stick blood glucose	N/A	N/A	$0.35
Creatinine	N/A	N/A	$3
Urine dipstick	100	$2.2	$0.02
Point-of-care HbA1c	20	$177.2	$8.86

B.5.2 Annual Regimen Costs Per Patient

Regimen	Components
Oral	Metformin 1000 mg 2x/d, Glibenclamide 5 mg 1x/d, Lisinopril 5 mg 1x/d
Mixte	Mixte 70/30 15 Units 2x/d, Lisinopril 5 mg 1x/d
Lente	Lente 15 Units 2x/d, Lisinopril 5 Units 1x/d
Lente + Regular	Lente 10 Units 1x/d + Regular 10 Units 2x/d, Lisinopril 5 mg 1x/d

Cost estimates	Medications	Clinic visits*	Lab testing†	FSBG‡	CHW salary	Total annual cost
Oral	$19	$18	$27	N/A	N/A	$64
Mixte insulin	$165	$36	$30	$20	$87	$338
Lente insulin	$176	$36	$30	$20	$87	$349
Lente + Regular insulin	$207	$36	$30	$20	$87	$380

* Clinic cost: $3/visit. If on oral therapy: 6 visits/year. If on insulin: 12 visits/year.
† Annual testing: finger-stick glucose at each visit; creatinine 2x/year, HbA1c 2x/year.
‡ If on insulin, 56 finger-stick blood glucose (FSBG) in the community per year (2 FSBG per day x 7 days, done 4 times per year).

B.5.3 Population Age Distribution and Case-Finding

Total population of catchment area	350,000
Percent of population over age 20 years (adults)	44%
Prevalence of diabetes in adults	1%
Case-finding rate	50%
Adults in catchment area	154,000
Adults with diabetes	1540
Cases found	770

B.5.4 Total Marginal Costs Per Capita

Regimen	Total cost		
	Proportion of patients on this regimen	Estimated patient load	Total annual cost
Oral	66%	505	$32,406
Lente insulin	13%	98	$34,315
Lente + Regular insulin	22%	167	$63,394
Total		**770**	**$130,114**
Annual Marginal Cost			**$0.37**

B.6 Hypertension Cost Models

B.6.1 Cost Inputs

Medication	Price per tablet	Goal regimen	Annual cost
HCTZ 25 mg tablets	$0.003	25 mg 1x/d	$1.03
Amlodipine 10 mg tablets	$0.01	10 mg 1x/d	$4.69
Lisinopril 10 mg tablets	$0.01	20 mg 1x/d	$7.37
Atenolol 50 mg tablets	$0.01	25 mg 1x/d	$0.97
Methyldopa 250 mg tablets	$0.02	500 mg 2x/d	$33.6
Hydralazine 25 mg tablets	$0.04	50 mg 3x/d	$83.9
Nifedipine 10 mg tablets	$0.01	20 mg 2x/d	$19

B.6.2 Annual Regimen Costs Per Patient*

Medication regimens	Annual cost per patient
1. **H:** HCTZ 12.5 mg	$0.59
2. **HN:** HCTZ 25 mg, amlodipine 10 mg	$6.57
3. **HNL:** HCTZ 25 mg, amlodipine 10 mg, lisinopril 20 mg	$16.04
4. **HNLA:** HCTZ 25 mg, amlodipine 10 mg, lisinopril 20 mg, atenolol 25 mg	$19.56

* H = HCTZ; N = amlodipine; L = lisinopril; A = atenolol

Hypertension stage	Projected yearly lab monitoring	Laboratory costs per patient per year
Stage I (140/90)	Urine dipstick 1x/y, creatinine 1x/y for 5%	$0.17
Stage II (≥ 160/100)	Urine dipstick 1x/y, creatinine 1x/y for 10%	$0.32
Stage III (≥ 180/110)	Urine dipstick 1x/y, creatinine 1x/y for 20%, chemistries 5%	$0.98

Hypertension stage	Regimen*	Total clinic costs**	Medication	Laboratory testing	Total costs
Stage I (140/90)	100% H	$3	$0.59	$0.17	$3.7
Stage II (≥160/100)	100% HN	$6	$6.57	$0.32	$12.9
Stage III (≥180/110)	70% HNL, 30% HNLA	$18	$17.10	$0.98	$36.1

* H = HCTZ; N = amlodipine; L = lisinopril; A = atenolol
** Clinic cost: Stage I (1 visit per year); Stage II (2 visits per year); Stage III (6 visits per year). $3/visit

B.6.3   Population Age Distribution and Case-Finding

Total population of catchment area (district)	100%	350,000
Percent of population over age 30 years (adults)	30%	105,000
Prevalence of stage I (>140/90)	7%	24,500
Prevalence of stage II (>160/100)	3%	10,500
Prevalence of stage III (>180/110)	1%	3,500

B.6.4   Total Marginal Costs Per Capita

Program costs by treatment threshold	140/90 threshold	160/100 threshold	180/110 threshold
Population at risk (# patients)	38,500	14,000	3,500
Total annual medication costs	$143,356	$128,856	$59,837
Total annual clinic costs	$199,500	$126,000	$63,000
Total laboratory costs	$11,014	$6,812	$3,437
Total supply costs*	$5,471	$5,471	$5,471
Total costs	$359,341	$267,139	$131,744
Average annual medication cost per patient	$3.72	$9.20	$17.10
Annual per capita medication cost	$0.41	$0.37	$0.17
Marginal annual per capita total cost	$1.03	$0.76	$0.38

* Automatic blood pressure machines (1 per 200 population @ $46.89 each).

B.7   Chronic Respiratory Disease Cost Models

B.7.1   Cost Inputs

Individual medication costs	Price per unit/tablet	Goal regimen	Annual cost
Salbutamol 100 mcg inhaler	$0.01	200 mcg 4x/d	$20
Beclomethasone 250 mcg inhaler, medium dose	$0.02	500 mcg 2x/d	$33
Beclomethasone 250 mcg inhaler, high dose	$0.02	750 mcg 2x/d	$49
Aminophylline 100 mg tablets	$0.00	200 mg 3x/d	$10

B.7.2   Annual Regimen Costs Per Patient

Asthma severity	Regimen
Intermittent	Salbutamol 200 mcg 4x/d
Moderate persistent	Salbutamol 200 mcg 4x/d, beclomethasone 500 mcg 2x/d
Severe persistent	Salbutamol 200 mcg 4x/d, beclomethasone 750 mcg 2x/d, aminophylline 200 mg 3x/d

Asthma severity	Medications	Clinic visits	Cost per clinic visit	Total clinic visit cost	Total cost per patient
Intermittent	$20	3	$3	$9	$29
Moderate persistent	$53	10	$3	$30	$83
Severe persistent	$79	12	$7*	$83	$211**

* Including transportation cost.
** Includes community health worker effort for directly observed therapy.

B.7.3   Population Age Distribution and Case-Finding

Total population of catchment area	350,000
Prevalence of chronic respiratory disease	2%
Case-finding rate	15%
Total cases of chronic respiratory disease (in those over 5 years of age)	24,500
Cases found	871

Severity classification	Estimated severity distribution	Patients	Total annual cost
Intermittent asthma	60%	523	$15,318
Moderate persistent	35%	305	$25,361
Severe persistent	5%	44	$9,213
Total	100%	490	$49,892

B.7.4 Total Marginal Costs Per Capita

Severity classification	Total annual medication cost	Total annual clinic costs	Total CHW cost	Total annual cost
Intermittent asthma	$10,612	$4,706	-	$15,318
Moderate persistent	$16,210	$9,151	-	$25,361
Severe persistent	$3,461	$2,615	$3,137	$9,213
Total	$30,283	$16,471	$3,137	$49,892
Annual cost per patient	$35	$19	$4	$57
Marginal annual per capita cost	**$0.09**	**$0.05**	**$0.01**	**$0.14**

APPENDIX C

Indicators for Monitoring and Evaluation

· ·

C.1   Heart Failure and Post-Cardiac Surgery Follow-Up

Demographics
Percent male and female
Median age
Number of new patients enrolled during reporting period
Total number of patients at the end of reporting period
Total number of patients at the end of reporting period by district and sector

Diagnosis and Case-Finding
Number and percent of patients without a cardiology consultation since enrollment
Number and percent of patients without a preliminary echocardiogram, preliminary diagnosis or both
Number and percent of patients referred each quarter to NCD heart failure clinic and confirmed not to have heart failure
Percent of patients without a creatinine check in the last 6 months
Percent in each diagnostic category (cardiomyopathy, pure mitral stenosis, other rheumatic heart disease, pericardial disease, congenital heart disease)
Number/percent with creatinine ≥ 200 µmol/L
Number of post-cardiac surgery patients

Interventions
In the cardiomyopathy subgroup, percent with heart rate ≥ 60 bpm at last visit not on carvedilol
In the cardiomyopathy subgroup, percent on lisinopril or captopril
In the mitral stenosis subgroup, percent with heart rate ≥ 60 bpm at last visit not on atenolol
In the rheumatic heart disease subgroup, percent on penicillin
In the subgroup of women < 50 years old, percent using modern contraception

Case-Holding/Retention
Percent and number of patients not seen in the last 6 months
Percent and number of patients not seen in the last 3 months
Percent and number of patients without a community health worker

Palliative Care
Percent and number of patients with reported pain score 0 or 1
Percent and number of patients with reported dyspnea score 0 or 1

Palliative Care (continued)
Percent and number of patients with improvement of pain score since the last reporting period
Percent and number of patients with improvement of dyspnea score since the last reporting period
Percent and number of patients prescribed morphine for symptom relief

Outcomes
Number and percent of patients enrolled in the heart failure program who died in the last reporting period
Of patients enrolled in the heart failure program, number of hospitalizations in the last reporting period
Of the patients with a mechanical replacement valve, the number and proportion whose INR has been between 2 and 4 the entire time since the last reporting period

Data Quality
Percent and number of patients without an intake form

C.2   Cardiac Surgical Referral and Case Selection

Demographics
Percent male and female
Median age
Number of new patients enrolled during reporting period
Total number of patients at the end of reporting period
Total number of patients at the end of reporting period by district and sector

Diagnosis and Case-Finding
Total number of cases referred for cardiac surgery evaluation since the last reporting period
Of the cases referred, the number and percent confirmed to be surgical candidates
Of the cases confirmed to be surgical candidates, the number and percent who have single valve disease
Of the cases confirmed to be surgical candidates, the number and percent who have disease of 2 or more valves
Of the cases confirmed to be surgical candidates, the number and percent who are labeled as requiring surgery within 1 year

Interventions
Of the number of cases referred for cardiac surgery, the number and percent who receive valve replacement
Of the number of cases referred for cardiac surgery, the number and percent who receive valve repair

Case-Holding/Retention
Of the patients on the cardiac surgery registry, the number and percent who have not seen a cardiologist in the last 12 months
Of the patients on the cardiac surgery registry, the number and percent who have not had a cardiologist echocardiogram in the last 12 months

Palliative Care
Percent and number of patients with reported pain score 0 or 1
Percent and number of patients with reported dyspnea score 0 or 1
Percent and number of patients with improvement of pain score since the last reporting period
Percent and number of patients with improvement of dyspnea score since the last reporting period
Percent and number of patients prescribed morphine for symptom relief

Outcomes
Number and percent of patients enrolled in the cardiac surgery program who died during the last reporting period

Data Quality
Percent and number of patients without a contact phone number

C.3   Renal Failure

Demographics
Percent male and female
Median age
Number of new patients enrolled during reporting period
Total number of patients at the end of reporting period
Total number of patients at the end of reporting period by district and sector

Diagnosis and Case-Finding
Percent and number of patients with documented proteinuria that have ever had a creatinine check
Percent and number of patients referred from HIV clinic that have HIV and proteinuria
Of those enrolled in the renal failure program, percent and number of patients with stage 4 or 5 CKD

Interventions
Percent and number of patients with proteinuria who are treated with lisinopril or captopril

Case-Holding/Retention
Percent and number of patients not seen in the last 6 months
Percent and number of patients not seen in the last 3 months
Percent and number of patients without a community health worker

Palliative Care
Percent and number of patients with reported pain score 0 or 1
Percent and number of patients with reported dyspnea score 0 or 1
Percent and number of patients with improvement of pain score since the last reporting period
Percent and number of patients with improvement of dyspnea score since the last reporting period
Percent and number of patients prescribed morphine for symptom relief

Outcomes
Percent and number of patients with hyperkalemia (K ≥ 5.0 mEq/dL)
Percent and number of patients with renal failure who have blood pressure controlled (≤ 130/80 mmHg)

Data Quality
Percent and number of patients without an intake form

C.4 Diabetes

Demographics
Percent male and female
Median age
Number of new patients enrolled during reporting period
Total number of patients at the end of reporting period
Total number of patients at the end of reporting period by district and sector

Diagnosis and Case-Finding
Percent and number of patients referred each quarter to NCD diabetes clinic and confirmed not to have diabetes
Percent and number of patients referred to NCD diabetes clinic and confirmed to have diabetes based on (a) fasting glucose ≥ 126 mg/dL, (b) HbA1c ≥ 6.5%
Percent without an HbA1c in the past 6 months
Percent without a documented foot examination in the past 12 months
Percent with a documented eye examination in the past 2 years

Interventions
Percent on any insulin
Percent on NPH + regular insulin
Percent on NPH insulin alone
Percent on Mixte insulin
Percent on metformin
Percent on glibenclamide

Case-Holding/Retention
Percent and number of patients not seen in the last 6 months
Percent and number of patients not seen in the last 3 months
In subgroup (on insulin) percent and number of patients without a community health worker

Palliative Care
Percent and number of patients with reported pain score 0 or 1
Percent and number of patients with improvement of pain score since the last reporting period
Percent and number of patients prescribed morphine for symptom relief

Outcomes
Percent with HbA1c ≤ 8%
Percent and number with 3 or more hypoglycemic episodes in prior 3 months
Percent and number of patients hospitalized for diabetes

Outcomes (continued)
Number of deaths in patients enrolled in the diabetes program in the last year

Data Quality
Percent and number of patients without an intake form

C.5   Hypertension

Demographics
Percent male and female
Median age
Number of new patients enrolled during reporting period
Total number of patients at the end of reporting period
Total number of patients at the end of reporting period by district and sector

Diagnosis and Case-Finding
Of patients referred to NCD hypertension clinic, number/percent confirmed to have hypertension
Of patients with confirmed hypertension, number/percent with stage I HTN
Of patients with confirmed hypertension, number/percent with stage II HTN
Of patients with confirmed hypertension, number/percent with stage III HTN
Of patients with confirmed hypertension, number/percent with proteinuria
Of patients ≤ 40 years old, number/percent without a recorded creatinine
Of patients with stage III HTN (SBP ≥180 or DBP ≥ 110), number/percent without creatinine

Interventions
Number/percent of patients with proteinuria on ACE inhibitor (or have documented contraindication)
Of patients with Stage III hypertension, number/percent on 2 or more antihypertensives

Case-Holding/Retention
Percent and number of patients not seen in the last 6 months
Percent and number of patients not seen in the last 12 months

Palliative Care
Percent and number of patients with reported dyspnea score 0 or 1

Outcomes
Percent and number of patients with last recorded BP ≤ 140/90
Number of deaths in patients enrolled in the hypertension program in the last year

Data Quality
Percent and number of patients without an intake form

C.6   Chronic Respiratory Disease

Demographics
Percent male and female
Median age
Number of new patients enrolled during reporting period
Total number of patients at the end of reporting period
Total number of patients at the end of reporting period by district and sector

Diagnosis and Case-Finding
Of patients referred to NCD respiratory clinic, the number/percent with confirmed chronic respiratory disease
Of patients enrolled in NCD respiratory clinic, number/percent with asthma/COPD
Of patients enrolled in NCD respiratory clinic, number/percent with brochiectasis
Of patients enrolled in NCD respiratory clinic, number/percent evaluated for tuberculosis with sputum analysis
Of patients referred for sputum analysis, the number/percent diagnosed with tuberculosis

Interventions
Of patients in NCD respiratory clinic, number/percent treated with salbutamol
Of patients in NCD respiratory clinic, number/percent treated with beclomethasone (any dose)
Of patients in NCD respiratory clinic, number/percent treated with aminophylline
Of patients in NCD respiratory clinic, number/percent treated with prednisone in the last 3 months

Case-Holding/Retention
Of patients in NCD respiratory clinic, number/percent not seen in the last 6 months
Of patients in NCD respiratory clinic, number/percent of patients with moderate or severe persistent classification not seen in the last 3 months

Palliative Care
Percent and number of patients with reported pain score 0 or 1
Percent and number of patients with reported dyspnea score 0 or 1
Percent and number of patients with improvement of pain score since the last reporting period
Percent and number of patients with improvement of dyspnea score since the last reporting period
Percent and number of patients prescribed morphine for symptom relief

Outcomes
Of patients in NCD respiratory clinic, number/percent who have improvement of severity classification over the last 6 months

Outcomes (continued)
Of patients in NCD respiratory clinic, number/percent who have worsening of severity classification over the last 6 months
Of patients in NCD respiratory clinic, number/percent who have an "intermittent" classification

Data Quality
Percent and number without an intake form

APPENDIX D
Forms

···

Here we provide a sampling of the forms used to follow non-communicable diseases (NCDs) at district hospitals and health centers at PIH-supported sites in Rwanda. All forms have both French and English translations. These forms are used both for clinical and monitoring and evaluation purposes. They have gone through many years of revision through input from all of the NCD clinicians. These forms are dynamic and undoubtedly will continue to change as the chronic care integration strategy expands nationally.

All forms are entered electronically into an electronic medical record. There is one data officer at each district hospital focused on form entry after clinical encounters. The data officer also works with the NCD clinicians to report on program indictors (see **APPENDIX C**).

D.1 Intake Forms

Each disease followed in the NCD or integrated chronic care clinics has a corresponding intake form. These forms generally take 15 minutes to complete. There is some variation in intake form length based on the complexity of the disease. Intake forms are meant to be repeated every 6 months to 1 year.

Here we give an example of an intake form used for heart failure patients in the district NCD clinics.

1. History of present illness	
A. **Patient referred from:** ☐ acute clinic ☐ hospital ☐ other clinic other_____	
B. **Chief complaint** _____	
C. **Duration of symptoms** ___ days /months / years	
D. **Ever hospitalized for these symptoms?**	☐yes ☐no
Total number of hospitalizations: ___	
E. **Has the patient had:**	
dyspnea on exertion?	☐ yes ☐ no
orthopnea?	☐ yes ☐ no
If yes, does the patient sleep sitting because of orthopnea?	☐ yes ☐ no
F. **Ever treated by a traditional healer for these symptoms ?** yes ☐ no	
Diagnosis: ☐ poisoning ☐ other_____	
Treatment: ☐ purgative ☐ other _____	
Cost: _____FRW	
G. **If female:** **Did the symptoms start around delivery?**	☐ n/a ☐ yes ☐ no
If a woman between 15–45 years old, does she use birth control? If no, why_____	☐ n/a ☐ yes ☐ no
H. **Does the patient have:**	
a. chronic cough (more than 3 weeks)?	☐yes ☐no
If yes : ☐ productive ☐ hemoptysis	
b. night sweats that soak clothing?	☐ yes ☐ no
c. a large weight loss?	☐ yes ☐ no
If yes, how much? _____ kg or ☐ clothing is looser	
I. **Does the patient smoke?**	☐ yes ☐ no ☐ past
If yes : ☐ traditional ☐ modern ☐ pipe	____ cigarettes or pipes/ day
J. **Does the patient drink alcohol?**	☐ yes ☐ no ☐ past
If yes : ☐ traditional ____ liters/ day	☐ modern____ bottles/ day
Document any other relevant history:	

2. Previous outpatient medications

Is patient on cardiac medications at intake? ☐ **yes** ☐ **no** ☐ Never taken cardiac medications

Medication	Dose	Frequency	Still taking?
☐ furosemide	____ mg ☐ oral ☐ IV	☐ 1/d ☐ 2/d ☐ 3/d	☐ yes ☐ no
☐ captopril			
☐ lisinopril	____ mg oral	☐ 1/d ☐ 2/d ☐ 3/d	☐ yes ☐ no
☐ aldactone	____ mg oral	☐ 1/d	☐ yes ☐ no
☐ atenolol			
☐ carvedilol	____ mg oral	☐ 1/d ☐ 2/d	☐ yes ☐ no
☐ amlodipine			
☐ nifedipine	____ mg oral	☐ 1/d ☐ 2/d	☐ yes ☐ no
☐ digoxin	____ mg oral	☐ 1/d	☐ yes ☐ no
☐ aspirin	____ mg oral	☐ 1/d	☐ yes ☐ no
☐ warfarin	____ mg oral	☐ 1/d ☐ 2/d	☐ yes ☐ no
☐ hydrochlorthiazide	____ mg oral	☐ 1/d	☐ yes ☐ no
☐ methyldopa	____ mg oral	☐ 1/d ☐ 2/d ☐ 3/d	☐ yes ☐ no
☐ isosorbide dinitrate			
	____ mg oral	☐ 1/d ☐ 2/d ☐ 3/d	☐ yes ☐ no
☐ hydralazine	____ mg oral	☐ 1/d ☐ 2/d ☐ 3/d	☐ yes ☐ no
☐ prednisolone	____ mg oral	☐ 1/d ☐ 2/d	☐ yes ☐ no
☐ penicillin V	____ mg oral	☐ 1/d ☐ 2/d ☐ 3/d	☐ yes ☐ no
☐ benzathine penicillin	☐ 600,000 IU IM		
	☐ 1.2 M IU IM	☐ 1x/month ☐ 2x/month	☐ yes ☐ no
☐ _____	____ mg ☐ oral ☐ IV	☐ 1/d ☐ 2/d ☐ 3/d	☐ yes ☐ no
Drug allergies _____	☐ yes ☐ no	If yes, explain: _____	

3. Past medical history

A.	Has the patient ever had an HIV test ?	☐ yes ☐ no
	If yes, result: ☐ positive ☐ negative Date of last test: ____ / ____ / ____	
	If positive: Last CD4: _____ Date: ____ / ____ / ____	
	Enrolled in the IMB HIV program? ☐ yes ☐ no	
B.	Has the patient ever been treated for tuberculosis?	☐ yes ☐ no
	If yes, how many times? _____ In what year(s) ? _____	
C.	Other history :	

4. Social history				
A. Occupation:	☐ unemployed	☐ retired	☐ farmer	☐ small child (< 5)
	☐ professional	☐ driver	☐ cleaner	☐ in school
	☐ school-aged, not in school	☐ miner		☐ _____
B. Too sick to work ?		☐ yes ☐ no		
C. Civil status:	☐ married or lives with partner			☐ partner in prison
	☐ single or child			☐ divorced or separated
	☐ widow (partner died of:_____)			☐ orphan
D. Transport :	☐ foot ☐ bus ☐ bike ☐ taxi ☐ other			
	Cost of transport (round-trip)			_____ FRW
	Time to travel to health center			_____ hrs

E. Socio-economic status:	
The patient's house has: _____ rooms	_____ occupants
Does the patient's family own a house? ☐ yes ☐ no	
Roof is: ☐ tin ☐ thatch ☐ cement ☐ sheeting	
The floor is: ☐ cement ☐ dirt	
Does the patient's family own land? ☐ yes ☐ no	**if yes:** _____ hectares
Does the patient's family have goats or cows?	_____ goats
	_____ cows
How many children has the patient had or if a child, how many siblings in the family?	_____ children
Are all the children still alive? ☐ yes ☐ no causes of death:_____	
Do all the school-aged children go to school? ☐ yes ☐ no ☐ N/A	
Other social information:	

5. Physical Exam		
Vital signs:		
BP: _____ / _____ mmHg	Pulse: _____ bpm	Weight _____ kg	Height _____ cm
Does the patient feel dizzy upon standing up? ☐ yes ☐ no		
If indicated : Temp: _____ °C	RR: _____	SaO2: _____ %

	Normal	Abnormal
General	☐ well-appearing	☐ cachectic ☐ obese ☐ tachypneic ☐ use of accessory muscles
HEENT	☐ JVP normal	☐ JVP high ☐ goiter
Lungs	☐ clear	☐ crackles (If yes, location:_____) ☐ wheezing
Heart	☐ PMI non-displaced ☐ regular rhythm ☐ no murmurs	☐ tachycardia ☐ irregular rhythm ☐ PMI displaced ☐ **murmur 1** location :_____ 　☐ systolic ☐ diastolic ☐ **murmur 2** location :_____ 　☐ systolic ☐ diastolic
Abdomen	☐ soft ☐ non-tender ☐ no hepatomegaly ☐ no splenomegaly ☐ no ascites	☐ splenomegaly _____ cm ☐ hepatomegaly : _____ cm ☐ pulsatile liver ☐ ascites: ☐ mild ☐ moderate ☐ abundant ☐ tenderness: ☐ RUQ ☐ LUQ ☐ RLQ ☐ LLQ
Extremities	☐ no peripheral edema ☐ no joint pain or swelling	☐ cold ☐ peripheral edema ☐ 1+ ☐ 2+ ☐ 3+ ☐ joints ☐ swollen joints
Neuro	☐ no abnormalities	☐ focal motor deficit
Other	_____	_____

6. Previous labs (including today)

	Date	Results
1.	___/___/___	
2.	___/___/___	
3.	___/___/___	**Chemistries** point of care Na: K: Cal: iCa : CO2: Urée: Créat: Glyc: Hgb:
4.	___/___/___	**INR/ PT** point of care INR : PT :

7. Previous studies

	Date	Results		
CXR	___/___/___	☐ normal ☐ cardiomegaly	☐ mild ☐ moderate ☐ severe	☐ Infiltrates (location:_____) ☐ pleural effusions ☐ small ☐ big (location:_____)
EKG	___/___/___	☐ normal ☐ LVH ☐ atrial fibrillation ☐ infarction (location:_____)		

8. Preliminary echocardiographic result:

Left ventricular function

☐ Normal	☐ mildly depressed	☐ markedly depressed
Ejection fraction estimate:_____ %		
☐ No mitral stenosis	☐ Mitral stenosis	
☐ Normal right ventricular size	☐ Large right ventricle	
☐ Normal IVC	☐ Large IVC	
☐ Other abnormalities _____		

9. Clinical Impression

A.	Summary

B.	Diagnosis

☐ Heart Failure

Type of Heart Failure:
- ☐ Cardiomyopathy
- ☐ Rheumatic heart disease ☐ Mitral stenosis ☐ Other
- ☐ Hypertensive heart disease
- ☐ Other type of Heart Failure: _____

Severity of symptoms (If between categories, mark both)
- ☐ **NYHA class I** (Asymptomatic) No limitation on activity
- ☐ **NYHA class I-II**
- ☐ **NYHA class II** (Mildly symptomatic)
  Symptoms only with moderate exertion, such as climbing a hill
- ☐ **NYHA class II-III**
- ☐ **NYHA class III** (Moderately symptomatic)
  Symptoms with even light activity but comfortable at rest
- ☐ **NYHA class III-IV**
- ☐ **NYHA class IV** (Severely symptomatic)
  Symptoms with all activities, may be symptomatic at rest

☐ **Renal Failure**
☐ **Liver Failure**
☐ **Other**

C.	Patient's fluid status:	☐ hypervolemic	☐ euvolemic	☐ hypovolemic

10. Final plan			
A. Labs, studies:	☐VS ☐HIV ☐ sputum x 3 ☐Chest X-ray ☐_____ ☐Albumin ☐SGOT ☐SGPT		

B. Medications

☐ No medications	MORNING	NOON	EVENING
☐ Furosemide (Lasix)	____ mg		____ mg
☐ Captopril	____ mg	____ mg	____ mg
☐ Lisinopril	____ mg		____ mg
☐ Aldactone	____ mg		____ mg
☐ Carvedilol	____ mg		____ mg
☐ Atenolol	____ mg		____ mg
☐ Amlodipine	____ mg		____ mg
☐ Nifedipine retard	____ mg		____ mg
☐ Isosorbide dinitrate	____ mg	____ mg	____ mg
☐ Hydralazine	____ mg	____ mg	____ mg
☐ Hydrochlorothiazide	____ mg		
☐ Potassium (600 mg tab = 8mEq)	____ mg		____ mg
☐ Prednisolone	____ mg		____ mg
☐ Aspirin	____ mg		
☐ Warfarin	____ mg		
☐ Penicillin V	____ mg		____ mg
☐ Benzathine penicillin 600,000 UI IM	☐ 1x/month	☐ 2x/month	
☐ Benzathine penicillin 1.2 M UI IM	☐ 1x/month	☐ 2x/month	

C. Other medications: _____

		☐ Follow-up ____/____/____
D. Disposition	☐ Admit to hospital ☐ Discharge home	

D.2 Flowsheets

Here we present a sample of the flowsheets used for each disease follow-up visit. The purpose of the flowsheets is to capture key clinical indicators while minimizing paperwork and allowing clinicians to easily assess a patient's progress over time. Each disease has a flowsheet for clinical findings (different for each disease) as well as an event and medication sheet, which are more or less the same across diseases. Each flowsheet has a cover sheet with summary and demographic information that is placed at the front of the chart.

D.2.1 Sample Cover Sheet

EMR	CLINIC	☐ Rwinkwavu	☐ Kirehe	☐ Butaro	
		☐ Other:			
	Change in clinic ☐ yes Date: ___/___/___ Clinic _____				

EMR	DEMOGRAPHICS	EMR	ADDRESS
	Date of birth:___/___/___	Province: _____
	Age:	District : _____
	Sex ☐ F ☐ M	Secteur: _____
	Daily CHW: ☐ yes ☐ not indicated Name : _____	Cellule: _____
		Umudugudu: _____
	Change in CHW ☐ yes Name :_____ Date: ___/___/___	Telephone: _____
		☐ patient ☐ other_____
	If a child: Name of parent or guardian _____	Change in address or telephone: ☐ yes
		Date: ___/___/___
	Telephone:_____	Go to page 2 to change

CARDIAC DIAGNOSIS					
Diagnosis or Problem	EF	Date of dx	Type		Clinician
		__/__/__	☐ preliminary ☐ confirmed		
		__/__/__	☐ preliminary ☐ confirmed		

NON-CARDIAC DIAGNOSIS AND PROBLEM LIST					
EMR	Diagnosis	Date	EMR	Diagnosis	Date
		__/__/__			__/__/__
		__/__/__			__/__/__
		__/__/__			__/__/__

☐ Cardiology consultation completed _____/_____/_____

Surgical candidate? ☐ yes ☐ no
If yes: Passport : ☐ yes ☐ not indicated
Visa : ☐ yes ☐ not indicated

D.2.2   Sample Events Flowsheet

HOSPITALIZATIONS				
EMR	Date of admission	Date of discharge	Hospital	Reason for hospitalization
	__/__/__	__/__/__		
	__/__/__	__/__/__		
	__/__/__	__/__/__		

SOCIAL ASSISTANCE OR ASSESSMENT					
EMR	Date	Type of assistance or assessment	EMR	Date	Type of assistance or assessment
	__/__/__			__/__/__	
	__/__/__			__/__/__	
	__/__/__			__/__/__	
(ex. Home visit, house construction, school financing, transport financing, food supplementation)					

CHANGE IN CHW, ADDRESS OR TELEPHONE		
EMR	Date	
	__/__/__	
	__/__/__	
	__/__/__	

NON-MEDICAL LIFE EVENTS SINCE DIAGNOSIS					
EMR	Date	Event	EMR	Date	Event
	__/__/__			__/__/__	
	__/__/__			__/__/__	
	__/__/__			__/__/__	
(e.g. marriage, divorce, pregnancy, births, death of family members, change in socioeconomic status, change in residence since diagnosis)					

D.2.3 Clinical Findings Flowsheet

Here is an example of how two rows from the clinical indicators page might look for a typical heart failure patient. Here, we see the patient was fluid-overloaded and tachycardic with class III symptoms at the first visit in the setting of missing her medications. A point-of-care chemistry panel was done. The patient was also not on birth control. On the next visit, it is clear that the patient's vital signs and symptom class improved and she had been taking her medications. She also had been started on birth control.

RENDEZ-VOUS/ CLINIC VISIT														
Date	Wt	BP	P	NYHA Class	Hemodyn.	Missed any meds ?	Na	K	CO_2	Cr	Hgb	INR	On birth control ?	F/up
	50	90/ 60	110	III	X hyper ☐ eu ☐ hypo	X yes ☐ no ☐ N/A	133	4	24	130	11	N/A	☐ yes X no ☐ N/A	2/9/10
2/2/10	Comments :													
	45	100/ 70	80	II	☐ hyper X eu ☐ hypo	X yes ☐ no ☐ N/A							X yes ☐ no ☐ N/A	2/16/10
2/9/10	Comments :													

In the section below, we show one line of the clinical indicators flowsheet for some of the other diseases followed in the clinics.

D.2.3.1 Asthma

CLINIC VISITS							
Date	# times/week awoken by dyspnea	# puffs/week of salbutamol	Peak Flow	Good inhaler technique	Asthma classification ☐ not asthma	Activity limitation due to shortness of breath	Plan and Follow-up
	_____ times	_____ puffs		☐ yes ☐ no ☐ brief coaching given	☐ well-controlled ☐ moderately controlled ☐ poorly controlled	☐ daily or almost daily ☐ several times per week ☐ less than once per week ☐ not at all	RDV __/__/__ ☐ group class : __/__/__ ☐ step up treatment ☐ continue the same treatment ☐ step down treatment
	Comment :						

D.2.3.2 Diabetes

CLINIC VISITS									
Date	Weight	BP	Pulse	Proteinuria	Na	K	CO_2	Cr	Missed insulin ?
									☐ yes ☐ no ☐ N/A
Glucose:		Glucose today :_____						☐ fasting	
Sx of low blood sugar ?		☐ yes ☐ no	When?: ☐ morning ☐ afternoon ☐ evening						
Comments									

D.2.3.3 Post-Cardiac Surgery

Date	Wt	BP	P	NYHA Class	Volume Status	Missed any meds ?	Na	K	Cr	Hgb	INR	On birth control ?	F/up
					☐ hyper ☐ eu ☐ hypo	☐ yes ☐ no ☐ NA						☐ yes ☐ no ☐ NA	
Comments :													

CLINIC VISIT

D.2.3.4 Hypertension

Date	Weight	BP	Pulse	Proteinuria	Na	K	Cr	F/up
Comments								

CLINIC VISIT

D.2.3.5 Medication Flowsheet

Below we give an example of part of a medication flowsheet. Like the clinical indicators sheet, this allows clinicians to see at a glance both which medications the patient is on and what changes have been made recently. This is particularly helpful for following patients with diseases such as heart failure, which require frequent dose adjustments.

MEDICATION LIST

Medication	Dose	Frequency	Start date	Stop date	Reason for stopping
			_/_/_	_/_/_	
			_/_/_	_/_/_	
			_/_/_	_/_/_	
			_/_/_	_/_/_	

D.2.4 Palliative Care Flowsheet

The following is a flowsheet included in each patient's chart to be filled out at the discretion of the clinician, depending on the severity of the patient's disease. The questions are based on the African Palliative Care Assocation's Palliative Care Outcomes scale, which has been validated in rural sub-Saharan African communities.[1]

ASSESSMENT OF SYMPTOM MANAGEMENT (To be done at intake and as needed thereafter)				
Ask the following questions with regard to **the last 3 days** Have the patient rate their answer on a **scale of 0 (none or not at all) to 5 (a lot or all the time)**.				
Date	_/_/_	_/_/_	_/_/_	_/_/_
1. Rate your pain				
2a. Have any other symptoms been affecting how you feel?				
2b. If so, please rate each symptom:				
Dyspnea				
Nausea or vomiting				
Constipation				
Diarrhea				
Incontinence				
Pruritus				
Fever				
Weakness				
Insomnia				
Foul Odor				
3. Have you been feeling worried about your illness?				
4. Have you been able to share how you are feeling with your family or friends?				
5. Have you felt life was worthwhile?				
6. Have you felt at peace?				
7. Have you had enough help and advice for your family to plan for the future?				
If family is present:				
8. How much information have you and your family been given?				
9. How confident has the family felt caring for the patient?				
10. Has the family been feeling worried about the patient?				

Appendix D References

1   Harding R, Selman L, Agupio G, et al. Validation of a core outcome measure for palliative care in Africa: the APCA African palliative outcome scale. Health Qual Life Outcomes 2010;8:10.

APPENDIX E
Common Normal Values

....

TABLE E.1   Normal Vital Sign Values by Age[1]

	Heart rate (beats per minute)	Systolic blood pressure (mmHg)	Diastolic blood pressure (mmHg)	Respiratory rate (breaths/minute)
0-3 months	120-160	60-80	45-55	35-55
3-6 months	90-120	70-90	50-65	30-45
6-12 months	80-120	80-100	55-65	25-40
1-3 years	70-110	90-105	55-70	20-30
3-6 years	65-110	95-110	60-75	20-25
6-12 years	60-95	100-120	60-75	14-22
Adult	60-80	90-140	60-90	14-18

TABLE E.2   Blood pressure ranges by age for children[2]

Age (year)		Blood pressure (mmHg) percentile (for 25th percentile of height)			
		50th percentile	90th percentile	95th percentile	99th percentile
1	Systolic	83	97	101	108
	Diastolic	36	51	55	63
2	Systolic	87	100	104	111
	Diastolic	41	56	60	68
3	Systolic	89	103	107	114
	Diastolic	45	60	64	72
4	Systolic	91	105	109	116
	Diastolic	49	64	68	76
5	Systolic	93	106	110	118
	Diastolic	52	67	71	79
6	Systolic	94	108	112	119
	Diastolic	54	69	73	81
7	Systolic	95	109	113	120
	Diastolic	56	71	75	83
8	Systolic	97	110	114	122
	Diastolic	58	72	77	85
9	Systolic	98	112	116	123
	Diastolic	59	74	78	86
10	Systolic	100	114	117	125
	Diastolic	60	74	79	86
11	Systolic	102	115	119	127
	Diastolic	60	75	79	87
12	Systolic	104	118	122	129
	Diastolic	61	75	80	88
13	Systolic	106	120	124	131
	Diastolic	61	76	80	88
14	Systolic	109	123	127	134
	Diastolic	62	77	81	89
15	Systolic	112	125	129	136
	Diastolic	63	78	82	90

TABLE E.3   Peak Expiratory Flow Rates For Women (L/min)[3]

Age (year)	140 cm	150 cm	165 cm	180 cm	190 cm
20	390	423	460	496	529
25	385	418	454	490	523
30	380	413	448	483	516
35	375	408	442	476	509
40	370	402	436	470	502
45	365	397	430	464	495
50	360	391	424	457	488
55	355	386	418	451	482
60	350	380	412	445	475
65	345	375	406	439	468
70	340	369	400	432	461

TABLE E.4   Peak Expiratory Flow Rates Men (L/min)[3]

Age (year)	150 cm	165 cm	180 cm	190 cm	200 cm
20	554	602	649	693	740
25	543	590	636	679	725
30	532	577	622	664	710
35	521	565	609	651	695
40	509	552	596	636	680
45	498	540	583	622	665
50	486	527	569	607	649
55	475	515	556	593	634
60	463	502	542	578	618
65	452	490	529	564	603
70	440	477	515	550	587

TABLE E.5   Peak Expiratory Flow Rates For Children[4]

Height (cm)	PEF (L/min)	Height (cm)	PEF (L/min)
109	147	142	320
112	160	145	334
114	173	147	347
117	187	150	360
119	200	152	373
122	214	155	387
124	227	157	400
127	240	160	413
130	254	163	427
132	267	165	440
135	280	168	454
137	293	170	467
140	307		

TABLE E.6   Normal Lab Values[5]

	Adults	Children
Na	135–146 mEq/L	135–146 mEq/L
K	3.5–5.5 mEq/L	3.5–5.8 mEq/L
Cl	95–112 mEq/L	95–112 mEq/L
CO_2	22–32 mEq/L	20–28 mEq/L
BUN (Urea)	7–25 mg/dL	5–18 mg/dL
Hgb	**Female:** 12–16 g/dL **Male:** 14–18 g/dL	**Child:** 10–14 g/dL **Newborn:** 15–25 g/dL

TABLE E.7   Normal Creatinine Values by Age[6]

Newborn	27–88 µmol/L (0.3–1.0 mg/dL)
Infant or preschool-aged child (2 months–4 years)	18–35 µmol/L (0.2–0.5 mg/dL)
School-aged child (5–10 years)	27–62 µmol/L (0.3–0.7 mg/dL)
Older child or adolescent (10–15 years)	44–88 µmol/L (0.5–1.0 mg/dL)
Age > 15–adult	**Female:** 0.6–1.2 mg/dL **Male:** 0.5–1.5 mg/dL

Appendix E References

1   Custer JW, Rau RE. The Harriet Lane Handbook: a manual for pediatric house officers. 18th ed. Philadelphia, PA: Mosby/Elsevier, 2009.

2   The fourth report on the diagnosis, evaluation, and treatment of high blood pressure in children and adolescents. Pediatrics 2004;114(2 Suppl 4th Report): 555–76.

3   Leiner GC, Abramowitz S, Small MJ, Stenby VB, Lewis WA. Expiratory Peak Flow Rate. Standard Values for Normal Subjects. Use as a Clinical Test of Ventilatory Function. Am Rev Respir Dis. 1963;88:644–51.

4   Voter KZ, McBride JT. Diagnostic tests of lung function. Pediatr Rev. 1996; 17(2):53–63.

5   Hay WW, Hayward AR, Levin MJ, Hicks JM. Current pediatric diagnosis and treatment. 15th ed. New York: Lange Medical Books/McGraw Hill, 2000.

6   Current medical literature : Nephrology and urology. London, England: Current Medical Literature, Ltd., 1994.

INDEX

· ·